D1238645

# coping with reality shock:
## the voices of experience

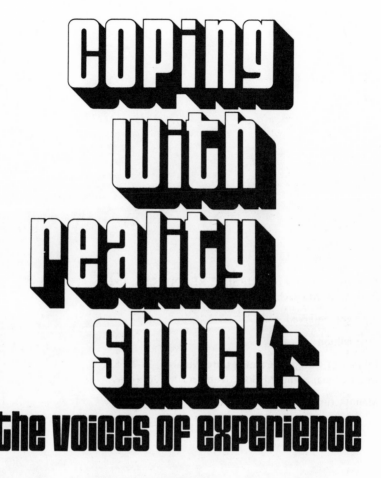

# Coping with reality shock: the voices of experience

**CLAUDIA SCHMALENBERG, R.N., M.S.**

Research Assistant and Project Director
Reality Shock and Conflict Resolution
   in Neophyte Nurses Research Grant
University of California
San Francisco, California

**MARLENE KRAMER, R.N., Ph.D.**

Professor, School of Nursing
University of California
San Francisco Medical Center,
San Francisco, California

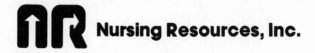 **Nursing Resources, Inc.**

Copyright © 1979 by NURSING RESOURCES, INC.
Wakefield, Massachusetts

All rights reserved

First edition

Library of Congress Catalog Card Number: 78-70683
International Standard Book Number: 0-913654-50-7

Manufactured in the United States of America

92434

BELMONT COLLEGE LIBRARY

RT
86
.534

*To New Graduates:*
*To those who were;*
*For those who are yet to come*

# Preface

When a new graduate enters the work force she* is looked upon as inexperienced. To the extent that experienced means being made skillful or wise by means of trial or observation while being engaged in a particular work, the label "inexperienced" holds true. However, if experience is looked upon as the skill or wisdom which results from the actual living through of an event, then the new graduates have a great deal of experience. It is the latter definition which is used here. This book reports "experienced" new graduates' adjustments to the work world.

In a previous research study, the effect of an Anticipatory Socialization Program in a school of nursing on easing the transition of the student nurse into the staff nurse role was described[1]. In the current research study, a Role Transformation Program instituted in eight medical center hospitals was found to be effective in easing the adjustment of the newly graduated nurse[2]. The Role Transformation Program consisted of a series of seminars, a series of individualized instructional materials, and a series of workshops. The program was instituted as a special orientation program through the inservice departments of the eight medical centers. The material to be presented here will describe the seminar portion of the Role Transformation Program. The instructional programs are contained in the book *Path to Biculturalism*.

Why are new graduate seminars needed? Chapter 1 provides an overview of the process of reality shock and the place of the seminars in dealing with this process. The theoretical notions, preparation of the leaders, and anticipated outcomes of the seminars are also discussed. Chapter 2 provides details on how to set up and conduct new graduate seminars. It describes medical centers where the seminars were held, the contract made with the participants, the actual procedure used in implementing the seminars, and the data analysis methodology.

---

* The female pronoun is used only because most nurses are women. No discrimination against male nurses is intended.

Chapters 3-6 present the content of the seminars. Subject areas will be described in four clusters—"the organization," "the individual," "the ambiguous, tenuous span," and "patients and patient care"—each with a different organizing framework. The frequency of occurrence and the patterning of the subject areas will be described.

Did the seminars work? How do we know if they worked? What affected the outcomes of the seminars? The answers to these questions as well as unanticipated outcomes of the seminars are presented in Chapter 7. The implications for the use of the data and suggestions for implementing seminars are given in the conclusion.

It is expected that this book will be of primary interest to nurses in service organizations. Directors of nursing service, inservice educators, head nurses, and staff nurses should find the material informative and useful. The seminars were conducted in hospital settings by personnel employed by each of the eight medical centers. The concerns voiced by the new graduates have a very special perspective—one that only a newcomer to an organization can have—perspective which allows the new graduate to see things, perhaps, which others no longer see or have come to accept. A number of the concerns of the new graduate are matters which concern all individuals working in nursing and which perhaps need reconsideration in light of new developments. As you read about the concerns of the new graduates, some of you will be thankful that such matters and conditions do not exist in your organization. Before passing judgment, we challenge you to take a fresh look at your organization—you may be shocked to find that similar problems do exist. The voices of the new graduates quoted in this book may provide thoughtful stimulation for future work with new graduates entering a service organization.

Faculty in schools of nursing will also find the concerns of the new graduate of interest. Many of the issues discussed in this book are perceived by the new graduate to be problems due to their lack of preparation. These perceptions may be somewhat distorted—or they may not. As you read this book, we suggest that you ask yourselves "How does our curriculum address the issues discussed?" Then talk to recent graduates of your nursing program and honestly seek to discover the problems they have. The concerns of the graduates of your program may be the same as or different from those expressed here but must be dealt with in some way. The suggestions in the chapters may be helpful.

Students and new graduates are expected to be among the major readers of this book. The reality of the concerns here may be overwhelming and act as a driving force. Let that force drive you to prepare yourself in the best way possible to meet the problems and concerns of the work world. It is hoped that the sharing of this information will be a beginning for your endeavors. The success and failures of those whose experiences are contained here will help you to be even more creative than those who preceded you in meeting the realities of nursing.

The research presented here was supported by a federal grant, NU 00505. This support is gratefully acknowledged. The support of many others was needed to complete this research. A special "thank you" goes to the hospitals who participated, the satellite directors who led the seminars and directed the research at their institution, and to the new graduates and their head nurses who participated in the research.

## REFERENCES

1. Kramer, M. *Reality Shock: Why Nurses Leave Nursing.* St. Louis, Mo.: C. V. Mosby, Co., 1974.
2. Kramer, M. and Schmalenberg, C. Bicultural training and new graduate role transformation. *Nursing Digest,* 5(4): 1–47, 1978.

# Contents

# Chapter 1
# Reality Shock:
# A Lonely Experience

For the new graduate, the movement from the yesterday of school to the today of nursing practice can create feelings of helplessness, powerlessness, frustration, and dissatisfaction. This turmoil can be labeled "reality shock." New graduate nurses do not have a monopoly on reality shock; it can and is experienced by people in many professions, and by the established professional as well as by the newcomer. As a group of nurses, however, new graduates experience reality shock more intensely and more homogeneously than do other nurses. Seminars or informal discussions with new graduates during their initial employment provide an opportunity for these new voices to tell of their experiences.

Although the phenomenon has been described previously, this chapter will begin with an overview of reality shock, both to provide a common framework and to place the seminars in theoretical perspective. The chapter will then discuss the purpose of the seminars as well as the role of seminar leaders.

## DIFFERING SUBCULTURES

Reality shock is the conflict resulting from the movement from the familiar subculture of school to the unfamiliar subculture of work. The two subcultures have their own values and behaviors. Generally speaking, in schools of nursing, the dominant values transmitted are comprehensive, total patient care with individualization and family involvement. Use of judgment, autonomy, cognitive skills, and decision making are strongly promulgated in this system. In the work subculture, the emphasis is on the value of providing safe care for all the patients. Organization, efficiency, cooperation, and responsibility are highly valued. In terms of behavior, the school's emphasis is on teaching general role behaviors or principles of behavior applicable in a wide variety of settings. This is in contrast to the role-specific behaviors demanded in the work setting. The differences between the values and behaviors of the two subcultures can result in incongruent socialization. That is to say, the individual may be a good student nurse and not a good staff nurse.

Within each subculture there is more congruence of values and behaviors than between subcultures. It is the *incongruency* of values and behaviors between the school subculture and the work subculture that leads to role deprivation or reality shock. Since the majority of school subcultures teach comprehensive, individualized care for one or two patients (whole-task system) and the majority of nursing service organizations function on the premise of a little bit for everybody, with a number of different people providing the care (part-task system), value and behavior discrepancies are encountered. Although the degree of discrepancy will vary depending upon which school an individual graduated from and which service organization or which unit within an organization the individual goes to work in, some discrepancy between systems is likely to be encountered and some reality shock will be produced.

## THE REALITY SHOCK PROCESS

The role transformation from student to staff nurse evolves in a fairly predictable pattern. The process usually consists of four phases[1]. In the first, the honeymoon phase, the world is seen through rose-colored glasses: the world is all good; everything is wonderful. The nurse receives a regular paycheck; she can pay her bills and buy new clothes. Because she is in the work scene for longer periods of time than during her training, she will probably get more positive feedback and recognition from her patients. And that feels good! You hear new graduates saying things like:

> My head nurse is just fantastic, really fantastic. I can talk to her about anything. She always has really great ideas.

Another one says:

> I've got so much energy. I'm moving like a snowplow.

And another says:

> Oh, it's just super; I love it; I really do. It's all so perfect. Everything. Better than I ever thought it would be.

It is evident that these perceptions are distorted, but this is the way many initially see the work world.

During the honeymoon phase, the graduate is concerned with two major activities. The first of these is mastery of skills and routines. Nursing educators can tell students ad infinitum:

Don't worry about skills. You'll learn them when you get out. The first six months will be a little hard, but if you know the theory, you'll readily learn the skills you need to know.

The fact is that many feel they have graduated with a bushel basket of theory and a paper bag of skills, and they quickly learn that the work subculture values mastery of skills. There is something readily measurable about skill acquisition. For example, in doing a catheterization, if the tube is in the right place and the urine comes out, success is achieved. Immediate reinforcement is built in. This is not true, for example, with making judgments. Often it is not until much later that the correctness of a decision is known. Positive reinforcement for skill mastery received from the nursing staff also contributes to the honeymoon glow.

The other focus during this phase is to become socially integrated into the unit or ward staff group. Considerable time and energy is invested into getting along, being part of the group. New graduates want to be liked, respected, and perceived as nurses.

It is also during this time of social integration that the graduate goes through a period of testing. She perceives this first job as a proving ground, a place to determine what kind of a nurse she is really going to be. She attempts to pass her own tests and at the same time be accepted and liked by the staff. Many times the sizing-up process consists of performing in a manner prescribed by others on the unit. The new graduate diligently strives to pass these informal tests and, generally, she meets with at least initial success in this area.

However, the second or shock phase is approaching. When the new graduate tries to achieve some desired and valued goal and the way is blocked either by her own inadequacies or by deterrents within the system, shock sets in. When one tries to accomplish something and finds that the nursing values taught in school are not valued by the work surroundings, one becomes shocked and learns that reality differs from expectations.

## Shock

There are four major characteristics of the shock phase: moral outrage, rejection, fatigue, and perceptual distortion. The moral outrage is expressed by an outcrying of values: "You should do things this way; everyone should really care about patients." There are numerous "should's" in the outrage, and frequently there is almost an evangelistic tone to the words:

It's awful! I can't believe it. I never thought it would be like this. I knew it wouldn't be a picnic, but this is ridiculous. The stupid way they do things around here. Sometimes I wonder if any of these girls have ever been to nursing school. They know nothing at all about care plans, or histories, or discharge summaries, and the aides are so mean to the patients. I hope I never get like that.

Rejection is another characteristic of this phase. It can take two forms: rejection of the schooling or rejection of the work scene. An example of the former:

I've been robbed! I didn't learn a thing in school! My instructors should have known what I needed to know to be a nurse. They should have taught me or seen that I learned what I needed to know.

Rejection of the work scene sounds like this:

I'm really disappointed because they don't care as much about patients as I had been led to believe. Nurses really don't make the decisions my instructors always said they would.

I'd just started, but immediately I thought the care was so bad that I didn't want to be a part of it. I was not able to effectively change the work in that environment to the degree that I had pride in what I was doing. I would go home every night and cry and cry and then be so exhausted that I had to go to bed.

This leads us to the third characteristic of the shock phase, fatigue:

And then there's the sleep syndrome. When you go home, all you want to do is sleep so you can get up and go to work the next day. Pretty soon, all you're doing is sleeping and working.

The last major characteristic is perceptual distortion. As globally positive as the graduate was during the honeymoon phase, she is now globally negative. Perceptions are distorted so that nothing is good; everything is bad. There is a marked tendency to polarize things, to be hypercritical. She tends to see the world as "we" and "they," as "good guys" and "bad guys." Two excerpts will illustrate this point:

I don't like the way they talk to the patients. They just go in and do the job as if they were dealing with a herd of cattle.

In the past, it has really been hard to motivate anyone to do anything because they have just been there so long. And I know that it's not hard to motivate new graduates to do things. In the past when you would tell the night nurse about something that should be done, you would just get this long line of defense, like you were talking to a brick wall. But somehow, I don't get that feeling when I talk to a recent grad. At least she will listen to me. She doesn't have that hard shell built up yet.

Not only are the we's, they's, and should's in these excerpts perceptible but also the faint tone of superiority. It says, "We've got the message and we're trying to give it to you, but you're not listening, you're not taking it in."

As a matter of fact, the graduate during this period is often so busy and preoccupied with emitting her own message (conveying strongly felt values and feelings) that she has some difficulty in receiving undistorted messages from others, as in the following excerpt from an interview:

> I had been on the floor six weeks and suddenly one day, I was told that a meeting was set up—the girl from inservice, the supervisor, one of the nurses, and myself. We're in this meeting and there were many charges and accusations made against me. This really bothered me because that was the first I had heard of it. I was amazed and dumbfounded to think I had been on the floor for six weeks and no one had bothered to tell me.

This view was expressed by the young nurse even though she had received a written evaluation attesting to the same thing and had signed it as having read it. The point is that the strong emotions of frustration, disillusionment, and anger can block and distort incoming messages.

The shock phase cannot go on forever. Moral outrage and active rejection are depleting. It is extremely exhausting to be continually upset, angry, frustrated, and to try to persuade others to accept your ideas when you do not receive input that you are making any progress. Sooner or later, some kind of recovery or resolution must take place.

Next in the role transformation process of student to nurse is the recovery phase. It is characterized by a return of one's sense of humor so that one can begin to laugh at some of the things that were so annoying and aggravating before. The graduate begins to discriminate between all good and all bad; the world doesn't look quite so bleak. An example:

> I have adjusted to my horror of cockroaches. I can laugh about them. One night I was assisting a doctor with a Pap smear, and a cockroach crawled right across the slide! Later, the doctor wanted to know how to get this urine specimen down real fast and asked, "What's the fastest mode of transportation?" And I answered, "Well, you could strap it on the back of a cockroach."

Cockroaches are not being condoned, but in some places they simply may have to be tolerated, and a stance of peaceful coexistence adopted. Prolonged righteous anger is unproductive. There is no point in getting upset over something that you can do nothing about. This is what is meant by a return of a sense of humor, a return of perspective, so that one can begin to differentiate things from a balanced viewpoint.

With perspectives in balance, there is a high probability of recovering and of moving into the last phase, resolution. There are many ways in which reality shock can be resolved; some are constructive and some destructive. There are two specific dimensions to constructive resolution of conflict. First of all, it must be growth-producing and self-actualizing for the individual as a person. Second, it must enable the individual to contribute toward improving the health care system and quality of nursing care.

There are several major ways in which nurses in the various research samples chose to resolve the conflict between school and work values. One is to "go native," throwing over the school values and behaviors and adopting those that are prized, valued, and rewarded in the work scene. With declining emphasis on individualized, comprehensive patient care, the person who does this becomes a competent, organized, efficient nurse, the epitome of the organization woman. The organization woman is the individual who, to a large extent, keeps the bureaucratic system functioning, status quo. This can be an effective way of resolving conflict for the individual, but it is not generally a constructive avenue for improving the quality of patient care and the health care system.

Another resolution is to renounce work behavior and values and return to school where these are prized. Performing what might be called a lateral arabesque, these nurses pirouette away from the patient's bedside back to the ivory towers of learning and then eventually into schools of nursing where they teach others to nurse the way they could not. Not all faculty in all schools of nursing have done this, but a good percentage have, particularly those who receive a B.S. degree in June, work for three summer months, return to graduate school in September, get another degree, and go directly into teaching without any additional work experience. It is highly probable that such faculty have chosen this as a way of resolving the conflict. Other nurse faculty with limited, unsuccessful, and unenjoyable work experiences who could not find satisfaction in nursing practice have also probably done lateral arabesques. This does not mean they are not good nurses according to school subcultural values; it means that in the work system they were not perceived either by themselves or by others as being successful. Their reaction is not a constructive mode of conflict resolution, either for the individual, or for the system. Teaching others to nurse the way you would like to, but found you could not, does little more than add another generation of frustrated nurses to a system already overburdened with them.

There are other options. One alternative is to say "A plague on both your houses. If you guys in school and work can't get it together on what I need to know and on what nursing is all about, the heck with both of you; I'm just going to become a rutter." Rutters are individuals who say something like this:

> Nursing is just a job. I'll put in my eight hours and then I'm going home. I know I'm in a rut, but that's fine—just leave me be. It takes too much effort and hassling to do anything else. This month I'm working for the stereo, next month for the washing machine. I'm going to stop work as soon as I can.

These are the equivalents to the incongruently socialized outcasts. The rutters resolve the value conflict between school and work by limiting their involvement or commitment to the lowest possible denominator. They do the minimum to get by. This may be a constructive avenue of conflict resolution for an individual whose emotional investment in nursing was not strong to begin with, but under no circumstances can this be considered beneficial in terms of improving the health care system.

Another option is to become a burned-out individual who doesn't really resolve the conflict but turns it inward. She walks around looking chronically constipated. On the surface, she may appear to have very good control, but underneath, there is constant ferment which may erupt at any time. A chronic griper and complainer, she frequently offers suggestions negatively with a tone of voice that says, "I know you won't listen to me or accept this change, but I'll tell you anyway." The burned-outs never resolve the conflict. Turning it inward creates a rather unhealthy state of affairs, obviously not constructive for the individual or for the system.

Another alternative for resolving the conflict is to become a job-hopper. Job-hoppers always see the other person's pasture as being greener; they change jobs often enough to remain perpetually in inservice orientation. That can be a very nice, comfortable existence—you're always being oriented, you might have more weekends free, and usually you have special work assignments. A doubtful way of resolving conflict for the individual, it is extremely costly for the system, (directors of nursing service report that it costs between $1,000 and $3,000 to orient one new nurse), and a person cannot make a contribution if she is not in the system long enough to earn informal power.

Another option is complete withdrawal: "I've had it! I'm leaving nursing altogether." The seriousness of this reaction is illustrated by what happened to the 220 nurses in one of the samples over a two-year period, from 1968 to 1970. In general, they had been working for three and four years by 1970. A little over 50 percent were still working in hospitals in 1970. About one-fourth were in public health nursing jobs, were teaching for "love of teaching," or were not working for marriage and pregnancy reasons. The remainder ($N = 72$, or 29.33 percent of the sample) had left nursing practice altogether. They stated during interviews that the major reason for quitting the profession was that they were frustrated, disillusioned, and fed up with it. What did these people do after leaving nursing? Many entered graduate school in other disciplines. They were going to be elementary school teachers, art teachers; they were pursuing occupations not requiring RN licenses. Some were working in travel agencies, or as librarians; two were horse trainers. This group constitutes roughly one-third of the sample. Abandoning nursing may be a constructive and healthy resolution for them individually, but the loss of their creative ideas and input certainly is potentially destructive for nursing and for improvements in the health care system.

The last method, chosen by a scant handful of nurses studied, but the one which the authors believe is the avenue toward which we must work, is called biculturalism. A bicultural individual has constructively resolved the school-work conflict in such a way that she has a foot in both camps. This does not mean she abjures or forsakes her beliefs and values, or forces her beliefs on others. A bicultural person works with the best of both worlds, knows and understands the rules, values, and norms of the work world, and deliberately breaks them when necessary for patient care. But most importantly she is willing to accept the risks and consequences of doing so when it is necessary for the improvement of patient care. Such an individual is frequently labeled a troublemaker by head nurses, supervisors, and directors of nursing. An often heard comment is: "Oh, Jane! She's a good nurse, but she's a troublemaker. She's constantly in there trying; she's always after something, but she really cares about the patient." There is always a tone of admiration and respect, and sometimes of exasperation; there is always the recognition that Jane is a good nurse. Involved and committed, she makes waves, but she doesn't swamp the boat. One nurse's experience with bicultural behavior will illustrate this method of conflict resolution:

At first my head nurse didn't see any need for all of the emotional and psychological support for the patients. And there was a lot of this business: "We've got to get all this work done; we've got to get these patients bathed by 9:30." And I'd say "Phooey." One of the other nurses who trained in a hospital program ten years ago had come to the floor. She was oriented in July and was told: "You have to have all the patients bathed by 9:30." I came to work in September, and in October we were sitting down to coffee when she said, "I just don't know if I can keep working; I can't keep up with all the work." I asked, "What's the problem?" And she answered, "I can't bathe four patients by 9:30 and get the meds out." I said, "So what? Bathe them at 11:00 or 1:00. What difference does it make?" Then I said, "Look, it doesn't make any difference. You have to set priorities and deal with them that way. If we get an amnio in, or if someone is upset and crying, it's more important to take care of that than to get baths done by 11:00." It blew her mind. She could not understand that you could do this—that when the administration said, "This is the way it is going to be," you could say, "OK, I accept that, but there are these other things." At first the head nurse was a bit taken aback, but I just joked it off and said, "I'm not very efficient; it takes me longer than 9:30 to do up my patients." But then she saw the kind of care I was giving, even if it was in the afternoon, so she didn't say anything more about it. Now she even tells others about it.

The bicultural troublemaker accomplishes both immediate and long-term goals, and does so in such a way that no dead or injured bodies are left in the wake of the boats she rocks. This avenue of conflict resolution would appear to be the most constructive both in terms of the individual as well as the system's improvement dimension. It is the mode of resolution that recent graduates (as well as old-timers) are challenged to adopt.

## ROLE TRANSFORMATION AS A CRISIS

The behavior adopted by individuals may be viewed as a means of resolving a crisis situation. The individual entering the shock phase of reality shock may be viewed as an individual experiencing a crisis. A crisis occurs when a person faces a block to important life goals and is unable to deal effectively with the block in her usual manner of problem solving so that a period of disorganization and emotional distress ensues[2]. For the new graduate it is the blocking of the attainment of the goals and ideals carried from school which catapults her into the emotionally distressing shock phase of reality shock. This crisis is a time when the new graduate experiences anger and frustration at the discovery of reality; a time when the evaluation of values and behaviors creates confusion and disorganization.

The precipitating event and subsequent emotional distress of crisis are often associated with a significant loss[3]. The loss for the new graduate is most evident in the "rejection" characteristic of the shock phase. There may be a rejection either of the school values and behaviors or of the work values and behaviors. The new graduate's loss could therefore be a loss of those ideals of nursing which were taught in school and the people associated with those ideals, or a loss of her own future life goals and plans if nursing cannot be practiced in the desired manner in the work world. Whichever form the rejection takes, a loss will be perceived by the new graduate—a loss causing disequilibrium, disorganization, and emotional distress.

A further factor in the dynamics of crisis is the inability to cope in the usual manner with the stressful event. The first obstacle faced by many new graduates is complete unawareness of what the problem is. There may be awareness that there are differences in what one is now expected to do versus what had been expected in school, but the newcomer often does not know what the difference is, why it exists, or what to do about it. It is difficult to reorganize when the source of difficulty is not clearly understood. Once she has identified causes and dynamics, the new graduate will frequently find that her usual support systems are no longer available. Often fellow classmates and instructors are not around. Friends outside of nursing may listen and do what they can but generally they cannot truly understand the predicament felt by the new graduate. To solve the situation alone is difficult because it is very hard to look at the work situation with a new and different perspective when one is emotionally involved in it and is all alone. For many newcomers, the usual coping maneuver is to apply oneself more diligently and to redouble one's efforts to practice nursing as one has been taught. But this will usually result in more frustration and distress because the incongruence of school-work values and behaviors becomes more pronounced. And if the new graduate decides to cope by conforming totally to the practice of nursing as she sees others practicing it, she lacks the necessary skills. (However, in time, this second option, if obtainable, will lead to some abatement of the distress felt.) Thus the new graduate finds herself in a "Catch-22" situation with neither the strategies needed to practice nursing as she was taught, nor the skills to practice as the work world demands.

The demands of the work world as perceived by the new graduate are obviously a part of the events precipitating the crisis state for the new graduate. The demands of the work world are transmitted by the work group with which the newcomer is now in daily face-to-face interaction. It is when the new graduate is in continuous contact with the work group that she becomes aware of the existence of differing outlooks and perspectives between the world of nursing as taught in school and the world of nursing as practiced in the service organizations. The way in which the new graduate was taught to perceive and order the world of nursing is no longer possible. Her unfamiliarity with the new values and her lack of appropriate behaviors necessary in the current situation cause confusion and conflict for the new graduate. An examination of referent group theory provides a framework for understanding this aspect of the new graduate's dilemma.

## REFERENT GROUP

The term "referent group" is commonly used to label a group which provides a perceptual perspective, a way of looking at the world[4, 5]. The former faculty and fellow students thus constitute the referent group of the new graduate. The way nursing is viewed, its values and behaviors are derived from the school socialization. When the new graduate enters the work world and quickly finds another view of nursing is operating, unfamiliarity and confusion result. However, the mere existence of different perspectives is not enough to create the severity and the extensiveness of the transition difficulty experienced by the newcomer.

A second common usage of the term "referent group" clarifies the difficulty; it refers to that group which assumes the functions of setting and enforcing norms, the group whose claims are paramount in a given situation[6, 7]. The newly entered ward unit group "reeducates" the new graduate by the use of rewards and punishments for appropriate and inappropriate behavior[8, 9]. The group uses positive and negative feedback and withholding of entrance to the backstage as rewards and punishments to shape the behavior of the newcomer. The more intimately involved in the group's activities and the more interdependent group members are for job performance, the greater the exposure to the group's norms and thus the greater the susceptibility to changing one's values and norms[10].

Likewise, the longer the separation from interaction with the group who originally guided the values and behaviors of the new graduate (faculty and student peers), the greater the loss of values espoused by that group[11]. Thus, the ability of the unit group to provide the rewards and punishments required to maintain conformity to certain standards of behaviors and attitudes makes their demands more critical for the new graduate who wishes to gain acceptance into that group. In time, the newcomer will modify her behavior to adopt values and behavior more like those of the group with whom she is constantly in interaction. There is tremendous conflict for the individual who is viewing the world from one perspective and experiencing demands to behave from another perspective. Because the new graduate's successful performance is tied to evaluation standards in accordance with the new group, there is little room to choose truly the perspective upon which she will operate.

Besides setting norms, the referent group also serves as a comparison group for making judgments[12, 13]. This is the third common usage of the term referent group—a group which serves as a reference point for evaluation. In any activity, those who are new to the role seek to compare themselves with others to determine how well they are performing in the role. This is true of the new graduate. When the newcomer first takes a job she establishes certain criteria for herself in role performance. She is also concerned about how well she does in comparison to others functioning in the same role. As the new graduate looks around at other nurses she is working with, she finds that her own technical competence is not as good as theirs. The other nurses do not seem to have the difficulty she has with skills such as starting IVs, catheterizations, making out patient assignments. Many other job skills such as setting priorities and making appropriate nursing judgments are not as difficult for others as they are for her. The attitudes and the values of the other nurses on the unit are also different from her own. The new graduate has less experience than the others and really cannot expect to perform as well; yet she has no one else with whom to compare herself. Additionally, since the new graduate has a different perspective on what nursing is and how one should nurse, the priorities she sets and the judgments she makes will be different from those with whom she is comparing herself. Thus, because the new graduate looks to her current group of associates as a reference for comparison, this same comparison creates a sense of insecurity and inadequacy.

The change in referent group from student peers to work peers thus creates a difficult situation for the new graduate. The new graduate experiences the turmoil and conflict of being surrounded by others who have a different perspective on the world of nursing and who have the ability to influence this perspective through the application of rewards and punishments for the enactment of behavior consistent with the norms of the group. The new graduate finds herself in a group that has more experience, and she thus develops a sense of insecurity and inadequacy when comparing herself to the others.

The change in referent group is perhaps the major factor in precipitating a personal crisis for the newcomer. In addition to the feelings engendered by the new referent group, the new graduate is also dealing with frustration, disequilibrium, and confusion resulting from the crisis state. In order for the new graduate to make an effective role transformation or transition to the work world, some form of crisis intervention is required.

## CRISIS INTERVENTION

Individuals in a crisis state, in particular those in a transition state, become highly emotional. The affective state must be dealt with before the individual can go on to effective problem solving. Thus the first step in working with new graduates in the normal maturational crisis of the first job as a professional nurse is to provide a general support system. This allows the new graduate to express her feelings and blow off steam in a safe arena[14, 15]. Since individuals in a transition state often develop a sense of marginality as well as distress due to a sense that there is something fundamentally wrong with them, the safest and most helpful arena for support is a temporary community of others in the same situation that can relate meaningfully to each other's experiences[16]. Therefore, it was concluded that temporary groups of new graduates brought together for discussion would most effectively deal with the frustration and other feelings of the newcomer in the shock phase.

The bringing together of these temporary groups of new graduates not only would provide the general support needed, but also would form a potential referent group. The new graduates would be likely to have similar values and attitudes and thus could support each other in the maintenance of these school-bred values. A certain amount of danger exists here in that a group like this could support the value system which is at odds with the prevailing values of the unit group. However, since most new graduates ultimately desire membership with the ward staff work group and since such a group of new graduates has no control over rewards and sanctions of behavior, it was thought that this would not constitute a major problem. And since all of the individuals in the temporarily constituted seminar group were now facing the reality of the work world, it was hoped that they would help each other to find ways to implement their school values in the work world. Thus the pure school-bred ideals would be tempered by reality.

A new graduate seminar group could also serve the social comparison function of a referent group. If a group of new graduates with approximately the same length of employment were brought together for discussion, then each new graduate could use the group as a standard of comparison for her performance. The comparison would be fair because the group members would all have about the same level of skill and judgment. Thus she would be ensured of a more successful evaluation of her performance.

A major portion of the comparison function was expected to occur as a result of the new graduates telling "war stories." Our new graduate had such a story to tell:

It was just terrible. I'd like to forget it but I can't. Three nights ago, Terry and I were working evenings. Only two of us; usually there's three. It was hectic. Kids screaming and crying, the IVs backed up and infiltrating, and I was late passing out the six o'clock meds because one kid in the diarrhea room kept needing diaper changes. Then right in the middle of passing meds, this one kid—a favorite of mine—comes up and wants to tell me about the new little sister he just got. I really wanted to listen to him, I know it's important, but I was just tearing my hair out. Well, anyway, about seven o'clock, Dr. Bradley, the resident, comes up to restart Ralphie's IV—I had called him earlier because it had infiltrated badly—and Ralphie is a holy terror. He's a real sick little kid—three years old. He's got some kind of blood problem, dyscrasia. It's rare, but he's a real fighter. Even just for a shot he screams and it takes two or three people to hold him down. You can imagine what it's like when you try and restart an IV. In the treatment room, it took all three of us, Dr. Bradley, Terry, and me. Terry starts to undo this tape that was holding the IV into the back of his hand— he's such a tiger that his hand was all taped down onto an armboard—and all you could see were the tips of his fingers. I'm holding the kid down, and the doctor and Terry start to pull the tape off, but there's so much tape and he's yelling so, that Bradley says, "We'll never get it off this way; let's cut it." So Terry pulls out her bandage scissors and starts to cut away the tape next to the little finger. And the next thing, Ralphie lets out the most blood curdling scream you ever want to hear—and there's blood all over and Terry looks absolutely panic stricken. At first, I couldn't figure out what happened, but finally the doc says, "Looks like you cut his finger off, Terry," but there was so much blood and tape and yelling that you really couldn't see. Bradley orders some phenobarb for the kid and tells me to get a suture tray. So I dash out to do this and about ten feet from the treatment room, guess who I run into? Ralphie's parents and his doctor. And the parents are looking really worried and the mother says, "Is that Ralphie I hear screaming? I know there's something wrong." And the doctor says: "Nurse I'm sure you can reassure Ralphie's parents that their son is all right." What was I going to do? Here, I stand with blood all over my uniform, screams echoing down the hall. I couldn't say that their kid was all right, because sooner or later they had to know about the finger. Yet, I didn't think it was my place to tell these parents that their kid's finger had been accidentally amputated. What was I going to do. I felt so bad for Ralphie, for Terry, and for the parents. I just wanted the floor to open up and swallow me.

When new graduates hear such a war story, many comment, "Oh, I wouldn't have known what to do either" or "I think I would have called the doctor" or "That was a good thing to do." This allows the new graduate who is relating the experience to evaluate her performance in terms of what her peers think would be an appropriate behavior. In addition to the benefit to the teller of the war story, there is also benefit to listeners. A type of "anticipatory" guidance occurs for them. The new graduates mentally rehearse and at times verbally indicate what they would do in the type of situation described in the war story. Thus should one of them encounter a similar situation, she is better prepared to deal with it.

New graduate seminars were designed as a way of assisting the newly entering nurse to deal effectively with the crisis and referent group aspects of the shock phase of reality shock. The seminars are intended to permit the new graduate to discharge the emotions felt with a group who shared similar experiences, gain support and confirmation for her school-bred ideals and values, and compare herself with a group of nurses having a similar level of experience.

As a result of the new graduates coming together then, it was expected that:

1. They would not feel that there was something wrong with them, but that reality shock was a normal, expected occurrence.

2. They would be better able to hold onto their values and ideals while tempering them with reality.

3. They would feel more secure about their abilities when able to compare themselves with others at the same level.

4. They would gain advanced knowledge of events which might occur and be better prepared for those events as a result of hearing about real experiences that cause shock, conflict in values and increased stress (i.e., war stories).

5. They would be better able to deal cognitively and rationally with the stresses and problems encountered as a result of having first dealt with them on an emotional level in a safe and supportive environment.

## Seminars

A number of decisions had to be made about details of the seminars. When should these seminars begin? How many should there be? Who would lead them?

The timing of the seminars was perhaps the most well-guided decision since it was based on previous research findings[17]. Since it was known that newcomers are generally quite happy and productive in the honeymoon phase, but that they experience most of their difficulty during the shock phase, it was a straightforward decision to hold the seminars after honeymoon, but before the newcomers were too deeply into shock. The shock phase usually hits when the new graduate tries to put into practice her school ideals and meets with resistance, when she is working on her permanent unit and shift, carrying responsibility for decisions and judgments on her own. Although the specific time at which the shock phase might be predicted will vary from place to place depending upon the length of orientation program, it usually occurs between four to eight weeks after beginning employment.

Keeping in mind crisis theory and group process theory, it was decided that six weekly seminars would be sufficient to allow the group to feel safe enough to open up and share with each other, yet long enough to give them a good start through the crisis period. Although six weeks is frequently estimated as the time by which some resolution must take place for a crisis to be surmounted, it must be remembered that in the case of the new graduate, crises often reoccur on a more or less daily basis. Therefore, it was not expected that this crisis would be resolved within the six-week period, but rather that the new nurse would experience sufficient emotional relief so that her usual coping mechanisms could take over, or new ones be developed, and so that some situational support could be built up through the peer reference group in the seminars. Thus, the seminars were held for an hour and a half per session, one session each week for six weeks.

## Role of Leader

Because the seminars were designed as a place where the new graduates could share and explore feelings and experiences, the role of the leader was one of facilitator rather than information-provider. The leader of the seminars must have a clear understanding of the reality shock process and of the common concerns of the new graduates. This knowledge provides a framework for the conceptual organization of the seminar discussions, and allows the leader to make sense out of the sometimes seemingly disjointed and rambling discourses of the participants.

As a facilitator of discussion, the leader need not have an *in depth* knowledge of group dynamics. Obviously, some understanding of group process will help, but the main purpose of the group is not to examine the dynamics of its movement nor to provide psychotherapy or group sensitivity training. It is not advisable for an individual to attempt to lead new graduate seminars without some clear-cut instruction and direction as to how to lead them effectively.

Although the authors have seen successful seminar leaders hold different positions in organizations (inservice, head nurses, assistant directors of nursing), a person in an inservice position does appear to be particularly suitable; because inservice personnel are usually in a staff position rather than a line position relative to the new graduates, they have more credibility in the nonintervention and confidentiality aspects of the contract to be discussed in the next section. Perhaps even more important than the specific position the leader holds in the organization is that the leader be a good listener, be sincerely interested in helping new graduates make their first job adjustment, be an individual who has had some previous staff nursing experience within that organization, and be a person with a strong ego and self-concept. The latter characteristic is important so that she can absorb the strong emotions and feelings discharged by angry young people, for often the leader herself has no support. Being equally bound by the contract of confidentiality, she is unable to utilize her usual support system. Previous staff nursing experience within the organization enables the leader to have both understanding and credibility when the new graduates describe and discuss actual events and situations on the units. With this brief overview of desirable characteristics of the leader, let us move on to look at how the leader functions.

The leader of new graduate seminars has four major functions: establishing the atmosphere and "setting the contract"; gatekeeping; facilitating the discussion; clarifying. Everything that goes on throughout the seminars affects atmosphere; the aim is to achieve an informal, comfortable one. A meeting place should be chosen which allows an informal discussion format rather than a classroom arrangement. A room in which refreshments or smoking are permitted is useful, and new graduates who find they need to eat their lunch or have a break while in seminar can relax and do so. The major concern of the leader in creating the appropriate atmosphere is to provide a comfortable and safe place for the discharge of emotion. Having participants introduce themselves so that they begin to get to know one another helps to do this.

"Setting the contract" with the participants also helps to establish atmosphere; this means clarifying the purpose and format of the group. The purpose of the seminars needs to be clearly stated as a means for the participants to share and explore their experiences—the good and the bad—in order to provide for emotional discharge and referent group development. Since the seminars are for new graduates, the content from week to week is generated by the group. No prepared content is brought to the seminar by the leader. Discharging the emotion associated with reality shock puts the participants in a position where they can then use reason to solve some of their problems. Promotion of referent group development encourages the formation of much needed evaluative and support systems.

In addition to explaining the purpose of the seminars, the contract must clearly establish the role to be played by the leader of the group. Besides acting primarily as a facilitator of the group's discussion of its concerns, the leader is a participant as well. It is expected that she will help the group to focus on and examine some of the problems brought to seminar but she is not there to intervene with the staff on behalf of the new graduates. A new graduate may present some difficulty in working with a particular staff member, or the whole group may focus on problems with the nursing administration. The group may then turn to the leader and ask, either directly or indirectly, what the leader can and will do about these problems. The leader's answer must be "Nothing." If the new graduates wish to consider what course of action they might take to deal with the situation, they should be encouraged and helped to do so. However, it would be counterproductive in assisting them to become effective workers if the leader accepts responsibility for taking the information provided and intervening. Nonintervention sounds simple and logical; however, on an individual basis, it is often difficult, particularly when the leader knows the system, knows that she could readily circumvent the system, and knows that she had worked successfully within the system in the past. To deny intervention to people who ask for it is difficult, but it's necessary to do so if the newcomers are to learn how to solve their own problems.

There will be many times when answers to the questions, problems, and concerns of the new graduates are not readily known either to the leader or to the other participants. It is important to make clear at the onset of the seminars that the leader does not have all the answers.

A word of caution is offered to leaders about listening behavior. For many of us, listening behavior includes the gentle nodding of one's head while the other person is talking or relating some difficulty or concern. Often an individual who is distressed, frustrated, or angry, interprets such nodding as agreement with what is being said, rather than as a sign of listening only. Leaders should take note that if nodding is part of one's listening profile, seminar participants should be warned that it does not signal agreement. In this way, considerable confusion can be allayed.

Since one goal of the leader is to establish a safe place for emotional discharge and for discussion to take place, it is important to stress the confidentiality of the seminars in the initial contract. The leader maintains the trust of the group by not discussing material voiced during seminar with anyone else. So too, the new graduates are expected to maintain the confidentiality of the group. On occasion, a new graduate returns to seminar with a remark such as, "I was talking to my head nurse about what Dorothy said last week and she was telling me what she thought about evaluation." A message such as this indicates violation of group confidentiality. Such violations must be immediately recognized by the leader and the contract reemphasized with the group. No one can continue to feel safe to express her feelings and experiences if there is a possibility that the information discussed will leave the seminar.

New graduates have also indicated that, at times, it is difficult not to share what happened in seminar when they return to their unit and that the head nurse or other staff nurses would ask, "What went on today?" Most new graduates find that an explanation of their reason for not sharing the information is well received by others on the unit. Occasional individuals will continue to press to find out what went on in the seminar. The leader's role is to help the new graduate learn to deal with any pressure exerted on her to violate the confidentiality of the group.

At times, seminar participants also report a sense of pressure either from themselves or from their coworkers to remain on the unit rather than to attend seminar. These feelings are understandable, particularly when the unit is quite busy or understaffed. Although the leader can empathize with the problem, she must clearly state the expectations for attendance. New graduates are expected to attend seminar each week for the six weeks they are held. In cases where more than one series of seminars is being conducted simultaneously, it is important that the new graduates understand that they are to attend the same seminar each week as it is detrimental to the group if a member moves from one group to another once the seminar series has begun. The support and cooperation of the head nurse and other unit staff is crucial in decreasing the pressure the new graduate feels to stay on the unit. If for any reason a participant cannot attend a session, a phone call to inform the leader is expected. If a participant does not attend the first or second seminar session, the leader can call the participant to find out why she was not at seminar and encourage attendance at the next session. The telephone calls are not meant to be punitive or to pressure the new graduate into attending seminars if she chooses not to go. The calls are meant to convey interest and concern and to ascertain whether, in fact, the new graduate knew that she was scheduled to attend the seminar. A new graduate may say, "I was 20 minutes late so I decided not to come." In answer, the leader can explain to the prospective participant that, although the seminars will usually start and finish on time, she is welcome to come for as much of the seminar as she can and that the leader understands that there will be times when she will get tied up with unit activities but to come for as much time as she can, as the seminars are important.

The final aspect of the contract that must be dealt with is any housekeeping details or ground rules. In most institutions there will be such details as how time is to be charged or handled if the new graduate is coming to seminar during off-duty time and what does the new graduate do if she is the only nurse on the floor? There is no set way to handle these details; each institution must make its own decisions in accord with its policies. The important thing is to follow through with the decisions and to apply them to all new graduates participating. If decentralization of administration dictates that different areas be handled in different ways, then this needs to be made clear. There is no reason why each new graduate cannot be given the responsibility to check out the details with her own head nurse if these decisions vary from service to service or unit to unit. If the leader wishes to set any particular ground rules for the group, she should do so when the initial contract is set. One particular ground rule or contract item useful to the leader is asking the permission of the group to tape record or make a few notes during the sessions. It needs to be explained to the group that this will allow the leader to review what happened during the seminar each week so that important issues discussed are not missed and so that the leader can analyze and improve her behavior. Tape recording or making notes is particularly important when the group is very talkative and addresses a large number of concerns. In reviewing the seminar session, the leader may become aware of issues which at first were not apparent. These issues can then be brought back to the group in succeeding seminars. Since tapes could be a source of potential confidentiality leaks, the tapes must be erased immediately after review by the leader.

Every attempt should be made to minimize the amount of time for housekeeping details and setting ground rules. So that the group can quickly begin discussion, whatever can be handled in written form (schedules, time accounting, etc.) should be. Contract setting usually requires as much as 15 to 20 minutes the first week. In succeeding weeks, little will need to be done in terms of contract setting, except to reiterate the confidentiality and nonintervention aspects.

Once the contract is set, it is time to get started. Getting the group started on time and finishing on time are a part of the leader's gatekeeping role. This may be a problem the first week; people are just finding out where to go and often they are late. Since it is important that all seminar participants are well aware of the contract, the start of the first seminar may need to be delayed until all arrive. Thereafter, it is important to start and finish on time so that participants need not lose time on their units. The leader must allow 10 to 15 minutes for summarizing and closing each seminar as participants tend to get restarted as the seminar discussion is summarized.

Another aspect of the gatekeeping role is to provide an opportunity for all participants to become involved. For the leader, this means watching out for either the unusually quiet or unusually talkative participant. In the case of the unusually quiet individual, the leader must watch for nonverbal signs which indicate that the individual has a contribution to make about a particular topic of discussion and provide the opportunity for this individual to talk. The leader may notice a rather silent participant nodding her head and break in to say, "I see you nodding your head, Sally. Does this strike a chord with you?" or "Did you have something you'd like to share with the group?" The exact words are unimportant as long as the opportunity to participate is provided. At times there may be no nonverbal signs that an individual has something to say. Depending upon the leader's style or particular feeling about the situation, she may point out the silence by a member. "You've been particularly quiet today, Betty. Anything you wanted to contribute?" or "Is there anything going on with you?" This will provide an opportunity for the silent member to contribute. If openings are provided and a silent individual does not wish to participate verbally, the leader should not force participation. As a matter of fact, some new graduates will come right out and say, "I'm quiet and I don't talk much. If I have something to say, I will." The right of the participant not to talk must be respected. The lack of verbal participation does not mean that the individual is not getting anything out of seminar.

The other type of participant who requires intervention by the leader is the one who monopolizes and dominates the discussion. This individual talks frequently, at great length, and often so much that other participants lose interest in what is being said and begin to show signs of boredom and restlessness. This type of participant causes others to lose the opportunity to talk. The role of the leader is to allow the participant to talk long enough so that the leader has an understanding of the issue or concern of the individual, and then to open up the conversation to the rest of the group. For example, the leader may listen and then say, "So what you are talking about is not having any control over what happens in the care of the patient despite the added time you spend with the patients? Does anyone else have similar experiences or feelings?" This prevents the concern of the individual from being lost but opens the discussion to all members of the group.

The leader's most important function is to facilitate the discussion of experiences by the new graduates, to achieve focus and direction with a lot of participant-to-participant interaction and a minimum of leader-to-member interaction. If the group is moving, the leader needs only to pay attention and listen to what is going on. If some direction is needed, the leader intervenes to provide what is needed and then turns the discussion back to the new graduates. The leader must be careful not to get into the habit of calling on the participants for contributions, thus setting up leader-to-member interaction patterns and controlling participation as in a classroom.

The kind of facilitation needed varies with groups. Some groups need encouragement and stimulus questions to get started and keep moving; others need someone to keep everyone from talking at once. The groups usually provide clues in their initial introduction as to what will be needed to facilitate their discussion. Some members merely state who they are and other participants indicate that they have a lot to talk about or that they jumped at the chance to come and share their experiences. In instances where the group members indicate that they have a lot to talk about, the leader can facilitate sharing merely by turning the discussion over to the members, saying, "A number of you have indicated that you have a lot to say, perhaps the best way to go is just to get started sharing your experiences." The leader then needs to be silent and provide the group with a chance to get started. At other times the leader may need to provide a stimulus question to get the group moving. There are a number of questions which can open the discussion and allow the group to move in a variety of directions. Some of these questions are as follows:

1. "Was nursing what you expected it to be?"
2. "Can you be the kind of nurse you want to be in your job?"
3. "What was your greatest surprise when you first started work?"

Such questions set the stage so that all experiences can be discussed. Although the majority of the experiences new graduates discuss in seminar tend to be negative (things that are going well generally are not of concern or bothersome to new graduates), any way of starting which provides the opportunity to talk about either positive or negative experiences is a good beginning. In the first seminar, a wide range of experiences should be discussed with little in depth exploration of any particular issue. Encouraging the preliminary exposition of a large number of issues and concerns provides the seminar participants with a wide range of choice for topics for deeper exploration in future sessions. It also increases the probability that the issues subsequently selected will be of interest to and meet the needs of the majority of the participants. The more issues that come out the better. (In extremely talkative or volatile groups, the first seminar can sound very much like a flight of ideas with new graduates hopping from one topic to another.) If a group narrows its focus too soon, there is a greater possibility of turning the seminar into a group interview situation where, with each group member, the leader successively questions and explores individual concerns or experiences.

To facilitate movement in succeeding seminars, it is a good idea when summarizing and closing a seminar session to provide food for thought for the next seminar. The leader summarizes and then asks the group if they want to pursue one of the issues further at the next seminar or if there is something else the participants would like to discuss. If the group has no particular desires, the leader may suggest one of the areas that came up during seminar or some other idea related to areas of new graduate stress that did not arise in that particular group. For example, the leader may suggest, "Next week let's look at particular experiences which are either satisfying or dissatisfying for you." It doesn't matter exactly what is to be discussed the next week as long as the participants are given something to think about for the next week. This saves a lot of time at the beginning of seminar trying to decide what will happen that day.

In successive seminars, the previously chosen topic need not always be discussed. Prior to beginning the suggested agenda, the leader can open up the seminar for participants to discuss anything that may have happened to them during the week or any items from the last seminar which may have stimulated some thought and further discussion. Any new happenings or discussion can be easily brought up. It is important, however, that if something more pressing takes precedence over the suggested topic, the leader clearly indicate that the group will get back to the earlier topic, if not during this session, then most certainly in the next. This follow-up and clarification is important as participants who have put a lot of thought into preparing themselves for the seminar will get frustrated if the item is not dealt with.

When the group begins to cool down after having discharged their emotional reactions in the first sessions, the leader can help the participants to identify common concerns and focus on them for more in depth exploration. Initial attempts to focus the discussion may be less than successful; when the group has strong emotion and a lot to talk about, the leader is often ignored. This can be frustrating for the leader, and yet as long as the participants are sharing their experiences with one another and not continually retreading the same ground without getting anywhere, the work of the seminars is under way. Usually by the fourth seminar, the group will be ready to look at issues and concerns in more depth.

At this point the leader's role is to help the group look at the issues in specific rather than general terms and to examine the issues from different perspectives. A frequent seminar theme is, "No one cares about the psychosocial needs of the patient." It is difficult even to know for sure what such a general statement means. It is, however, possible and helpful to deal with the problem of whining Mrs. Smith whom the staff ignores and doesn't care about. Thus, it is the function of the leader to bring the discussion of such a general theme down to a more specific level. This can be accomplished by asking an individual participant to describe a situation which exemplifies the theme.

Once the new graduates begin to give specifics, exploration of perspectives is possible. After the participant has had a chance to talk about a situation from her own perspective, the leader can introduce ideas or questions to help her look at other perspectives. For example:

> You described a situation in which you were feeling pretty bad about what you were doing and didn't really know what to do next. What did the other staff say when you called for help?

The participant may reply:

> Well you know, that was really funny. The other nurses couldn't understand what I was so upset about. They said they thought I was doing okay and handling the situation real well.

or:

> I really felt deserted. I mean the patient died and the family was there and I didn't know what to do and no one helped me out. It was as if they just dumped this patient on me and left.

The participant just quoted went on to talk about her own experience in more detail. When she had expressed her feelings, others in the group shared similar experiences in which the staff had left them in situations they didn't know how to handle. The leader further explored by saying,

> You know, a number of you have indicated that you didn't know what to do and felt that someone else should have been there to help you out. What do you suppose it is like for the other nurses?

The participants do not always respond in a way that indicates they have any sense of what is going on for the other person, yet it is important to help them look at perspectives other than their own. At times the participants have differing perspectives on issues. Sharing their different perspectives allows participants to challenge each other's views and learn from one another. For example, when one participant said,

> No one does nursing care plans. Or if they do, no one ever reads them. Why do they teach us these things in school if no one does it out here in the real world?

another participant responded,

> But nursing care plans are important. A couple of weekends ago I had this patient who was being discharged. And she didn't speak English very well . . .

When differing perspectives come from within their new peer group, it forces the new graduates to stop and take a look at what they are saying and at the implications of their individual perspectives. The peer group tends to carry more weight and credibility than the leader, who is not a peer. It is much more powerful for a fellow new graduate to say care plans are important than for the leader to say that care plans are important. Likewise, the participant who hears from a fellow new graduate, "Look, you can't come to work expecting it to be like school. It isn't. And my head nurse is not my teacher," is more likely to pay attention. The new graduates do not expect such admonitions from one another and thus are somewhat stunned to hear them, whereas they expect a certain amount of "preaching" from the leader. While the new graduates can readily challenge each other, it is more difficult for the leader to challenge participants since they often interpret any direct statements as a defense of the way things are rather than a different perspective on the situation. For this reason, the leader can best introduce the idea of differing perspectives through questioning rather than by direct challenge. Even if the new graduates are unable to recognize any other perspective to an issue or concern, the leader does not have to accept the new graduates' perspective, however. She is free to disagree, although it is not a good idea to argue with the participants. Arguing tends to convey to the new graduate that the leader is not listening and that she will automatically defend the perspective of the organization. Arguing also tends to entrench both parties in their isolated perspectives so that the goal of entertaining alternative perspectives is not achieved.

In exploring issues and concerns, sometimes new graduates have a tendency to get stuck on what is wrong, disapproval of how other staff members perform, or what they have to do rather than what they want to do. There are a number of questions which can assist the new graduate to look beyond what is happening to what they would like to see happen or what could happen. For example:

1. What is it you would like to see happen? What is it that you would like to do with your patients that you don't do now?

2. What keeps you from doing what you want to do or being the kind of nurse you would like to be?

3. What are others doing that makes you feel that way?

4. How could you let others know about your problems or ideas in a way they could accept it?

Another function of the leader in helping the new graduates identify their real concerns is keeping tabs on a participant's contributions throughout the series of seminars. Sometimes a new graduate will talk about a situation in the first seminar, then in the fourth and fifth seminars will add a little more about the same situation. It is only when the three pieces are pulled together that the real issue becomes clear. The leader must be able to help a participant link these pieces when necessary. One new graduate described the following situation:

1st week—
I'm having trouble with this aide. She won't do what she is supposed to do and sleeps most of the time. It really makes me mad. And the supervisor knows it.

2nd week—
I don't know why, but this aide is giving me more trouble than she gives any of the other new grads. She seems to leave you all alone but she sure gives me trouble.

3rd week—
Well you know, Sarah knows she can get my goat. She gets at me until I blow and then just laughs. I've tried to control myself but I can't take it.

When all the pieces were out, it became clear why the new graduate was so disturbed by the situation and what was really bothering her. Once the problem was identified, the group could further explore and work with the issue.

Once the issue has been examined, the new graduate can begin to look at alternatives to what is going on. It is important to help them free their minds from the "either/or" mode of thinking—"It has to be *either* the way I learned in school *or* the way it is done here at the hospital." Although this may sometimes be the case, usually it is more helpful to stimulate new graduates to generate other alternatives, to help them see the consequences of different behaviors, so they can make informed choices as to what to do. The leader must introduce the possibility of negative as well as positive consequences, e.g., "If you chose to do that you may find that no one will talk to you again," or "We've talked a lot about all the things that could go wrong for you if you try that idea. What might go well?" So the leader's role is to help the individual look at the situation fully and then allow the new graduate to choose the best alternative for herself (even though the leader may not agree with the choice). Some questions which may be of help to the leader in getting the group to look at alternatives are as follows:

1. Does it have to be all their way or all your way?

2. Let's take a look at all the possible things you might do. What else could you do in this situation?

3. What's the worst that could happen to you if you did that?
4. What's the best that could happen to you?

Ultimately, the new graduates must be allowed to make their own choices and solve their own problems.

The leader must exercise discretion in helping new graduates delve into matters in depth which are common concerns and not unique to a particular new graduate. Although the terms of the discussion should be specific the leader should consider the general applicability of situations. For example, if a new graduate in obstetrics talks about how difficult it is to gain a certain skill for labor and delivery, the leader can point out the common element of the problem and seek specific input.

> We've all had situations in which we didn't have the skills we needed and had difficulty gaining them. Have any of you met up with this problem? What did you do about it?

As long as an issue has general applicability and concern, the new graduates can identify with it and focus their energy on it.

In the process of exploring concerns in depth, there are times when the new graduates "wind down" in discussing an issue or a related issue is brought into the discussion. In either case, the leader will need to provide a mini-summarization of the discussion that has taken place as a recap of the points raised and as a last chance for participants who have something more to say about an issue before the seminar moves in a new direction.

In facilitating the discussions, whether to identify or to solve problems, it is sometimes necessary for the leader to provide clarification. When indefinite references are used, when inaccurate or contradictory information is presented, and when the issue is unclear, clarification is required.

In their discussion, new graduates often refer to "we," "they," and "everyone." These indefinite references are particularly noticeable in situations in which there is polarization of issues. Vague references such as the following should be clarified:

> And these people come on the unit and they ask a few ridiculous questions, look around, and leave. They never do anything to help you.
>
> I'm really trying to be a good nurse and do the things I know are best for the patient but they won't let me.

In some seminar discussions, new graduates seek information from each other on factual matters. The new graduate may want to know where to go to straighten out a problem with a paycheck, or who to see to correct a problem regarding health insurance. Peers at times don't know and spend considerable time trying to figure out this information. Or peers may provide inaccurate information regarding the appropriate channels for handling a problem. In either case it is useful for the leader to provide accurate input regarding these factual concerns. There is little point in allowing new graduates to spend time on these kinds of issues.

A slightly different situation involves contradictory information. The new graduate says one thing, and then later says something completely different. A certain amount of confusion ensues. Contradictory information must be handled carefully, particularly if the information in the first or second seminar is in direct opposition to information shared in later seminars. Often the information is not truly contradictory but is the individual's perception at a point in time. For example, when the new graduate is in shock, the information shared is the reality at the time. By the later seminars the reality for the new graduate, who is now less emotionally upset, has changed. However, if contradictions occur within the same seminar or between later seminars, say the fourth and sixth, the leader may wish to clarify such contradictions with the participant.

At times as the new graduates talk about their experiences, it is difficult to understand what is meant even though the description is not contradictory. The leader may wish to clarify an issue further by asking a question such as: "Well now, is the issue you are raising that there are other nurses who are incompetent?" This question gives the new graduate the chance either to confirm the issue as restated by the leader or to describe the real issue some other way. Putting an unclear issue into a few words is particularly helpful if it has taken quite a lengthy statement for the new graduate to put her experience into words.

In attempting to lead any group, there are certain problems which develop for the leader. The two most common problems for beginning leaders are missing cues and piggybacking questions. Initially, lack of familiarity with the reality shock dynamics and phenomenon and the accompanying concerns of the new graduates causes the leader to miss important messages. The second common problem, piggybacking questions, occurs when the leader asks several questions without giving the participants a chance to answer one question before asking the next. Piggybacking is usually the result of tension on the leader's part or is an attempt to clarify the initial question. Piggybacking tends to cause confusion because no one knows which of the questions to answer, if any at all. It is advisable for the leader to think a question through before posing it, so that it can be stated very clearly initially and to ask just one question at a time, giving the participants a chance to answer. Occasionally, the group members will not answer quickly and it seems that the silence is forever. If you expect an answer to a question which requires thought, then "thinking time" must be provided.

Besides these common problems the most difficult problem for leaders tends to be the leader's own feelings and reactions to the new graduates' discussion. The new graduates' perceptual distortions and discussion of backstage reality which paint the organization as all bad often spark defensive reactions in the leaders. If the new graduates are to feel safe and comfortable, the leader must control her own reactions—both verbal and nonverbal. Nothing will be gained by the leader declaring, "It isn't so!" When their anger cools a bit and their perceptions become less distorted, the new graduates will see for themselves that some of what they perceived earlier is probably true, and some is probably not.

A related problem occurs if the seminars do not meet the leader's expectations. The leader knows that, although there are goals, there is no set behavioral objective for each seminar. Nevertheless, after a leader has led several series of seminars, she may begin to have some general expectations of how they will go. She may expect that in the first couple of seminar sessions the group will hopscotch all over the place and touch on many concerns only superficially, in the third and fourth session they'll focus in on one or two particular concerns, and by the last two, they'll begin to solve problems. But the leader must remember that each new graduate seminar group is unique. Although new graduates have many difficulties and concerns in common, they express them differently and deal with them at different times. In some seminar series which the authors have led, the participants have been so vocal, volatile, and emotional that they never were able to focus and solve problems. The leader may feel that somehow she has failed but she must realize, for example, "It's OK if they don't get into problem solving." The group derives a great deal of benefit from simply having a safe place to dissipate accumulated emotion and relate shocked observations. As an older staff nurse said to one of the members of a volatile group: "I don't know what goes on at your group meetings, but whatever it is, it's helping you. You're so much easier to live and work with after you've had a meeting."

In other seminar series, the leader's expectations may be unmet for the opposite reason; she may be confronted with such a quiet group that she feels she has to pull teeth to get anything out of the members. One of the hardest groups to deal with is the sad and depressed group, whose members are so down that the emotion hangs over the room like a heavy curtain.

All groups are different, so the outcomes will be different and the leader must learn to live with her unmet expectations. The worst thing to do is to try forcing each group into some common mold.

One final word of advice should be mentioned to prospective new graduate seminar leaders. Ideally, two people from an organization should be trained to lead seminars together. Although the actual leadership is centered in one, the other person can be extremely helpful in noting the flow of the discussion, drawing in the silent members, observing the reaction of the group, and, most importantly, in providing a sounding board for a debriefing session for the primary leader after the seminar session is over. The leader absorbs a great deal of the emotion and she needs to talk about it afterwards. Because of the contract of confidentiality, she cannot do this within her usual support system. A coleader helps immensely also in validating the leader's observations and recall of what went on in seminar.

## SUMMARY

Reality shock can be a lonely experience for the new graduate in a crisis state. Frustrated by her inability to put into practice her school values, the newcomer becomes angry and disillusioned. To become an effective and productive worker, the new graduate nurse needs to express and explore her feelings. New graduate seminars can provide a temporary community for the sharing of these experiences and feelings with others. Through this community new graduates can come to understand the almost universal nature of the process they are experiencing. They can begin to develop an awareness of the perspectives of others. The new referent group that develops can provide ongoing support for the newcomer and an appropriate standard for self-evaluation. Reality shock need not be a lonely experience; it can be the stimulus for growth and effective role transformation.

## REFERENCES AND NOTES

The following description of the first phases is taken from

1. Schmalenberg, C. and Kramer, M. Dreams and reality: Where do they meet? *J. Nurs. Admin.,* 6(5): 35–43, 1976. Reprinted with permission.
2. Caplan, G. *An Approach to Community Mental Health.* New York: Grune and Stratton, 1961, p. 18.
3. Morley, W. E. Theory of crisis intervention. *Pastoral Psychol.,* 21(203): 16, 1970.
4. Shibutani, T. "Reference Groups as Perspectives" in Hyman, Herbert H. and Singer, E. (Eds.), *Readings in Reference Group Theory and Research.* New York: The Free Press, 1968, p. 104.
5. Sherif, M. "The Concept of Reference Groups in Human Relations" in Hyman, Herbert H. and Singer, E. (Eds.), *Readings in Reference Group Theory and Research.* New York: The Free Press, 1968, p. 86.
6. Morley, W. E. 1970, p. 104.
7. Kelley, H. "Two Functions of Reference Groups" in Hyman, Herbert H. and Singer, E. (Eds.), *Readings in Reference Group Theory and Research.* New York: The Free Press, 1968, p. 80.
8. Hackman, R. "Group Influences on Individuals" in Dunnette, Marvin (Ed.), *Handbook of Industrial and Organizational Psychology.* Chicago: Rand McNally College Publishing Co., 1976, p. 1462.
9. Jackson, J. M. "Structural Characteristics of Norms" in Biddle, Bruce and Thomas, Edwin (Eds.), *Role Theory: Concepts and Research.* New York: John Wiley and Sons, Inc., 1966, p. 124.

10. Hyman, H. et al. *"Reference Groups and the Maintenance of Changes in Attitudes and Behavior"* in Hyman, Herbert H. and Singer, E. (Eds.), *Readings in Reference Group Theory and Research*. New York: The Free Press, 1968.
11. Jacobson, G. F. Crisis intervention from the viewpoint of the mental health professional. *Pastoral Psychol.,* 21(203): 388, 1970.
12. Hyman, H. et al. 1968, p. 388.
13. Shitubani, T. 1968, p. 104.
14. Kelley, H. 1968, p. 81.
15. Morley, W. E. 1970, p. 17.
16. Jacobson, G. 1970, p. 28.
17. Weiss, R. S. "Transition States and Other Stressful Situations: Their Nature and Programs for Their Management" in Caplan, Gerald and Killilea, Marie (Eds.), *Support Systems and Mutual Help: Multidisciplinary Explorations*. New York: Grune and Stratton, 1976, p. 216.

## BIBLIOGRAPHY

Aguilera, D. and Messick, J. *Crisis Intervention Theory and Methodology*. St. Louis: The C. V. Mosby Co., 1974.

Charters, W. and Newcomb, T. "Some Attitudinal Effects of Experimentally Increased Salience of a Membership Group" in Hyman, Herbert and Singer, E. (Eds.), *Readings in Reference Group Theory and Research*. New York: The Free Press, 1968.

Eisenstadt, S. N. "Studies in Reference Group Behavior" in Hyman, Herbert and Singer, E. (Eds.), *Readings in Reference Group Theory and Research*. New York: The Free Press, 1968.

Hall, J. E. and Weaver, B. (Eds.). *Nursing Families In Crisis*. Philadelphia: J. B. Lippincott Co., 1974.

Hartley, R. "Norm Compatability, Norm Reference, and the Acceptance of New Reference Groups" in Hyman, Herbert and Singer, E. (Eds.), *Readings in Reference Group Theory and Research*. New York: The Free Press, 1968.

Janken, J. K. The nurse in crisis. *Nurs. Clinics North Am.,* Vol. 9. No. 1, March 1974.

Kardener, S. A methodologic approach to crisis therapy. *Am. J. Psychotherapy,* 29(1), 1975.

Kramer, M. *Reality Shock: Why Nurses Leave Nursing*. St. Louis: The C. V. Mosby Co., 1974.

Krech, D. et al. *Individual and Society*. New York: McGraw-Hill, 1962.

Kuhn, M. "The Reference Group Reconsidered" in Manis, J. and Meltzer, B. (Eds.), *Symbolic Interaction: A Reader in Social Psychology*. Boston: Allyn and Bacon, Inc., 1967.

Parad, H. (Ed.), *Crisis Intervention: Selected Readings*. New York: Family Service Association of America, 1965.

# Chapter 2
# The Setup

The new graduate seminars reported in this book were implemented as a part of a nationwide research study on bicultural training and role transformation[1]. This chapter details a description of the participating medical centers, how the leaders were prepared for seminar leadership, anticipated concerns of the new graduates, implementation of the seminars, and procedures for data analysis.

## DESCRIPTION OF MEDICAL CENTERS

The seminars were conducted in more than eight different medical centers. The medical center hospitals ranged from 300 to 1,500 beds with a 65 to 99 percent occupancy range. The operation of the medical centers was divided approximately equally between the public and private sectors. All of the institutions served as training facilities for a variety of allied health personnel, including medical students and residents, nursing students, physical therapists, occupational therapists, and dietetic students. All the medical centers provided outpatient as well as inpatient services. The clientele varied from lower to upper class, with most of the medical centers serving the middle class population. The medical centers hired from 65 to 150 new graduates a year. The graduates' average term of employment ranged from 8 to 15 months.

New graduates in the participating medical centers were given both general orientation and unit orientation. The general orientation always presented the philosophy and objectives of the hospital, policies and forms, functions of other departments in the organization, legal aspects of nursing, medications, admission and discharge procedures, cardiopulmonary resuscitation, intravenous therapy, and teaching patients. The medical centers varied somewhat in other procedural and patient-related topics. Some medical centers included tracheotomy care, catheter care, and postmortem care, whereas others included neuroassessment, cardiac monitoring and defibrillating, and chest tube care. The general orientation varied in duration from 15 to 56 hours of classroom instruction.

In all the medical centers the new graduates were also involved in unit orientation, varying in duration from two to six weeks. Some of the unit orientations were structured, carefully delineating how and what was to be done with the new graduate; others were less structured, with the unit or service deciding how the new graduate was to proceed. The combined time span of the general and unit orientations usually placed the new graduates in the orientee category from 4 to 12 weeks. Thus although there were similarities in the orientation of new graduates, differences also existed between medical centers.

## PREPARATION OF SEMINAR LEADERS

Each of the medical centers participating in the research study was asked to select an individual who would serve as a satellite director for the Role Transformation project. This person would be responsible for conducting the seminars and for implementing the research protocol at the particular medical center. The satellite director would be an individual who was successful in the organization, held informal power, was respected by the nurses, and knew the organization well. No stipulation as to the actual position held within an organization was made. The idea was that a nurse with respect and influence could obtain the cooperation of the rest of the staff in encouraging the participation of the new graduates in seminar, and her knowledge of the organization would be beneficial in understanding the new graduate discussions during seminar. The satellite directors held a variety of positions—administrative, head nurse, and inservice educator—within the medical centers.

Because the satellite directors needed instruction, they were brought to San Francisco for explication and discussion of the research protocol, instructional programs[2] and seminar leadership. Knowledge of the instructional material was essential so that any questions arising about the material during the research could be handled by the satellite directors. In addition, the instructional materials provided the satellite directors with an understanding of the reality shock process and the role transformation of the new graduate. This understanding was to serve as a conceptual framework for understanding the new graduates' seminar discussions.

In a one-day leadership training session the role of the leader in new graduate seminars was discussed. This discussion was similar to that presented in the preceding chapter. After the discussion of the content, the satellite directors were paired off for purposes of leading a series of three new graduate seminars. The new graduates for these practice seminars were obtained through the help of Bay Area hospitals. All prospective new graduate participants were sent a letter giving them an introduction to the seminars and some questions to think about before coming to seminar. Each of the leader pairs led three one and one-half hour long seminars, all of which were videotaped. Immediately following the seminar, the leader pair had a critique session with one of the authors. The purpose of this critique session was to provide the satellite directors with immediate feedback on their leadership behavior and to suggest changes and improvements prior to the next seminar session. Three mornings a week during the two-week time period were devoted to general group sessions during which the total group observed and discussed specially selected clips of the TV tapes depicting problems or styles in seminar leadership. This broadened the learning for all of the participants.

In addition to allowing them to examine their leadership behavior, the practice seminars provided the prospective leaders with exposure to common new graduate concerns and topics. This helped the satellite directors not only to master the cognitive material, but also to recognize topics in the way that new graduates express them.

## ANTICIPATED CONCERNS

Over the past decade, the authors have worked extensively with new graduates both on an individual basis and in groups. Together they have led or have attended many new graduate seminar discussions. Based on input from these extensive contacts with new graduate nurses the following areas of discussion were anticipated:

*Professional-bureaucratic conflict.*   School had prepared the new graduates to function in a whole-task way; when they came to work it wasn't at all as expected.

*Proving ground.*   The new graduates expected themselves to be able to perform certain tasks or activities in order to really earn for themselves the title of nurse. Others were watching and testing the new graduates to see what they could and couldn't do.

*Delegation.*   It is difficult to delegate tasks to others because what has to be delegated is what the new graduate wants to do herself. Moreover others may not accept orders from the new graduate well so rather than delegate, the new graduate does the work herself and never seems to get done working.

*Interpersonal problems.*   New graduates experienced hassles with coworkers on the same shift and different shifts as well as between nurses and physicians and between nurses and other departments. At times, race became a point of conflict.

*Competency.*   New graduates found that they were unable to perform some of the skills required by the job. They lack not only manual-technical skills but also interpersonal and management skills needed to do the job.

*Backstage reality.*   The practices that the new graduates encountered were, at times, shocking. People gave meds without orders and started IV's using the same needle to stick a patient three or four times.

*Staffing.*   There is not enough staff to do the job especially on the weekends.

Although this list does not exhaust all of the concerns which new graduates might discuss, these anticipated concerns provided the leaders with common points of discussion and orientation as to what they might expect in their own medical centers.

## IMPLEMENTATION OF THE SEMINARS

The medical centers were expected to provide the time for the new graduates to attend seminars. The satellite directors set the day and hour of the seminars to obtain the best results in terms of new graduate participation. (Because of research protocol, all series of seminars began during the fifth or sixth week of employment.) Seminars were held in early morning, midafternoon, and late night to accommodate new graduates on different shifts. Seminars were held late morning and during visiting hours when new graduates would be less busy. Even with the best of planning, some new graduates had to attend seminars on off-duty time. The medical centers determined how this time was to be handled. For the most part, either compensatory time or overtime was utilized depending upon the contractual agreement the hospital held with the nurses.

Once the day and hour of the seminars were set, the satellite directors informed the project directors so that a debriefing session could be arranged. The purpose of the debriefing session was to provide an opportunity for the satellite directors to talk about what had gone on in seminar, to ask any questions they might have about leadership behavior on topics discussed. To facilitate effective intervention by the project director in the leadership behavior of the satellite directors, a contract was set with the new graduates for the audio recording of the seminar sessions. These tape recordings were made for the purpose of weekly review by the satellite directors and the project director, for compilation of common themes, and, in some medical centers, so that new graduates who missed a seminar could listen to what had happened. The tape recordings were mailed to the project director after each seminar. The project director then listened to the tapes and in the telephone debriefing sessions provided direct feedback regarding topics which had been adequately explored, topics needing more exploration, cues picked up or missed, and general leadership behavior. Also, because the satellite directors could not discuss the seminars with anyone in their own hospitals, the telephone sessions allowed them to talk about the seminar sessions and their reactions.

## DATA ANALYSIS

The tape recordings of 86 seminars were transcribed and typescripts prepared. Ten additional tapes were not transcribed as three were lost in the mail and seven had extensive background noise. These seven tapes were coded directly from the tapes using the same process as described below. Content analysis was chosen as the most appropriate means of analyzing the data obtained from the tape recordings of the seminars. Content analysis is a "research technique for objective, systematic, and quantitative description of the manifest content of communication"[3]. The purpose for performing such analysis on the seminar typescripts was to 1) describe the trends in the communication content, 2) examine regional differences in the content of new graduate seminars, and 3) explore the relative timing of content occurrences in the seminars.

As a preliminary step, all of the typescripts were read through and a beginning subject area categorization system was set up. This category system began with the list of anticipated concerns described earlier, but it was not bound by or limited to this list.

On the second reading of the typescripts, a more definitive category system was constructed. Sixteen subject areas of content were thus identified in the seminar typescripts. These subject areas and their description are as follows:

*Competency.*   Relates to new graduate's ability (or inability) to do the job. Besides skill and knowledge components, it includes interpersonal abilities in dealing with other staff members.

*Backstage reality.*   Relates to new graduate's discoveries of impression management. "The way things are taught in school is not exactly the way things are done in the work world." Other staff take "short cuts" and make adaptations and modifications in norms and practices. The modifications many times fall below the standards of practice the new graduate believes are and should be in operation.

*Role expectations.*   The new graduate expects certain behaviors of self and others in role functions. Discrepancies exist between set expectations and behavior enacted.

*Floating.*   Pleasures or conflicts resulting when nurses are requested to temporarily move from a permanent ward unit to another unit. Most frequently the floating is for one shift, but may be longer (does not include transfer to another unit).

*Responsibility.*   Realization by the new graduate that she is "it," the one directing and deciding about patient care. This sense of aloneness in responsibility is frequently accompanied by a feeling of either too much, or too little, or just the right amount of responsibility.

*Boredom.*   Relates to the dull, routine, and monotonous types of work to be done. New graduates sometimes found work repetitious and unstimulating.

*Feedback.*   A desire to know how one is doing in his jobs. Subject area incorporates all types of feedback, received or not received by the new graduate.

*Friction.*   Subject area relates to interpersonal "rubs" and hassles with other staff members or other departments. Blaming or fault-finding seems to pervade discussion. No real attempts at objectivity or problem-solving evident.

*Patient care.*   Major focus is on the patient or patient's family. Deals with the kind of care a patient is or is not receiving and the characteristics of the types of patients new graduates care for.

*Physical labor.*   Relates to the "hard work of it all." The type of physical labor and resulting fatigue as well as mental fatigue is included here.

*Competing interests.*   Nonwork interests and activities are interfered with by the job. A sense of being consumed or swallowed up by the work of nursing.

*Change.*   The new graduate perceives the need for change activity. Factors influencing change or influence attempts are encompassed.

*Death.*   The central focus is on death or the dying patient and his family. The concerns of the nurse and her experience with the dying patient are included in this subject area.

*Fairness.*   Relates to the new graduate's perception that rules or policies are not applied equally to all or that the treatment received is unjust.

*System.*   The central focus of this subject area is the organization— the rules, regulations, policies, and physical environment which have an impact on the new graduate in her role as a nurse.

*Self-concept.*   Relates to how the new graduate feels about herself in her nursing role. Reflects new graduate's responses and reactions to discoveries about her personality and performance as a nurse.

Within each of the overall subject areas, subcategories existed. For example, some of the new graduates talked about their lack of competency as being a lack of knowledge; others indicated that they had the knowledge but lacked the manual-technical skills needed to do the job;

still others found the technical competencies to be no problem at all but lacked the skill to deal with the interpersonal aspect of the job. Since there are three separate aspects to the new graduate's competency in the job, smaller units of analysis were needed within this subject area, as within other areas. The "theme" was chosen as the unit of analysis.

The definition of theme, for our purposes, is a "sentence (or sentence-compound), usually a summary or abstracted sentence, under which a wide range of specific formulations can be subsumed"[4]. For each subject area, themes were formulated to deal with the subcomponents. For example, the aspects of competency previously described were captured in themes such as "I don't have the skill I need to do the job"; "I lack the interpersonal skill required to deal with the staff." Themes were kept in the simplest form possible so as to decrease the possibility of errors in categorization of the content. All seminar typescripts were subjected to subject area and theme analysis. As the analysis proceeded, new themes were added or old themes altered if content segments could not otherwise be classified.

The typescripts were independently read and classified by two coders. Initially, the coders met after the coding of each typescript to make sure their categorizations of content by subject area and theme were consistently the same. During the process of analysis, there were times when the coders classified content passages differently. When this happened a discussion as to the essence of the content and the determination of the appropriate classification ensued. In areas where the two coders could not agree on the coding of a passage, a third reader read the typescript and coded the material. Discussion then ensued among the three coders until agreement was reached. In all of the analyses, care was taken to code passages within the context of the current and preceding seminar discussion. In most instances when discrepancies occurred between coders, it was the content (or poor tape quality) that caused the problem. Usually one of the coders had not gone back far enough in the seminar discussion to understand the context references of the passage to be coded.

When the coding of all the typescripts was complete, a tabulation of the themes was done. How frequently did a theme occur? Did the subject area occur in all medical centers? Was the theme discussed in early or late seminars? These questions formed the basis for the examination of the patterning of occurrence of the subject areas and themes. The tabulation of the patterning of the sixteen subject areas across the series of six seminars appears in Table 2-1. As can be seen in Table 2-1, almost twice as many subjects were discussed in the first two seminars as in the last two (44 percent as compared to 21 percent). This is understandable and is due largely to the pattern noted in Chapter 1; in the early seminars, the participants tended to discharge emotion and frequently hopped from sub-

TABLE 2-1. FREQUENCY AND PERCENTAGE OF OCCURRENCE OF SUBJECT AREAS ACCORDING TO TIME OF DISCUSSION

| Subject Area | Early Seminars (1 or 2) | | Middle Seminars (3 or 4) | | Late Seminars (5 or 6) | | Total | |
|---|---|---|---|---|---|---|---|---|
| | No. | % | No. | % | No. | % | No. | % |
| Role Expectations | 193 | 45.84 | 159 | 37.77 | 69 | 16.39 | 421 | 100 |
| Competency | 119 | 45.59 | 85 | 32.57 | 57 | 21.84 | 261 | 100 |
| System | 115 | 48.32 | 71 | 29.83 | 52 | 21.85 | 238 | 100 |
| Self-concept | 95 | 43.18 | 81 | 36.82 | 44 | 20.00 | 220 | 100 |
| Feedback | 55 | 28.06 | 75 | 38.27 | 66 | 33.67 | 196 | 100 |
| Patient Care | 65 | 46.10 | 53 | 37.59 | 23 | 16.31 | 141 | 100 |
| Responsibility | 64 | 53.78 | 39 | 32.77 | 16 | 13.45 | 119 | 100 |
| Backstage Reality | 61 | 54.46 | 34 | 30.36 | 17 | 15.18 | 112 | 100 |
| Change | 45 | 40.90 | 28 | 25.46 | 37 | 33.64 | 110 | 100 |
| Friction | 45 | 42.45 | 45 | 42.45 | 16 | 15.10 | 106 | 100 |
| Fairness | 25 | 40.98 | 24 | 39.35 | 12 | 19.67 | 61 | 100 |
| Death | 21 | 35.59 | 18 | 30.51 | 20 | 33.90 | 59 | 100 |
| Floating | 10 | 29.41 | 11 | 32.35 | 13 | 38.24 | 34 | 100 |
| Physical Labor | 15 | 46.87 | 11 | 34.38 | 6 | 18.75 | 32 | 100 |
| Competing Interests | 13 | 43.33 | 8 | 26.67 | 9 | 30.00 | 30 | 100 |
| Boredom | 11 | 47.83 | 9 | 39.13 | 3 | 13.04 | 23 | 100 |
| Total | 952 | 44.01 | 751 | 34.72 | 460 | 21.27 | 2163 | 100 |

ject to subject, whereas in later seminars, they tended to focus more and to discuss a topic until problem-solving or other resolution had occurred. There were some noticeable exceptions to this pattern, however. The topic of feedback increased in frequency as the seminar sessions progressed. Floating did also, but to a lesser degree. The subject area of death is notable because of its sustained and almost equal frequency as a topic of discussion throughout the seminar. Differences in patterning of occurrence will be discussed more fully when the subject areas are presented in detail.

Based upon the frequency and extensiveness of occurrence, subject areas were classified as either major or minor. Major subject areas tended to have a high frequency of occurrence in all the medical centers while the minor subject areas occurred infrequently or in relatively fewer medical centers. The major subject areas were explored to determine their rank relative to the other areas. In addition to the overall rank, the rank of the subject areas as compared to the other areas within a given medical center was determined. Table 2–2 presents the subject areas, the frequency of occurrence, overall rank, and the ranks for the medical centers. As can be seen in Table 2–2, although there were exceptions, there was an amazing amount of similarity among the medical centers in terms of the amount of discussion that the major subject areas (the first ten subjects) in particular aroused. The five highest-ranked subjects for the overall group also ranked within the top five for four of the nine medical centers; in three additional medical centers, only one of the overall top five subjects did not rank in the medical center's top five; and in one other medical center, only two did not. In fact, only one medical center (G) appears to be somewhat inconsistent with the general pattern of frequency of discussion. In this medical center, there was a tremendous amount of internal upheaval going on during the time of the study (Friction ranked second); and an unusually large number of new graduates worked in ICU/CCU in this medical center which accounted for the heavy focus on death (third rank).

If it is assumed that the new graduates talked about those things that concerned them most, then frequency of occurrence of a topic can be equated to its importance as a concern. It can readily be seen that four subject areas accounted for well over 50 percent of the subjects discussed. New graduates are most concerned about Role Expectations, Competency, the System, and Self-concept. Interestingly, two of these topics are focused on others or on the environment, while the other two (competency and self-concept) are directed more inwardly. In reporting and discussing the subjects and themes of the new graduate seminars, separation of the subject areas along the lines of major or minor areas will not be done. Rather, the subject areas and themes will be clustered into four logical major groups. Cluster 1, entitled "the organization," centers around the *system* as the place in which the work of the nurse is

TABLE 2-2. FREQUENCY AND RANK ORDER OF SUBJECT AREAS BY MEDICAL CENTER

| Subject Area | Frequency | | Overall | Rank by Medical Center | | | | | | | | |
|---|---|---|---|---|---|---|---|---|---|---|---|---|
| | # | % | Rank | A | B | C | D | E | F | G | H | I |
| Role Expectations | 421 | 19.46 | 1 | 1 | 1 | 2 | 1 | 1 | 3 | 1 | 3.5 | 1 |
| Competency | 261 | 12.07 | 2 | 4 | 2 | 1 | 4 | 5 | 1 | 8 | 2 | 3 |
| System | 238 | 11.00 | 3 | 5.5 | 3 | 6 | 2.5 | 3 | 2 | 6 | 7.5 | 2 |
| Self-concept | 220 | 10.17 | 4 | 3 | 4 | 3 | 5 | 4 | 5 | 4 | 3.5 | 5 |
| Feedback | 196 | 9.06 | 5 | 5.5 | 10.5 | 7 | 6.5 | 2 | 4 | 7 | 1 | 4 |
| Patient Care | 141 | 6.52 | 6 | 9 | 5 | 4 | 6.5 | 6.5 | 6 | 5 | 11 | 9.5 |
| Responsibility | 119 | 5.50 | 7 | 2 | 6 | 9 | 2.5 | 11.5 | 9.5 | 11 | 7.5 | 9.5 |
| Backstage Reality | 112 | 5.18 | 8 | 11 | 10.5 | 5 | 8.5 | 6.5 | 9.5 | 11 | 5 | 6 |
| Change | 110 | 5.09 | 9 | 8 | 10.5 | 8 | 8.5 | 8 | 7 | 9 | 6 | 8 |
| Friction | 106 | 4.90 | 10 | 7 | 10.5 | 12 | 11 | 9 | 8 | 2 | 11 | 7 |
| Fairness | 61 | 2.82 | 11 | 14.5 | 8 | 14.5 | 10 | 11.5 | 11 | 11 | 11 | 11 |
| Death | 59 | 2.73 | 12 | 11 | 13 | 10.5 | 12 | 13.5 | 12 | 3 | 14 | 15 |
| Floating | 34 | 1.57 | 13 | 14.5 | 7 | 14.5 | ... | ... | 14 | 13 | ... | ... |
| Physical Labor | 32 | 1.48 | 14 | 14.5 | 14 | 14.5 | 13.5 | 15 | 14 | 15.5 | 9 | 12 |
| Competing Ints | 30 | 1.39 | 15 | 14.5 | 16 | 10.5 | 13.5 | 10 | 16 | 14 | 13 | 13 |
| Boredom | 23 | 1.06 | 16 | 11 | 15 | 4.5 | ... | 13.5 | 14 | 15.5 | ... | 14 |
| Total | 2,163 | 100.00 | | | | | | | | | | |

carried out. This cluster, which accounted for 19 percent of the discussion, includes such system concerns as *floating, boredom, fairness, physical labor,* and *competing life interests.* Although the individual is not forgotten in this cluster, the emphasis is on how the system and its needs press in on or cause concern for the individual.

Cluster 2, entitled "the individual," is in many ways exactly the opposite of Cluster 1. Here the major concern and focus is on the person as an individual, her *competency, self-concept,* the *responsibility* she feels, and the *feedback* she does or does not receive. This does not mean that the environment of the individual is ignored, but rather that the problem is of major concern from the perspective of the individual. This cluster contained 37 percent of the discussion themes identified.

"The ambiguous, tenuous span" is the title of Cluster 3, which consisted of almost 35 percent of the themes discussed. It encompasses four subject areas: *backstage reality, role expectations, friction,* and *change.* These four subject areas focus almost equally on the individual and the organization and are concerned primarily with how problems and discrepancies between the two are spanned, articulated, and dealt with.

Cluster 4, which accounted for about 9 percent of the discussions, was entitled "patients and patient care." It encompasses the subject areas of *quality of patient care* and *quality of dying.* Here the primary concern and focus was on the patient and/or their relatives and what was happening to them.

## SUMMARY

A series of new graduate seminars was conducted by trained nurses designated as satellite directors for a nationwide research study. Typescripts of the 96 audio-taped seminar sessions were prepared and subjected to content analysis. The tabulation of the 16 subject areas showed that some concerns of the new graduate were major and other concerns were minor. A detailed presentation of the subject area clusters will be done in succeeding chapters.

## REFERENCES AND NOTES

1. For a more detailed report of the research study, see Kramer, M. and Schmalenberg, C. Bicultural training and new graduate role tranformation. *Nurs. Digest,* 5(4): 1–48, 1978.
2. The instructional programs referred to here constituted the cognitive element of the Role Transformation Program. These instructional materials are published in their entirety in Kramer, M. and Schmalenberg, C. *Path to Biculturalism.* Wakefield, Massachusetts: Contemporary Publishing, 1977.
3. Berelson, B. "Content Analysis" in Lindzey, G. (Ed.), *Handbook of Social Psychology,* Vol. I. Reading: Addison-Wesley Co., 1954, p. 489.
4. Berelson, B. 1954, p. 508.

## BIBLIOGRAPHY

Argyle, M. and Rendon, A. "The Experimental Analysis of Social Performance" in Berkowitz, L. (Ed.), *Advances in Experimental Social Psychology,* Vol. 3. New York: Academic Press, 1967.

Cartwright, D. and Zander, A. *Group Dynamics Research and Theory,* 3rd ed. New York: Harper and Row, 1968.

Knowles, M. and Knowles, H. *Introduction to Group Dynamics.* New York: Associated Press, 1959.

Luft, J. *Group Process: An Introduction to Group Dynamics,* 2nd ed. Palo Alto: National Press Book, 1970.

Marram, G. *The Group Approach In Nursing Practice.* St. Louis: C. V. Mosby Co., 1973.

Schein, E. and Bennis, W. *Personal and Organizational Change Through Group Methods.* New York: John Wiley and Sons, 1965.

# Chapter 3
# The Organization

The focus of this chapter is the system, that is, the hospital or other nurse-employing organization viewed as an entity. To maintain its survival and to foster its growth, the organization must ensure that its needs are met and must induce its participants to make contributions to its functioning that are commensurate with the inducements the employees receive. An organization's needs often compete with the individual needs of the employee. When this happens, some realignment of these needs is mandatory if the organization is to survive and if the employee is to derive any job satisfaction. To realign needs, the organization can increase the nurse's "zone of indifference" concerning required organizational activities. By increasing the number of activities that the employee accepts unconditionally, the organization can be assured of greater compliance to its rules, regulations, and procedures.

Following a presentation of the major theme—the system—five minor themes, each related to the major ideas of individual versus organizational needs, and increasing the zone of indifference, will be presented. Floating is a prime example of the clash between organizational and individual needs. Fairness, on the other hand, is of concern to the new graduate because of the inconsistency in which the rules, regulations, and procedures are utilized to meet the organization's needs. Physical labor, boredom, and competing life interests are themes that reflect incidences in which an organization's needs press in upon individual needs of the new graduate.

## THE SYSTEM

I still haven't got my priorities straight. What do you do when you have four things to do at once? Do you admit the patient? Do you count narcotics? Do you clean the bed full of you know what, or do you make sure that all of the slips are with all the bloods? . . . Which are you there for? I want to be for patient care, but I don't—I'm sure that that's the first priority here. It's a difference of priorities, you know. Counting narcotics is a hospital priority and getting blood slips out is a hospital priority and you can just let people sit. People come second. (5:2B:7)

In the course of performing her role, the new graduate just quoted found that her priorities for what was to be done for the patients were at times different from her perceptions of what the hospital viewed as the priorities of work to be done. The differences between the individual's priorities and what she perceived as the hospital's priorities often produced frustration and conflict for her. This chapter will examine the patterning and occurrence of the system subject area, the relationship between the organization and the individual, and will conclude with some suggestions regarding the system as an area of concern for the new graduate nurse.

The patterning of occurrence of the system subject was similar to that of the other major subjects. The greatest number of discussions related to the system (48 percent) occurred early in the seminars, with the percentage decreasing to 30 in the middle seminars and to 22 in the late seminars. This decrease would seem to indicate that at least some of the system concerns of the new graduates were alleviated as the newcomers got to know the system better.

The medical centers were about equally divided between low and high ranking of the system subject. Of the four medical centers with low rankings for system, three were of small size. Although not always true, it would make sense that the smaller the medical center, the less administrative structure required, and the less impersonal the atmosphere. One of the large medical centers also had relatively few discussions of system. This center had a higher percentage of diploma graduates than any of the other centers. Since it has been shown[1] that diploma nursing graduates tend to have a stronger concept of and loyalty to bureaucratic organizations than do other new graduates, this may account for the lower amount of concern and discussion relative to the system in this medical center.

An unexpected result was that in the one medical center in the study which had a markedly decentralized nursing administration, there was more than the usual frequency of discussion of system. One might expect that in a decentralized organization, where the formal structure of the organization tends to be flatter, there would be much less concern with the system than in other medical centers. This, however, was not true. A number of reasons for this finding are suggested by Alderfer[2]. It is not uncommon that following decentralization, top management personnel are left in a vacuum. Accustomed to controlling, checking on, and closely supervising personnel, middle and top management are now left in unfamiliar roles. The result is often to continue the close supervision (which is upsetting to employees in a decentralized administration) or to "stay out of the way and in their offices," which is personally distressing to them, and hence inconsistently done. The results could predictably be much discussion of the system by the nurses.

Another factor which might account for the plethora of discussion of the system in the decentralized medical center is the new graduates' unfamiliarity with the decentralized system of hospital organization. Yet another possible explanation is the "buck stops here" phenomenon. In a decentralized organization, if there are problems with the system, it is expected that for the most part, they will be handled on the unit level. There are no longer several management levels above the unit level to which one can refer the problem.

All of the themes in the system subject area could be consolidated into two major groups. One group was concerned with lack of knowledge of or dislike for the characteristics of the system. This group will be discussed under the theme, "It defies all logic." The other group, entitled "Me and it," dealt with the concerns emanating from differences between individual and organizational needs.

The "Me and it" theme accounted for the larger proportion (64 percent) of the system discussion. Within this group, three subthemes accounted for 108 of the total of 152 discussions. They were:

The staffing is so low; there aren't enough people or time to do the work.

The ineffectiveness of the system results in poor care.

I'm caught in a bind between doing all the tasks that have to be done and talking with the patients.

The remaining 36 percent of the system discussion were on the theme "It defies all logic," expressing concern because of lack of knowledge of or dislike for the characteristics of the system. Of the total frequency count of 86, 72 of the concerns mentioned were accounted for by these two subthemes:

I don't know the routines and I can't find the equipment and supplies I need.

The rules, regulations and policies bug me.

## Theoretical Concepts

As formal organizations hospitals and medical centers have certain properties and characteristics:

1. Explicit rules and regulations
2. Task specialization

3.  Formal status structure

4.  Line of authority[3, 4]

These characteristics provide principles and guidelines by which decisions and actions are carried out; they define the tasks to be accomplished and the expertise required to perform them; they explicate the roles, rights, and obligations of those working in the organization as well as their relationships to one another; and they define the structure required for the coordination, control, and direction of the organization. These characteristics allow the organization to attain goals economically.

The hospital as a formal organization exhibits the same characteristics as other formal organizations[5] and has as its major goal or objective the care and treatment of patients. Rules and regulations guide procedures and actions in the performance of the work. A variety of individuals with differing skills and abilities work interdependently in a hierarchical structure to achieve the overall goal. Performance and role functions are defined by the hospital for the role incumbents. In some instances, the limitations set by the hospital constrain those performances.

The hierarchical structure exists to influence workers to comply with the rules, regulations, and procedures that the organization considers to be necessary for its own survival and effective functioning. For each new worker entering an organization, there exist three groups of activities: 1) those which are required and which are clearly acceptable to the person, 2) those which are required but which are barely acceptable or barely nonacceptable (neutral), and 3) those which are required but which are clearly unacceptable[6]. The "zone of indifference" delineates those activities which are clearly acceptable. From the employee's perspective, indifference means that, because there is preexisting internal commitment on the part of the employee, she will automatically comply or adapt her behavior in these areas within the zone of indifference to the standards of the organization. In so doing, she is indifferent to the fact that required behavior is a rule. She does it because she already intended to do it all along.

To promote its life, stability, and growth, an organization seeks to increase this zone of indifference so that the employee will accept the rules and procedures of the organization and make what for the organization is a maximum contribution. The larger the zone of indifference, the more integrated is the individual into the organization.

For a nurse entering the employ of a hospital for the first time, there are required activities which fall into differing categories of acceptability. Rules and procedures such as those governing sick pay, how to order supplies, the necessary paperwork, and the routines for providing patient care, have varying degrees of acceptability and thus compliance.

The more congruent the required activities are with the new graduate's role expectations and hence the larger her zone of indifference, the more compliance will be attained. However, the more incongruent the rules, regulations, and procedures with the new graduate's conceptions and expectations, the smaller the zone of indifference, and the lower the level of compliance. Let us examine some new graduates' reactions to some of the rules, regulations, and procedures they encountered when they entered hospital organizations.

*It defies all logic.* The vast majority of the required activities encountered by the new graduates when they entered the system were in the neutral or barely unacceptable/barely acceptable category. There were few instances in which the organizational requirements were clearly acceptable or clearly unacceptable. Some comments in the neutral category were as follows:

> Sometimes you can work somewhere and feel as if you're a necessary and a valued part of the system. But here you don't feel that way. Maybe it's because it's so big, I don't know. You're just one of the whole herd of people. (3:6A:22)

> We really get chilly in the mornings. We used to be able to wear sweaters. Now we're not allowed to wear sweaters. All we have are those paper flimsy things. They're not very warm. So we did get some isolation gowns to wear. Now we're not so cold. We're not allowed to drink coffee at the bedside, because it doesn't look nice. (6:5B:7)

> And they have things in all different places. Half the dressing stuff is in the nurses' station, half the dressing stuff is in the IV closet, and a couple of things are in the utility room. You have to run all the way over. I mean, why don't we keep these together with these? Oh well, every floor has to be uniform and that's how it is on every floor. That's the reason. (3:1A:31)

> I think those reports are a waste of time. And money. I think the daily census sheets are the biggest waste of money. You fill them out every day and we don't get any better staffing or anything. You can put "total" on everything and you get the same number of people. (2:6A:39)

> There's something I really can't understand. It's about evening and night shifts. The staffing is so short and it's really uneven between shifts. (7:1B:25)

The neutral area of acceptability covered a wide range of subject matter. The new graduates discussed their treatment as individuals, the informal and formal policies, as well as routine requirements and staffing. The consensus of the excerpts is that the new graduates are bothered by what they meet, it doesn't make sense to them, and yet there is no indication that matters are quite bad enough to warrant corrective action to deal with the matters.

The possibility exists that sooner or later required activities with neutral acceptability will move into either the acceptable or the unacceptable categories. In many ways this is a desirable movement for the organization because the nurses' behavior becomes more predictable, and the areas where the nurses may cause some problems and require some sanctions can be anticipated. If the movement is from the neutral to the acceptable category, the newcomer's zone of indifference and hence compliance increase.

The neutral category is troublesome when there is *no* change or movement, for the organization can never quite be sure of reliable performance. At one time, the staff of a unit may consider it acceptable that a unit is slightly understaffed; another time it may not. Thus the probability of situational determination of acceptability exists, and periodic disruption and disequilibrium may result.

Organizational equilibrium is more stable when the neutral items move to the acceptable category or if the required activities are considered acceptable from the outset by the new graduates. The following excerpts indicated acceptable requirements:

> We've been promised inservice for a long time now and it's never come . . . Now they say we'll get it when we move. I don't know if we'll ever have it. It seems futile to say anything at all to anyone in nursing administration because nothing is going to happen.   (9:2B:33)

> I was used to thinking about everything that has to be charted in so many different places. Intakes and outputs on the sheet on the patient's door, on the clipboards, on the graphic sheets, and I don't think it's such a bad idea if it is put in the nurses' notes. There is so much repetition; there's plenty of room for error. You know, you were saying that you are doing every nit-picking thing you can think of, and I found that I'm doing all that stuff too. I don't know, we're getting more used to it now.   (1:4C:6)

These are examples of subsequent acceptance of areas which were initially neutral or even unacceptable. It's not really all right to have no inservice, but it is apparent that that's the way it is and there is no point in doing anything more about it. And now "I'm doing all that stuff too." Acceptance doesn't always mean liking. But the fact is that these new graduates are now going along with the organization, as indicated by their remarks that inservice will come with the move and that you need to chart in many different places.

Sometimes the requirements encountered were acceptable from the beginning:

> Oh, you know, we have to fill in all these little things all over the place. Make sure the mother's blood type is on everything, and make sure if she's allergic to something that it's on all the sheets so everyone will notice. You have to fill the mother's name and her number, and the baby's number on

everything. They have to be down there. There's no way around it. There's a logical reason for everything being down there. You still don't like it, but at least there's a reason. (2:6B:15)

You really learn to improvise and that's what is good. I mean I walked out on a ward and I'd never seen a ward. You've got radiators down the middle of the hall; you've got beds with curtains; $O_2$ tanks that you're rolling around. You give your own IPPB, which I never did. You do everything. You scrub beds. As a team leader, you are expected to do every one of those things. (9:2A:11)

In areas that are clearly acceptable, such as the work that the nurse must do in providing care or the paperwork that is required, the organization can count on the new graduate to comply with the requirements allowing for the effective and efficient performance of the organization.

Those areas which fall into the category of clearly unacceptable practices disrupt the smooth running of the organization, as the employee is likely not to comply.

The charge nurse wouldn't give the doctor a suture set because we have to keep track. I gave him one and he brought it back but she wasn't worried about the patient, she was worried about the suture set. One suture set down the drain; it could have been a life. We keep the good suture sets locked up. (7:3C:31)

It seems to me that incident reports are to document what happened for everybody's protection and concern. This place is incident report happy, and man, do they love to get an incident report on somebody. I mean I hear the doctors brag, "I've got five incident reports on that chart so far. Let's see if we can get another one and set a record." I'm not saying that incident reports are not warranted, but when the ward clerk says "Well an incident report has to be made out right now," then to me you're putting that above the patient. And boy that's one thing that I just really get ticked off with. Really! A couple of times I've found errors with some of the other shifts, and if we overlook them, we get written up. If we don't overlook them, we get written up. (2:4B:37)

These excerpts indicate that the practices the new graduates encountered were unacceptable. Although the newcomers don't indicate that they are doing anything about it, the probability is that the new graduate will be less careful with the suture sets than desired or will attempt to avoid writing incident reports even when they are warranted.

In the following excerpts two new graduates are more specific about the consequences of unacceptable requirements:

This is my big complaint. It's the whole thing. And that's what will drive me out of nursing, out of what I have wanted to do all my life. It would be that they are unfair as far as their time scheduling goes, and furthermore, they are doing it unnecessarily. (5:2B:8)

This is the thing with this whole hospital system. They're built on this guilt trip: you're *expected* to stay over and you're *expected* to do all this stuff. If you run a little over, and you put in overtime on it, boy do they come down on you. Really! I have a suggestion if you've got the guts to do it. I know what our unit secretary did. We got bombarded with admissions one evening and we only had three nurses on, and it was ridiculous, post-ops and the whole bit. She called down to her supervisor, and said, "Look, you'd better send me somebody; you know, I'm in a lot of trouble." They told her,"No, we can't send you anybody." She answered, "OK, I'm going home." And you bet in two seconds they had somebody up there. So if you've got the guts, and everybody picks up everything and calls in sick and says "We're leaving," you watch and see if anything happens.   (9:3B:21)

As the two new graduates indicate, the consequences of unacceptable requirements are either leaving the organization or attempting to sabotage its quest for its goals. The more unacceptable the activities required, the more likely the undesirable consequences for the organization as well as for individual new graduates, because the new graduate does not become integrated into the organization. Another area interfering with integration that was discussed by the new graduates in seminars was not knowing the organizational requirements. There were times when inefficient job performance resulted, not because the procedures were unacceptable to the new graduate, but because she simply did not know what to do.

All kinds of things are ordered for the patients. And you think, my goodness, how do I do that, how do I order it, what do I do? And you call everybody and finally you find out how to get him his x-rays or whatever you're supposed to get him. Boy, it can be a hassle.   (8:4:30)

Sometimes you get to wondering who designed the system to be so complex. There's a lot of nit-picky things that they haven't told me about. You just have to find out on your own and you have accidents and by that time it's too late. They're all ready to jump on you. There's a lot of things they haven't told me.   (1:4C:8)

In the situations described by the new graduates in the foregoing excerpts, the integration of the employees into the organization was interfered with by their not knowing the procedures and routines. It is possible and even likely that the new graduates would comply with these requirements if they knew what to do. The failure of the organization to transmit these requirements effectively prevents these activities from entering the newcomer's zone of indifference. When practices are unknown, ineffective and inefficient performance results from ignorance and not from willful nonconformity.

In other instances, organizational practices existed which acted as a barrier to the integration of the individual.

When I was hired, the nursing administrator down in the office said, "If you can make it on this ward you've got it made." The ancillary help had run off all the nurses. The head nurse quit, and this and that. *If* you make it there, you've really got it made. What a neat thing to confront you with in the very beginning. It turns out to be true! But why had the hospital ignored it? (9:2C:19)

I'm a new graduate and I know I have a whole lot to learn. But when I see someone who has been here for four or five years and they've been on probation and they are still here, I wonder what is going on. (7:3C:34)

I think that one thing that's important in an institution is just to prove the institution cares. You know, I could care less about the hospital if I call in sick, and I mess up the supervisor . . . I could care less. I don't call in sick because of the people I work with 'cause I know the institution doesn't care about me. I'm just a body on that floor. And if you can show them somehow that the institution does care about them as a person, just by meeting with them or whatever, that in itself is a motivating factor. To know people know that you're there as a person and not just as a body or a number to take care of so many patients. Maybe that's part of the reason that you're feeling the way that you do. Just come in and think of this as a job and stuff. Maybe if more of the institution cared about you as an individual, that could be a motivating factor in making people want to come and do their work, and be more careful in their work. (9:3C:33)

The impersonality of the organization and the allowing of staff members who are a problem to continue to work even when the organization is aware of the problem create a questioning, a disbelief that the organization really cares about what happens. The new graduates' discovery of these practices tended to establish a very negative attitude toward the organization, which can lead to high turnover or to cost and waste[7].

To accomplish the integration of the individual into the system, the organization must seek to increase that individual's zone of indifference. When the organization fails to do this, a discrepancy exists between what the organization asks of its employees and what the employee will in fact do, and conflict will result.

### The Individual and the Organization

Through the process of socialization, an individual comes to value and to desire an occupational identity. Formulating such an identity is influenced not only by the formal socialization process, but also by the inherent needs and strivings of the individual personality. Not infrequently, the new graduate nurse enters the hospital work force only to discover that her personal goals for the provision of comprehensive patient care are not congruent with the goals of the organization. She may also find her own individual striving to be in opposition to the organization's structure for the provision of care. Getzel[8] provides us with a model for examining this interaction between organizational and individual needs and for understanding social behavior which inevitably must function within the context of a social system.

A social system can be conceived of as involving two classes of phenomena, the publicly mandatory and the privately necessary. The publicly mandatory deals with organization, roles, and expectations, while the privately necessary deals with the individual, personality, and need-dispositions. The publicly mandatory dimension of the social system explicates the organizational element of the social system, while the privately necessary dimension expresses the individual element of the social system. The elements of both of these dimensions can be seen in the Getzel model depicted in Figure 3–1. To understand the nature of social interaction and behavior, it is necessary to examine the nature and relationship of the elements in this model. Let us examine the organization first.

FIGURE 3–1
PUBLICLY MANDATORY (NOMOTHETIC) DIMENSION

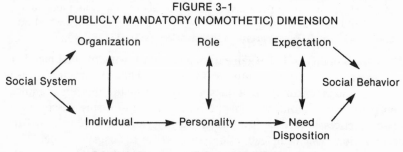

Privately Necessary (Idiographic) Dimension

Organizations are established to achieve goals. To achieve its goals, an organization requires that certain functions be carried out in more or less routine patterns. These patterns of behavior are invested into roles. Roles within an organization establish the position and status of the incumbent of the role, as well as that person's rights, obligations, privileges, and expected behaviors.

Individuals bring their unique personalities to a role. Getzel defines personality as "the dynamic organization within the individual of those need-dispositions that govern his unique perceptions and reactions to the environment and its expectations" and need-dispositions as the individual's "tendencies to orient and act with respect to objects in certain manners"[9].

All acts can be viewed as an interaction between the publicly mandatory and the privately necessary elements of a social system. When discrepancy exists between the formal requirements of the organization and the individual's need-dispositions, conflict will occur[10]. The individual finds himself in the position of having to choose whether he will meet the organization's needs or his own personal needs. If the employee chooses to meet the organization's needs, he is frustrated and dissatisfied because his own needs are not being met. If he chooses to meet his own individual needs, he is inefficient and ineffective from the perspective of the organization.

For the new graduate, the major conflict results from an incongruence between organizational and individual needs primarily because of difference in role definition of two reference groups, the nursing school and the hospital work group. The new nurse may quickly find that the two sets of expectations are contradictory. Meeting one set of expectations may make it impossible or at least difficult to meet the other set of requirements[11].

The voices in the new graduate seminars expressed concerns regarding the conflict between individual and organizational needs in three major areas: 1) performance of tasks versus total patient needs, 2) lack of time or staff to do the total job, and 3) interference in doing the job. The new graduates were well aware of the importance of doing tasks; however, it was the sheer magnitude of the tasks that prevented them from doing other things which they felt needed to be done for the patients.

> Paperwork! It's monumental! really. The way it's set up around here, there's always somebody that has to do it. The charge person spends her whole time doing that kind of thing unless an IV needs to be started and an LVN or an aide has the patient. Then she does that. It's really frustrating to be constantly aware that this particular paper has to be filled out and that pink slip number three or number five has to be sent for that. It takes away from the things that you want to do.  (9:3C:8)

> You can go in and get the tasks done that are ordered but now they are emphasizing looking at the patient as a person and not as a disease or illness. I find that I don't have the time to go in there and talk to the patient even when I know that patient is upset about something. If she has other things that are ordered and you really have to do them—it's a hassle.  (6:2B:4)

> Yeah, it's very frustrating because you've been taught and you really want to do the whole total job. But you find you can't because there are other things physically that need to be done. You know, the basics, and then the extra icing on the cake only comes when you can do it.  (3:3C:2)

The new graduates found that pressure on them from formal requirements to do the tasks, to fill out the forms, was in opposition to their own needs to do the total job of patient care. Other new graduates found that the pressure to do tasks emanated from others with whom they worked:

There's just no good old nursing going on. It's "Get the beds made. Get the temperatures done. Get everything charted. And get everything cleaned up." . . . You know what the first thing a nurse told me this morning was? "Make sure you get all the weights." And I told her, "I'm not doing any weights!" She said, "Well I'll do them. You start on my vital signs." But I said, "No, I'm going to start on my patients. I have a patient going home and I have to teach her about her meds first." And she looked at me as if I was crazy.   (6:4B:28)

Well, it seems like a lot of information I have is such a surprise to these people when I give them report . . . I like patient care and I just find out so much stuff. It's just amazing. When I casually mentioned some of these things throughout the evening I get all these looks, and I go, "Well, you've been in to see them, haven't you?" And they go "Well sure, but he didn't say anything about that." . . . The maximum number of patients I take is six, but when you're an RN and you have six patients, it seems like it takes a hell of a lot longer than if you're an aide and you have six patients . . . Talking to them and constantly thinking of all the things that are going on. And my team leader looks at me and says, "Do you have time to give me a report?!" I kept thinking, well after I have more experience, I'll be able to do this faster. But it's not true, because I really like to talk to people, and you talk to one person, and then you're so far behind . . . I feel better talking to them and being later, but then everyone looks at you like, "God, you must really be a goof-off to be still doing that."   (2:3A:8)

The new graduates find that many of the people they work with are task-oriented. Consequently they interpret this to be the way they should organize and do their own work. If the newcomers chose to go ahead and do the total job, they were made to feel crazy or at least inefficient. Frustration and conflict resulted from the formal and informal organizational pressures being at odds with the new graduates' desired ways of providing care.

The second area of discrepancy between organizational and individual needs was caused by the shortage of time or staff to allow for doing the total job of patient care. New graduates made these comments:

We have a lot of family meetings and patient meetings, and all the things that I consider will make your job more rewarding and give better patient care. And you don't have time for that. You carry bedpans for patients. That's no big deal. But that's why it's so dissatisfying for me when it gets really hectic. Because the days I leave and I'm really dissatisfied, I just think about what I've done. And it's been vital signs and meds and stuff like that.   (3:1A:17)

I don't have time to chart at all during the whole evening. So at 12:30 when I sit down to chart, I don't care much what I write down. By that time I'm hungry and I'm tired. I find myself—I don't check everything to make sure that it's all right. I just don't get back to the patients that had surgery two days ago. They may not even get their blood pressure taken during the evening. It scares me. I don't like it. That adds to my being mad at the end of the shift.   (6:6B:14)

It frustrates me when I don't get time to teach [the patients]. I feel it's important and I just think how I would feel going into something not knowing. I would really be frightened and I don't think that it's fair to the patients. At times I have a tendency to internalize the frustration and start to think it's my fault. If I could do things faster then I wouldn't be in this mess—I would be able to get a lot more done. Then at times when I'm feeling more together, I can sit back and say "But there's only three of us working today and there is this much to do, so it's really impossible and I'm expecting too much of myself." Sometimes I never even get to that point and I start feeling really crummy and I start feeling like I'm never going to be able to do this and I'm never going to learn how to be a good nurse. It really depresses me.   (7:2B:4)

It's just a lot of running. You don't have time to sit down and talk to people. You don't have time to get to know them or do what you're supposed to do for them. They make ten requests in a half hour and what's really bugging them? You fill those requests and they're still lying there with something wrong.   (3:1A:17)

Similar conflicts arose when there was inadequate staffing:

It's a real struggle when you have a lot of patients and not enough people. Thinking of my own individual care plans that I would like to have for a patient and I'm lucky if I have any time to think about that on certain days.   (5:2B:3)

I agree we have direct patient contact but you are so bogged down with charting, which I know is important. But with the staff that you have it is really impossible to spend all the time with the patient that you think you should—especially when it comes to teaching.   (6:2B:3)

Hospitals don't staff their floors, according to needs of patients, other than physical. Nine times out of ten, when you call, they want to know the census. How many are total patient care. Everything is wrapped around the patients' physical needs, and that's how floors are staffed. They don't think of the time when you might want to go in an hour and sit and talk with a patient 'cause . . . maybe he's very anxious about his surgery the next day and he needs somebody to spend half an hour, 45 minutes.   (9:3B:31)

I don't think it's that we are not emphasizing the patient as a person, I just think that if you are not staffed you can't really go in and utilize it. There are patients you can have that just want to talk. They really have something they want to talk to you about and you don't have the chance to do it. It's really kind of frustrating.   (6:2B:4)

Ultimately a shortage of staff results in the same problem as not enough time. The same frustration and conflicts between organizational demands and individuals' needs ultimately develop.

The last area discussed by the newcomers was interference which prevented the individual from providing care in a manner consonant with
her own needs. Much of the interference came about because the
coordination with other subsystems was less than ideal. In some cases the
new graduates found that there was no one else to carry out an activity
which had to be accomplished.

We've had real problems with the transporters. And today was the worst. I
finally had to go get one of my patients. He'd been sitting in medicine for
about 45 minutes. The transporters are really terrible. If you don't have the
patient ready to go right when they decide to walk in . . . Yet today, we
didn't have any wheelchairs or stretchers to put anybody in. So appoint-
ment times come and you can't get anyone ready to begin with. And the
transporters are supposed to see that you have the means to put them in.
They won't touch the patients. To move them from the bed to the wheelchair is just something they won't do. When you're running trying to watch
IV's and pass meds, somebody's coming back from surgery, somebody else
is vomiting, a patient's colostomy bag fell off in the hall and went all over,
and then you have to find a wheelchair and get the patient in it and figure
out how to transport them.   (4:2:4)

I find that I'm doing a lot of "non-nursing." Just stupid things that take
time. The big problem is linen. We're going around the whole hospital trying to find linen. There's one person giving linen out and one person going
to find linen. So all of us scatter and it's like a rat race. And it's just a waste
of time. I spent 15 minutes looking for a towel yesterday. How about the
two weeks without washcloths? We're putting blue plastic on all the beds
and running out of gowns. We make gowns out of pillow cases and towels.
We don't have anything. It's kind of sad though. You end up putting just
bathrobes on the patients, and when those get dirty, they don't have anything. These are just examples of things that take a lot of time, and it takes
time away that you have to spend with the patients.   (5:2B:14)

In order for weights to be valid, they say they are supposed to be done
before breakfast. Well, we have one big scale for the entire floor, which is
90 patients. We get out of report at 7:30 and the trays are done at 8:00.
How are all three units going to use the scales? It's just one of those things.
You think, "Now what?"   (6:5A:32)

The new nurses described incidents in which failure of the system or
ineffective functioning of some part of the system interfered with their
ability to provide care in accord with their own needs. In most instances
frustration and unhappiness resulted.

The consequences of such conflict and frustration to both the organization and the individual can be very serious. The more frustrated and
unhappy the worker, the more ineffective her performance. Thus the
individual may choose 1) to leave the system, 2) to accept the care as it is
given, or 3) to expend energies fighting the current practices. Whatever
the choice, the end result is less than ideal patient care. This result would

seem to impede both individual and the organizational needs in the long run. For both the individual to achieve success in need satisfaction and the organization to achieve success, attempts to decrease the discrepancy between the individual and the organization are imperative.

## Suggestions for Decreasing Discrepancy

One can infer from the new graduates' remarks about the system that they need to be more fully integrated into the system in order to provide for effective and efficient attainment of organization's goals. To integrate the newcomer more fully, there are three areas which require examination and perhaps change: 1) policies and procedures which affect integration, 2) work and staffing required to do the work, 3) enlargement of the job to provide increased congruence between organizational and individual needs.

The first requirement for achieving a better integration of the new graduate is to review existing policies and practices thoroughly. Does the hospital have policies which are clearly unacceptable to the newcomer? Organizations which fail to deal with the ineffective or incompetent employee, or which foster a sense of impersonality in the system, are less likely to be able to integrate the incoming employee. Unacceptable policies and practices must be altered if at all possible to allow the new graduate to become a committed and effective employee. Which policies tend to alienate and discourage entering newcomers can be discovered through questionnaires and interviews with individuals leaving the organization. It would be helpful if the information could be obtained from individuals within the system, but they may be reluctant to reveal their true thoughts and feelings if the possibility for sanctions is present.

Preservice organizations can be of assistance in helping future employees to understand the characteristics of formal organizations and the need for survival. The interface of students with the necessary aspects of hospital organization tends to be minimal. Without structure, the hospital would not survive long enough to be of any value at all to patients.

Employees' incomplete knowledge or understanding of the hospital's procedures and practices always interferes with the effective functioning of the hospital. In some way, all of the medical centers in this study presented their policies, procedures, regulations, and interrelations of their subsystems in orientation. But this means of transmitting essential knowledge of functions of the organization obviously was not sufficient. A more effective means of communicating and making this knowledge available is needed. The more the new graduate can master about the how's and where to's, the more time available for other activities and the less error in the provision of necessary care for the patients. Perhaps some kind of manual or two days of ward clerk duties would sufficiently acquaint the newcomer with the routines and procedures so that they would not continue to be a source of difficulty.

The newcomers indicated that a large portion of their time is taken up by non-nursing activities. Although in the past years ward clerks and other ancillary personnel have taken over many of these non-nursing functions, these improvements do not seem to have alleviated the amount of paperwork done by nurses. A reexamination of the effectiveness of the ward manager and ward clerk concepts may shed light on the exact nature of the problem. It may be that the support personnel actually are providing the necessary relief from non-nursing functions, but that the new graduates' overwhelming sense of not being able to accomplish what they feel to be necessary for patients makes the paperwork activities seem less appropriate. Increasing the possibility for the realization of the newcomers' individual needs may decrease the seeming inappropriateness of the other tasks they must do.

By increasing the possibility of successful accomplishment of their own goals, the second area of suggestions, a redefinition of the work to be done and the staff required to do the work, may help in alleviating the new graduates' sense that much of what they do is non-nursing in nature. The excerpts drawn from the new graduate seminars indicate that the major focus of the work of nursing continues to be on tasks. For some time now the concept of total care of the patient as a whole individual has been espoused, and yet the overwhelming pressure felt by the new graduates from their environment is for task completion. New graduates must come to accept that the technical tasks required in the care of the patients are extremely important. This emphasis is less evident in preservice settings than is needed. Preservice socializing agencies must equip students with the means necessary to place tasks in their proper perspective.

Equally important is that service organizations also place tasks in proper perspective. Tasks are important but nursing also requires attention to the psychosocial aspects of care. It is not enough to institute practices which decrease the patient load for nurses. Policies and routines which enhance the total care orientation must accompany any such changes in the organization of work. Twenty-four-hour reports that require an indication of the psychosocial aspects of a patient are needed. Supervisory follow-up on the psychosocial aspects and on teaching as well as on the physical condition of the patients will force this orientation. Acuity reports that account for the teaching and support needs of patients further the change from a task orientation to a total patient orientation.

Total care is difficult to achieve when the time and staff are insufficient. Many attempts to determine appropriate staffing to meet the needs of patients for quality care are documented in the literature. Each hospital must experiment to determine what formula will allow for the provision of quality care while at the same time insuring survival of the system. Whatever the arrangement is, for effective patient care it must provide not only job satisfaction for the nurse but also cost effectiveness for the hospital itself.

The third means of increasing the integration of the new graduate into the organization is to enrich or enlarge the job so that more congruence exists between organizational and individual needs[12]. One way of enriching the job is to move more to a whole-task way of work assignment. The move to primary nursing in recent years is a way of increasing the scope of the nurse's job so that more of the skills and abilities of the nurse are utilized in providing care. One of the difficulties with this way of enriching jobs stems from organizational philosophies and objectives. If a nurse is to move into a whole-task way of operating, then the nurse needs to play a more active role in the decision making relating to the policies and practices of the hospital. Mathews, in a study of administrative philosophy and climate, found that hospital administrations (including nursing administrators), while they believe that the staff ought to play a role in decision making, also desired supervisors to maintain close control over the staff and maintain somewhat impersonal relationships with them; they believed that the goals and work of the organization were top executive decisions; and they felt that workers should function according to rules and procedures[13]. Administrations which espouse this type of philosophy make it nearly impossible for nurses to exhibit the appropriate behaviors for whole-task care. However, Mathews also found that if the philosophy of the hospital administration was consistent, the turnover and absenteeism rates were low[14]. The implication of this finding is that, no matter whether the structure was participative or controlled, as long as it was consistent, the nurses tended to stay longer than if inconsistencies existed. Some nurses prefer a more traditional structure; any change in the structure would thus tend to decrease this group's congruency with organizational needs. It would appear that there will always be some individuals who will have some degree of discrepancy in needs. The question is, to what degree and how many?

To achieve more congruence between individual needs and organizational needs, a different type of structural organization may be desired, such as matrix organization. The hospital viewed as a matrix organization has a dual structure—a hierarchical coordination structure and a horizontal coordination structure. "The role of the professional nurse in this type of structure is to integrate and coordinate the efforts of a variety of functional team members to accomplish—1) the therapy and treatment prescribed by the physician, 2) the specialized psychosocial needs of the patient, and 3) the physical, nonclinical care of the patient''[15]. The nurse becomes the individual who coordinates and communicates with the team so that services on behalf of the patient are provided. This brief picture suggests the possibility that matrix organization structure can allow more autonomy and control for the nurse in providing patient care. This would increase the congruence of needs and lead to more satisfaction for the nurse as well as better patient care.

In summary, fostering the integration of new graduates into the system—the hospital organization—is necessary if better patient care is to be provided more efficiently and effectively. Hospital practices which are unacceptable and thus create a discrepancy between individual and organizational goals must be eliminated. It is mandatory that the newcomer to an organization acquire an increased understanding and tolerance for the necessity of structure. However, the structure for provision of care to patients must incorporate the total scope of patients' needs if new graduates are to find satisfaction in their work and patients are to receive the kind of care which the health care system is capable of providing.

## FAIRNESS

> We're probably going to split up into four teams because everybody getting oriented needs to get oriented to team leading. Here are these people who just came in but I have to wait three months.   (1:4B:9)

The new graduates in the eight medical centers at times perceived the treatment they received as different from the treatment of others in the organization, as unjust or as unfair. It was not uncommon for the new graduates to feel that they had received "the short end of the stick." This section of the "organization" chapter will focus on the new graduates' perceptions of their treatment by the organization. The section will begin with a discussion of the frequency of occurrence of this subject area, then discuss some concepts regarding fairness, the new graduates' perceptions of unfair practices, and will conclude with suggestions.

Fairness was a minor subject area, comprising only 3 percent of the total new graduate seminar discussions; about equally distributed in the early (41 percent) and middle (39 percent) seminars, the frequency of occurrence of the topic dropped in the late seminars (20 percent). It was discussed in all medical centers even though the frequency count was relatively low. Only one medical center had a high frequency count (medical center B); no particular reason was apparent for this finding.

### Causes of Concern Over Fairness

"Justice is a matter of human expectations; when the expectations are unrealized, men are apt to feel angry . . ."[16]. Injustices often occur in relation to the distribution of organizational rewards[17]. The rewards received for work done can be examined through an inducement-contribution schema.

Inducement-contribution theory indicates that organizations provide rewards or payments to employees in return for their contributions or work[18]. Inducements include wages, benefits, social acceptance; the contribution of the employee is the service or product produced. As long as the inducements offered are equal to or greater than the contribution made, the employee will continue to participate in the organization[19].

In nursing, as in many other professions, it seems that the opportunity to participate in the services rendered may be as much an inducement as it is the nurses' contribution to the organization. Research has indicated that some of the inducements important to keeping nurses working and satisfied are their having the opportunity to provide patient care, having adequate staff, receiving recognition from others, and having congenial working associates[20, 21]. As long as nurses can receive these rewards they will continue to be productive participants in the hospital organization.

The new graduates expected to receive certain inducements from the hospitals in which they worked. They expected to receive wages and benefits in accord with the work done and equal to the rewards and benefits received by the other staff[22]. (Although the equality of their performance may be questionable, the stance adopted here is to operate from the perceptions of the new graduates which formed the basis for their reality.) In the event that their expectations are not met, they perceive injustice. When new graduates perceived that others who came after them were being treated differently than they, the result was a sense that the inducements offered to others were greater than the inducements offered to them. For the newcomer, this was unacceptable.

You will recall that when the individual perceives that the organization deliberately creates unacceptable requirements, barriers to her integration into the organization ensue. When graduates perceived that the organization did not always distribute rewards equally, an unacceptable requirement and a sense of injustice were created which interfered with their integration into the hospital system. Let us examine the reward systems of the hospitals as perceived by the new graduates, looking first at wages:

> I've got a friend who opens mail and answers the phone and makes as much money as I do . . . I don't think the pay equals the job. I don't. (2:6B:8)

> I was talking to some people who are not in the medical field last night and they were talking about getting out of school. A lot of them don't have jobs, so we're lucky in that way. But a lot of them don't deal in life-threatening situations. It sounds heroic, but it does make a difference. And I just don't think that we are getting paid enough. We ought to get hazardous duty pay! It's not like checking groceries or being a librarian. I don't think we're paid for what we're trained to do. (8:5:1)

> You know, nursing is really good to start off with. I'm sure anybody just out of school would be really happy starting at this salary. But the thing about it is that in 20 years from now, it's just about the same.   (1:6B:13)

There would seem to be consensus that as a career, nursing does not receive a wage inducement equal to the contribution made.

A more dominant discussion among the new graduates related to the negative sanctions and consequences they felt or feared would result from their not knowing how to handle certain routines or situations for which they had not been prepared by the organization. The newcomers believed that in such situations they were being punished for factors beyond their control. As a result of these actual or feared negative consequences, they tended to develop resentment toward the hospital and those responsible for their orientation. This did not induce them to make a productive contribution to the organization. They commented:

> When I was orienting on days, they said, "You'll learn that on nights." And then when I got to nights, they said, "I'm sure you learned that on days." Wait a minute! Somewhere along the line somebody is going to have to tell me something, because everyone is assuming that someone else has done it.   (2:1B:15)

> "Oh, you've worked here before as a student," and so they expect you to know all kinds of things that you really don't know. You know they expect you to automatically know, and I don't, but they expect me to.   (3:1A:5)

> We have a procedure book for certain things, but it's by no means what we really need. Anyway, we had this kid who cut his eye and had to go to ER and he was well taken care of. He was doing OK. I left at 1:30 that night and when I got back the next day the senior staff was all over me because I hadn't called them. And there's nothing on the floor that says you have to call the senior staff or head nurse.   (4:6:9)

> I was on meds and I hadn't been oriented to the cart or the med closet. I didn't know where things were kept, so I was asking everybody, and all day it was: "It's right there. Can't you see it? Right in front of your face!" It was awful, but I'd rather ask than make mistakes.   (3:1A:13)

> The charge makes me angry, for one thing. I'm left by myself. And I'm in charge all the time. I've never been oriented and I don't think I could handle it if things weren't really slow.   (7:6B:2)

The new graduates found that they could not accomplish the job they were expected to do without hesitancy and difficulty because they had been insufficiently oriented. The patient care they provided was hampered by their lack of knowledge, and the staff at times gave negative feedback. The new nurses perceived these consequences as unjust.

Although the unfair expectations evoke anger from the new nurses and disrupt the effective functioning of the organization to a degree, their discovery that some employees call in sick when they really are not creates more far-reaching consequences for the hospital. Often the informal policy of the work group says that it is "OK to call in sick when you aren't" although official policy does not sanction it. The lack of punitive action by the organization says to the new graduate that it is an acceptable behavior within the organization to conform to this practice. Gradually the new graduate enters into the informally accepted practice. Thus a practice which is not acceptable by stated policy becomes acceptable behavior and enters the individual's zone of indifference. Unwittingly, the organization works against itself.

> Well, you know, it's predictable around holidays that people try to get more time off by calling in sick. And everyone knows. (4:6:25)

> Well our sick leave policy is changing and a lot of people have sick days they're going to lose. So everyone is calling in sick because they want to use their days up by September. (2:4A:11)

> When the floor is really hectic or when there are nights that are slow and a nurse will have to float, people will call in sick. And they tell each other, "I'm going to take my turn and call in sick." And people know about it, but nothing is done. (9:1B:16)

> There's two of us on call now and the other girl is sick, so I'm going to be the one coming again tonight. I know for sure that the other girl isn't really sick, but there is nothing that can be done about it. I think it's really unfair. (4:4:9)

The practice of calling in sick seems prevalent. Equally prevalent is the lack of action on the part of most of the organizations to stop the practice.

New graduates discovered other hospital practices which interfered with their integration into the organization. One such practice was unequal distribution of the rewards of the organization. For some this inequity produced additional motivation. For others it had the opposite effect.

> I was so upset because I was sure that the head nurse had lied to me. And after the investigation there was proof . . . I really started getting mad. They couldn't do what they did to me. And you know what? They did it. I can't function when I'm ticked off and full of resentment! (2:4B:45)

> I talked to the supervisor, and she told me that it was solution IV number 1 that was up. So, I asked her why she didn't tell me that before. Before, she had agreed that it was solution number 2, so I put the medication in it. And she said, "No, I didn't say that." Well, I asked her when she had found out different information. She said at one o'clock when she talked to the P.M. supervisor. When I asked her why she hadn't told me, she said, "I thought you understood me." So I told her that an incident report needed to be filled out because a different medication was supposed to have been in IV number 1. And she says to hold off on the incident report. So, since the supervisor was involved, there was a "cover-up" deal. (9:3C:23)

The two preceding excerpts indicate that there is differential application of rewards according to one's status within the organization. The higher one climbs, the greater the reward—you can get away with more if you have a higher status. This may act as a factor to motivate new graduates to work in consonance with the organizational policies so that higher status, and thus higher rewards, can be attained. However, the incidents quoted indicate that a negative attitude in the new graduate is probably created by the unfairness of the situation.

In other instances the new graduates perceived that lower status personnel received more preferential treatment than the new graduates.

> We have this aide, and she wanted to have next Tuesday off rather than Wednesday and Thursday, which were her usual days off. So she said she would call in sick. She got a leave of absence. It really burns me up because when an RN wanted a half-day off they refused to give it to her.   (2:5A:24)

> Well when you talk about gripes, there is something I just don't understand. I've been the only RN on lately and I find I'm running back and forth and sometimes I get so dizzy I just have to sit for a minute. I find that the other girls, the LVNs and the aides, take an hour break.   (2:3B:19)

> When I first started I really got to know the floor and the procedures. And I suppose my nursing skills weren't any better than other graduates. And we had our choice of shifts. I had wanted to work days, and that is really impossible when you first start anywhere, so evenings was my second choice and nights my third. So here I am on nights. Two new grads who just came two weeks ago wanted evenings as their first choice and they got it. It's unfair. I got really upset about that.   (7:2C:11)

The new graduates found that it was more advantageous to be an aide or an orderly than it was to be an RN when it came to getting promised breaks. Equally distressing was that more recent graduates were more able to get the shifts they desired than they were. From the perception of the new graduate, the contribution they made to the organization exceeded the contribution which either the aides or the more recent graduates made, and yet the rewards were less. The new graduates were puzzled and upset by the inequities of this inducement system. Again, these situations are likely to create a negative attitude and negatively influence the integration of the new graduate into the organization.

Other incidents described by the new graduates also indicated differential application of rewards, but no indication as to why this occurred was contained in their descriptions of the events. For example:

> You can see things happening around the head nurse. You sort of feel that some of the girls are teacher's pet. I can't say it happens all the time but I've seen it. I'm not comfortable talking to the head nurse because I feel that others have her ear more than me.   (2:4B:40)

> Some people can call the supervisor for more help and they get it. We call; we don't get any help.   (7:1B:19)

I finally said to the head nurse, "How come so-and-so works four, is off two, works three, is off one?" I'm working six- and eight-day stretches and I'm tired of this.   (9:1B:21)

It's not fair that one person has to work all of the nights.   (7:6C:5)

Although the emotional tone is not as strong in these last excerpts, the implication that the new graduates did not agree with the practices is present. If the integration of the new graduate is to proceed in an orderly fashion, the inequities perceived must be dealt with.


## Suggestions

Establishing appropriate systems of inducement and reward for the work done is a difficult task. We do not mean to imply that the rewards and inducements offered must be the same for all employees. What is important is that the inducements and rewards be equal to the contribution, and the first step for establishing equitable rewards is to formulate a system for their distribution.

It is not uncommon in many organizations that the rewards increase as the status of the organizational member increases since usually as status increases so, too, the responsibility increases and the contribution is greater. When the staff nurse becomes a head nurse or the head nurse becomes a supervisor, some inducement to entice individuals to take on the increased responsibility is offered. For the head nurse, one reward is having a primarily straight day schedule in conjunction with a pay increase. However, the reward that the new graduates perceived for the head nurse or the supervisor is that a person with that status can now lie or cover up and get away with it. The perceptions of the new graduates may be somewhat distorted, yet perceptions provide the basis for understanding reality. If the new graduates' perceptions are correct, then the organization's rewards do set a basis for unjust practices. If the new graduates' perceptions are incorrect or distorted, then the communication of the system of rewards needs to be more open. In some way it should be explicitly communicated that rewards increase due to increased responsibility; thus, much of the negative reaction of those in lower status positions might be alleviated.

The new graduates' finding that aides and more recent new graduates received better treatment than they themselves did would seem to contradict the rule that rewards increase as status and responsibility increase. Obviously the responsibilities for the RN (whether new or not) are greater than the responsibilities of the ancillary personnel. There may or may not be a basis for difference in rewards for the more recent new graduates, but in terms of reward by status, the rewards should be equal. If status does form the basis for increased rewards, then the new graduate, in her position, should receive more rewards than the nurse's aide or orderly. Since research has shown that wages are not the most important inducement, receiving a higher salary is not enough. Recognition for the work done, or getting some relief so the RN can sit down for a 20-minute break and not worry about the condition of her patients or have to stay late, would be rewards that registered nurses indicate are fair and satisfying. Attaining these rewards may alleviate the feeling that others in a lower status position are getting more rewards.

Another common basis for the allocation of rewards is seniority. Distribution of rewards should also be equitable and consistent when this basis is used. Inconsistencies of distribution of rewards engender suspicion and dissatisfaction that interfere with effective participation in the organization. Policy and practice must be consistent with each other, too.

It is important for the organization to determine if those who carry more responsibility do in fact receive more inducements. If this is not the case, some revision in the distribution to provide increased reward for increased contribution will create greater cooperation, integration, and effectiveness of the workers.

The effectiveness and the integration of the new graduates were affected by one other area of perceived injustice. The new graduates perceived that some of the employees ignored and even acted to abuse organizational policies, as by calling in sick when they really were not. In time, many new graduates joined in the practice, as it seemed as if their organizations really did not mind the practice since no action was taken to stop the abuse. To induce employees to comply with the demands of the organization, action to counter the impression that the "unacceptable is acceptable" must be taken. For the organization this means making it more rewarding to comply with the policies than to abuse them. It is for this reason that hospitals are beginning to institute practices whereby sick leave is returned at a given rate in the form of compensatory time or pay for those who do not use sick leave. This rewards the more conscientious nurses, rather than those who stay home when they are not ill. Another alternative for the hospital is to apply negative sanctions to those who abuse the sick leave privilege. This can be more difficult as it is hard to identify the offenders with certainty.

Although hospitals need to examine their practices relative to the distribution of rewards, the existence of apparent inequities in the reward system does not excuse the new graduate from the moral obligation to produce a fair day's work for a fair day's pay. Because some employees abuse the sick leave or get by with cover-ups, it does not mean that the newcomer is necessarily justified in joining in. Needless to say, two wrongs do not make a right.

New graduates perceived inequities in the inducements received for contributions made to the organization. These perceptions ultimately resulted in a negative attitude about the organization and made it difficult for the organization to increase the new graduate's zone of indifference. This failure on the part of the organization interferes with the integration of the new graduate into the system, and anything which interferes with this integration also interferes with the effective functioning of the hospital. Hospitals must correct the inducement-reward system in order to create a willingness in the new graduate to comply with appropriate hospital requirements.

## FLOATING

Nursing service organizations throughout the country need personnel to staff hospital units. The number and type of personnel needed changes daily and even from shift to shift because of fluctuations in census and changes in acuity of patients, and so, it is difficult to plan for adequate staffing. Moreover, staff numbers and composition may change due to emergency leaves, absence, or illness of staff scheduled to work. When either increased workload or absence of staff require additional staff for the day or shift, the organization must accommodate these demands by acquiring the necessary staff. Staffing adjustments are usually accomplished through the use of "floating," the temporary assignment of an outside person to a preformed, preestablished group. Floating can be achieved by reassigning personnel from another unit or bringing in help from the outside. The concerns of the new graduates were with the former and thus this section will center around the use of reassigning personnel from other units to adjust for staffing requirements. This section will describe the extent of floating discussed by new graduates, present information regarding the concept of floating and the Voices' experiences with floating, and conclude with suggestions and ideas about the reassigning of personnel.

Floating was a minor area of discussion, accounting for only 2 percent of the total discussion of the new graduates. The subject area held the overall rank of 13 and was highly regional. A discussion of floating occurred in only five of the nine medical centers and was most heavily concentrated in the privately operated facilities.

Unlike the majority of the other subject areas, the discussion of floating had the lowest frequency (29 percent) in the early seminars, increased to 32 percent for the middle seminars and 39 percent for the late seminars. The increasing concern is not unexpected as many medical centers do not immediately float new staff. Moreover, it is possible that until a newcomer becomes a part of the work group and comfortable with the skills required for the job, the prospect of leaving the unit is not as disfavorable as it might be later on. Additionally, new graduates wish to have many new learning experiences. The highlight of the day is learning, and floating would be an excellent source of new experiences. Thus the new graduates' concern about it may not have been great until they began to perceive floating as a negative event.

The fact that floating occurred more frequently in the private medical centers is also not particularly surprising. Often, because private facilities do not have the same financial resources as state-supported institutions, they must shift their own personnel around rather than using on-call per diem help.

## Theoretical Concepts

Floating, or the reassigning of personnel, is a practice used to compensate for shortages of staff on a unit that result in increased workload or staff absences. The most common means of making staffing adjustments is to move nurses from a less busy unit to a more heavily taxed unit[23], and it is a clear-cut case of an organization's meeting its own need in the most cost-effective manner.

Advantages and disadvantages exist for the "floating" individual. Floating allows an individual to have new experiences continually, thus preventing boredom and monotony in the work performed. It also permits maintenance of a variety of nursing skills and knowledges which normally suffer due to lack of use when an individual nurse works in only one area[24]. While many nurses find the variety which floating offers challenging, other nurses find that not knowing the routine and the floor is a disadvantage. Insecurity is also created for those nurses who have been on one unit for some time and find that they don't know much about the diseases and the problems of patients in another area, a disadvantage for the patients, as well.

A mismatch between the abilities of the nurse reassigned to a unit and the needs of that unit can compromise the quality of patient care. Manual-technical skills as well as clinical judgment skills of the nurse may not be equal to the patients' needs in the new area. The discrepancies are further magnified if the nurse is not oriented to the unit and does not know the supplies needed and the routines of care.

Disruption created by mismatched knowledge, organizational ability, and attitude is less likely for the new graduate than for those who have been employed for a longer period of time. The new graduate has not been in one area of practice long enough to lose contact with the other areas of practice and thus has forgotten less. The new graduate's organizational ability is generally not as good as that of more experienced staff, and thus the degree of upset between abilities on one's home unit and the float unit is not as great as for the other staff. Thus the newness of the routines and procedures is less bothersome to the newcomer. Moreover, the new graduate's desire to learn new things makes her a willing worker on the float unit, whereas the attitude of a longer-term employee is less positive.

However, the discrepancy between technical and judgmental abilities possessed and those required is greater for the new graduate. The new graduate's basic technical skill level and clinical judgment level are not as high as the more experienced nurse's. While an experienced nurse moving from an obstetrics unit to the adult surgical ward would require some help and assistance in translating her judgment abilities to the surgical patient, her judgment is developed and she already has many of the technical skills needed. For the new graduate, who has never exercised the particular judgments required or performed some of the technical skills before, translation is not enough. The new graduate often requires more assistance than the experienced nurse. Obviously this compromises the care of the patients.

To the extent that the individual nurse sees the advantages she can gain from floating rather than the disadvantages, there is congruence between the organization's needs for adequate staffing and the individual's needs. The new graduates seemed to indicate that although there was some matching of individual and organizational needs in floating, there was also some discrepancy.

> I got my patient assignment and then had to go to another floor for three hours. Then I went back to my own floor to find that my patients had been just lying there for three hours.   (7:3C:11)

> Well, one time I got pulled. I did vital signs and that was it. We have an aide on our unit who stays and we get pulled to do aides' work. You can use the time if it is slow for some continuing education or inservices. It doesn't have to be wasted, and that's what I feel. It's a total waste to pull someone just to make the areas look even in the books.   (1:6C:7)

For other new graduates, the discovery was not so much that they disliked floating but that the others on their unit strongly resented having to leave their unit to go to another unit.

> When the day shift came on and there were too many day nurses on the unit and they found out that somebody was going to have to float out, boy, did they put up the flak. Who was going to float? It's okay to float somebody in but when somebody's got to float out they were practically in hysterics fighting over who had to do it.   (2:5B:12)

Despite the fact that the older staff's needs seemed at odds with the organization's needs, many newcomers found that floating met their needs to learn new things.

> What happened is someone called in sick and they were really super short—two on the floor for 15 kids. So I went and worked eight hours in peds. I had a very good time. It may have been the change or just that I wanted to

get away for a night. I had six little kids and three of them were fresh post-ops. I had all my peedie drips and my volutrols. Junk I hadn't seen in a long time. I really enjoyed it. I mean, I wouldn't want to do pediatrics for 40 hours a week, but to float in, I enjoyed it.    (2:4B:25)

Everybody really seems to be out to help you find where things are and they know you don't know their routines. And there are really a lot of new things to learn.    (1:1B:6)

Other new graduates found that the floating from their own unit to another unit created difficulty for them and prevented their own needs from being met.

It burns me up but they take me from our unit up to somewhere where I know nothing about it. From orthopedics to metabolics. It's ridiculous!    (2:4A:14)

I got pulled to respiratory one day and I had no idea what to do with the respirator, because I had never been exposed to one. And then they even asked me to special a patient and I told them I couldn't because I didn't have any experience. I think it would be fair to give us a critical care course if they expect us to float to other units where there are critical care patients.    (6:4B:1)

Those new graduates who found that being floated to another unit meant not knowing how to take care of the patient with a different disease process from what they had become accustomed to often felt dissatisfied and frustrated. However, for some of the nurses, the fact that they were appreciated by the other staff brought satisfaction of their need to have recognition. The recognition they received offset the frustrations due to not knowing what to do for a certain type of patient.

Another area of "not knowing" which created difficulty for the new nurses was not knowing the structure or environment of the unit.

It's very hard to take somebody that's never been there and say "Here's the utility room and here's the —." But I said, "Hey, I don't know what I'm supposed to be doing." Everybody was helpful and they really appreciated me. It was just: "When do I do this and where am I supposed to write it?"    (2:4B:27)

I floated and they were glad to have me, but they wanted someone who knew the floor and the routines.    (7:3C:21)

"Not knowing" the unit meant that the new graduate spent more time trying to figure out where to go or what to do, which took time away from giving patient care. In one instance the new graduate seemed to feel bad because she wasn't just what the unit had wanted. The more the not knowing interferes with the nurse's ability to meet her own desired needs, the more the frustration she feels.

The new graduates did not seem overly concerned with floating to other units. It was as if being appreciated and learning new things balanced the satisfaction they felt in providing quality care to patients they knew how to take care of in a more familiar setting. However, the potential for a discrepancy between the organization's needs and the individual's needs exists. The suggestions will focus on decreasing the possibility of opposing needs.

## Suggestions in Regard to Floating

The need for the organization to readjust staffing patterns to fulfill the workload needs of a unit will likely always exist. Staffing plans and patterns will always have to compensate for absences of staff, yet the first suggestion is that floating should be used only when absolutely necessary. The new graduates indicated that at times they had the sense when they were floated that the change in unit was only done to "even out the books." At times hospitals tend to float staff from a less busy unit to a busier unit to even the workload although the busy unit already has its full complement of staff. Providing staff beyond the normal requirements of the unit provides relief for the staff, but it is not particularly helpful in stimulating the staff to perform at their optimum capacity. The practice of augmenting the usual staff can also hinder the staff from developing the ability to cope with their usual workload. The practice can also have detrimental effects on the floated nurse's "home" unit as well as creating resistance to floating because both the nurse and her unit feel that the disruption was unnecessary.

One of the major factors creating resistance to floating is the floated nurse's not knowing the layout or location of supplies on the unit or the diseases of the patients. There are currently in practice methods for partially alleviating this difficulty, such as the uniformity of supply location throughout the hospital, to which new graduates tend to object. Hospitals have also instituted steps to decrease the lack of knowledge regarding the types of patients the floating nurse must care for. Hospitals attempt to float nurses within the same service. Other hospitals have instituted a "sister" or "companion-unit" concept[25] whereby nurses are oriented to two units so that the staffs of the two units can be interchanged to cover shortages. Other hospitals have new graduates rotate to all units in a given service during orientation so that they are familiar with the units. Although this particular practice alleviates the resistance to floating that is caused by lack of knowledge of patients and routines, it increases the length of time that it takes for the new graduate to become a part of her work group and to achieve identity as a worker. All of the aforementioned practices will decrease the discrepancies for the floating nurse. Perhaps at the basis of all these practices is a certain amount of familiarity with the unit to which the nurse is floated. Even under circumstances where no particular strategy is used to deal with the knowledge discrepancy, there is no substitute for a sufficient orientation to the unit to which the nurse is being floated. It is the responsibility of the host unit to see that the nurse temporarily entering their work force knows where to obtain the supplies needed to care for her patients and the routines of the floor. A sense of welcome as communicated by the staff's willingness to orient the individual and help the individual goes a long way in offsetting her insecurity in not knowing the routines or the patients' diseases. Practices which decrease the insecurity of the employee not only decrease the resistance of the individual to the organization's need to float but also benefit the patient who receives care.

Another step to secure the meeting of the patients' needs for care, individual employee's needs, and the organization's needs is to match the abilities needed for the float unit with the abilities possessed by the nurse required to float. The supervisory person responsible for filling a staffing gap must know exactly what kinds of abilities the understaffed unit needs to manage its workload. Then the supervisor must determine where the workload is not as acute and who within that area possesses the abilities needed. Because the supervisor will not always know the staff well enough, the charge nurse or head nurse may need to be consulted to determine who among her staff has the particular abilities needed. For example, which staff member can best handle IV treatments and medications? Or who can make rapid judgments under pressure? This is quite a contrast to the usual "Send one of your RNs over to 3 East for the evening shift." By floating staff whose abilities match those required by the unit, the unit's needs are met; the individual's needs to use her abilities and feel secure in her work are met; the organization's need to provide adequate staffing to manage the workload is met; and the patients receive the best care possible within the situational constraints.

Instead of equalizing workload by moving personnel, another way to deal with an overload of nursing activity is to alter the activity load[26]. This may be accomplished by the nursing staff of the too busy unit paring their activities to the bare essentials, giving priority to completing the most essential activities. This means of dealing with a work overload can work temporarily, but it cannot go on for any extended period of time without affecting the staff's levels of fatigue and satisfaction and thus compromising patient care. A more acceptable system for dealing with fluctuating staffing needs is required.

A long-term method of adjusting the unit workload is to control the placement of patients on the units at the time of admission[27]. This requires nursing control in the assigning of beds as well as knowledge of the status of the nursing units. If a choice of units exists in terms of meeting a patient's needs, then the unit with the lower activity status would receive the patient. Although establishing such a system, and the criteria for determining acuity and unit status might take some time, in the long run this system may provide the best means for meeting the patient's, individual nurse's, and the organization's needs.

## PHYSICAL LABOR

The back-breaking, leg-aching work of it all was a minor area of discussion by the new graduates in seminar. This section will detail the pattern of occurrence of the physical labor subject area, discuss factors relating to work and fatigue, and conclude with suggestions.

The total frequency count for the subject area, physical labor, was 32, accounting for a little more than 1 percent of the total new graduate concerns discussed. The pattern of occurrence for the early, middle, and late seminars followed the major overall pattern of higher percentage in the early seminars (47 percent), lower in the middle seminars (34 percent), and decreasing further yet in the late seminars (19 percent).

The themes represented by most of the new graduate discussion in this area were as follows:

Working long stretches before a day off is tiring.
It's difficult to adjust to changing shifts.
The work is physically and mentally exhausting.

These themes as areas of discussion are not particularly surprising. Although many students realize that they will work long hours and have to rotate shifts, little, if any, experience in actually working full eight-hour shifts and working evenings and nights is obtained while in school.

### Factors Relating to Fatigue

Not surprisingly, as a review of the literature discloses, there are physiological as well as psychological factors which contribute to a sense of fatigue. Physical energy is expended in the work of the nurse. The size and set-up of the unit's physical environment and the type of patients that nurses care for affect the amount of physical energy expended. The larger the unit, the more energy expended. The heavier the patient, the more energy expended. Obviously, the nurse should eat well and get enough rest if she is to have sufficient energy. New graduates indicate that often they miss coffee and lunch breaks; thus needed energy sources may not be maintained at the appropriate level, creating a sense of fatigue.

It is also becoming increasingly evident that the nurse's biological systems are affected by her rotation to different work schedules. In rotating shift work, biological rhythms go out of phase with environmental demands[28] most frequently resulting in sleep deprivation, loss of appetite, and constipation[29]. These system disturbances are most apt to affect the worker who rotates to night duty. Loss of appetite and sleep deprivation seem to create the greatest difficulty. When the appetite is lost, the raw materials needed for sheer physical energy are decreased and fatigue becomes more pronounced. On an average, the night shift worker gets two hours less sleep and sleep of poorer quality than does the day worker[30, 31]. Thus individuals who work nights tend to experience more fatigue.

Readjustment of the biological systems once a worker changes shifts can take from one to four days or longer[32, 33]. Therefore, immediate relief is not experienced when the nurse leaves the night shift and returns to the day shift. The worker on an evening shift is the one who tends to get the most, and best quality, sleep so that the rotating day-evening pattern is not as disruptive as the day-night pattern[34].

In addition to the physiological bases for fatigue, an number of psychological factors correlate with fatigue. The more stress an individual experiences, the greater the fatigue level. Stresses result from life adjustment changes[35], inadequate resources to do a job, and inconsistencies in organizational demands[36], decreased motivation and incentive[37], and problems of job satisfaction[38]. To a certain degree, new graduates experience all of the stresses listed. The new graduate is in the process of making various life adjustments; in the seminars new nurses indicated that there are problems with time, supplies, personal competence, and staff so that adequate resources are not always available to do the job; and their incentive and satisfaction in the shock phase of their adjustment process tend to be quite low. As a result of stresses, the new graduate can be expected to experience psychological or mental fatigue.

The consequences of fatigue are great. Psychomotor function as well as information processing and handling are impaired by fatigue[39]. Consequently, performance of physical activities as well as judgments will be of lower quality when one is fatigued than when one is not. It is probable that medication errors and errors in judgment are most apt to happen when the nurse is fatigued[40]. Therefore, to prevent errors in the execution of patient care, hospitals must exhibit concern for the fatigue levels of their nurses.

An additional consequence for the organization is not a direct result of fatigue but rather a consequence of one of the factors producing fatigue. Hospitals need workers twenty-four hours a day. To the extent that the organization's need is congruent with the individual's needs, there are no consequences. However, as we have noted, shift rotation does interfere with worker's physical needs. Working off-shifts also interferes with the individual's social needs. Workers find that shift work interferes with normal social patterns such as family life, interaction with others, and even grocery shopping[41]. It can be expected that the more shift work interferes with the individual's personal needs, the more dissatisfied the worker will be with the work. New graduates were no exception.

The new graduates indicated a sense of both physical and mental fatigue.

> I'm on a six-day stretch right now. This is my fifth of six days and I'm really tiring. If I hadn't had such a heavy load maybe it would be different, but you'd think maybe after working this many days they could taper off the load a bit. (1:2B:29)

> I'm really tired. I just finished an eight-day stretch. I only had one day off before I started. And I move like molasses in January, as one of the nurses put it. And I feel terrible. I don't even know what I did yesterday. I was so exhausted. (6:3A:13)

> When we need staff, they call people to do a double shift. You really get rundown and tired. It makes for poor communication because it's just too much work. It's hard to deal with it. (9:3A:26)

The possibility for error was increased by long stretches and double shifts. Changing shifts also produced adjustment problems for the new workers.

> It's really hard for me to adjust to nights because I'm not sleeping at all during the day and therefore, I'm not working well at night. I have to stop and think "Now what did I come here for? What was I going to do?" It gets me really paranoid because I know I'm not functioning as well as I could be. (2:2B:35)

> I worked Monday night—my first night. And then I was off last night [Wednesday]. So I can't get into a pattern. I couldn't sleep all day Monday, and then all night Monday I was tired. So yesterday I thought I'd sleep real good. Then I had to go back to bed again last night. So I'm not going to sleep any today again and I'm going to get really sleepy tonight. You'd think they would give me three or four nights in a row to start. And every week is going to be different. Next week it's 3:00 P.M. to 11:00. (1:6B:17)

> I don't like nights. I feel the time I spend on nights just stagnates me. My mind doesn't function at its optimal level. I also find that I don't use my nursing skill. I haven't started an IV since I went to school. I feel like I've lost a lot of my nursing skills. (2:1B:17)

The new graduates found that adjusting to night work was difficult enough, and having to switch from one shift to another created more problems. The lack of sleep, poor functioning, and inability to use one's nursing skills, which are the consequences of changing shifts for the nurse, also are consequences for the organization. The diminished mental functioning is likely to result in errors, and there is a conflict between the nurses' personal desires to use their skills and abilities and the organization's need to have the night shift covered.

Newcomers reported fatigue existing for reasons other than long stretches or changing shifts of work.

> It's a real strain to care for this lady physically, she weighs 200 pounds. And for the first two nights, she just moaned real loud. You know, you're on the unit and you can't get away from it. When you leave, you're depressed and exhausted. (1:2C:7)

> I felt kind of torn at first. Trying to adjust to work and maintaining my home life. I really got into a rut. I got to where I would come to work, go home to bed; get up and come to work and go home to bed. My days off were fantastic. I'd sleep half of it away. (8:4:10)

> I was thinking that when I was having problems with shifts, I was really tired. And it was hard to keep a smile on my face and it was hard to be nice to everyone. There's a lot of mental fatigue that goes along with this job. (7:2C:1)

The new graduates became just plain tired from the amount of activity involved in doing their work—both physical activity and mental activity.

**Suggestions**

Not all difficulties related to the physical labor of the new graduates can be completely dissipated. As long as hospitals require 24-hour labor force, there will be some discrepancy between individual needs and the organization's needs. However, as is true with floating, steps can be taken to minimize the existing discrepancies.

Schools of nursing could help to alleviate some of the difficulty associated with the rotating of shifts by providing students with real exposure to this aspect of the work. A short tour of duty, as little as three days, can acquaint the student with the soon-to-come difficulty of working the night shift and still having to cope with the other activities of living. Having to figure out how to attend classes and work nights and missing out on the social activities of college life, would parallel the after-graduation work situation. Once exposed to the dilemma, students can constructively and meaningfully discuss with faculty ways of handling the conflicting demands posed by working the various shifts.

Hospitals can provide a valuable resource in helping individuals cope with night work. Within most hospitals there are a number of nurses who work nights and who enjoy working nights. These nurses can be an asset to faculty-student discussions as well as providing insights to the new staff nurse on how to cope with the night work life style. Although the problem cannot be eliminated, at least it can be lessened.

Biological rhythms differ for individuals. Indeed some nurses can cope with night duty or evening duty better than others. It is difficult both for the nurse entering the system and for the staff scheduling the work to know from the onset who can best cope with what shift. Once a nurse has worked through a rotation pattern, it becomes easier to determine her fitness for different shifts of work. Nurses who cannot adjust to the night shift are sometimes forced to give up their jobs because others are not willing to accommodate an exchange of shift. It would be more helpful to the individual and to the organization if new employees were not assigned a permanent rotation pattern upon employment. This would allow the organization and the individual to adjust the more permanent rotation patterns after the nurses had experienced working the various shifts. The development of criteria to assess the relative ease of adjustment could be done on the basis of physical and social-psychological indicators already known to be determinants of adjustment. The final rotation pattern is likely to end up in a more congruent fit between individual and organizational needs. Initially, there is no question that there may be added work and expense for the hospital.

Since adjustment to a change in shifts may take anywhere from one to four or more days, the pattern of changing shifts every week or two weeks is likely to result in a continual sense of fatigue. Certainly changes in shift which require the nurse to move from one shift to another without adequate time off will increase the sense of fatigue. Systems of scheduling such as block or cyclical scheduling may be an answer to the problem of constant shift adjustment. The worker who stays on a shift for a longer block of time will experience a better sense of adjustment than the employee who frequently changes shifts. Prior to starting a new shift, an increase in the number of days off may facilitate the adjustment to the new shift[42].

In conjunction with overall scheduling, having the night shift worker work fewer hours may also decrease the overall fatigue level[43]. One of the difficulties encountered by the night worker is the timing of getting to sleep. If sleep can begin prior to the biorhythm's heading toward an upward peak, the quality of sleep will be increased. It may be that a change in the starting and ending time of the night shift could achieve the desired goal without a decrease in the overall number of working hours. Much experimentation with new work schedules has been and is going on in nursing. Perhaps one other area to examine is how schedules can be altered to improve the quality of life for the night worker.

Most hospitals are attempting to make the work of shift rotation more palatable by using either a day-night or day-evening rotation rather than rotating to all three shifts. However, three shift rotation plans are still quite common. Evidence also indicates that it is the evening worker who gets the most sleep[44]. Therefore, it may be that the nurse completing night duty might do better if rotated to evening duty rather than day duty because of the possibility of quicker recuperation from the effects of the night shift sleep deprivation.

Physical fatigue can be alleviated by ensuring that the worker who is the only registered nurse on the floor does get the opportunity to have breaks and eat lunch. A nurse cannot obtain the energy she needs without consuming enough food. At times this can be a difficult task for the supervisor who has no one to help relieve the nurses.

Many of the psychological factors which create the sensation of fatigue have been dealt with in the sections on the system and fairness. It is enough here to say that correction of the adequacies of the resources to do the work and the distribution of inducements will decrease the stress which contributes to the feeling of fatigue.

Feelings of fatigue are somewhat inevitable in the work of nursing. The physical labor is at times heavy. The stresses associated with the work which produce mental fatigue cannot all be eliminated. Steps taken to alleviate the sources of fatigue due to both physical and psychological factors will help the organization to attain more effective productivity while at the same time increasing the overall well-being of the individual nurse.

## BOREDOM

> I'm thinking about going back to school. Some jobs are nice, and then some jobs are so awful. Like this one now. On our floor right now the work consists of doing jigsaw puzzles and playing cards with the patients. (3:6A:28)

When a job is unchallenging, it is awful. The new graduates' comments indicated that lack of challenge in jobs created boredom. As might be suspected, this was not a major discussion theme. Only 1 percent of the new graduate discussions dealt with the subject area of boredom. Most discussion occurred in the early seminars (48 percent) with the percentages decreasing in the middle (39 percent) and late seminars (13 percent). The highest frequency count was in medical center B, where the new graduate nurses had a prolonged on-the-unit orientation program. It may be that these new graduates did not progress as rapidly as other new graduates or as rapidly as they expected to, and hence experienced more boredom.

### Causes of Boredom

Boredom can be expected when a job or task requires minimum mental challenge or when an assigned task can be accomplished with little effort, skill, or thought[45]. Some tasks in any job are bound to be routine and unchallenging. When the new graduate found herself doing tasks which were repetitive or unchallenging, boredom resulted. The new graduates wished to make full use of their full capabilities in the performance of their work. When the work which they had to do was not taxing, they found their jobs boring. In order for the nurse to find satisfaction in the work done, her own needs must be met to some degree. When the individual's needs remain unmet, the individual will likely seek a means to increase the meeting of her needs. Like the new graduate who indicated that perhaps leaving the organization would help, other new graduates indicated search behaviors.

> You feel bad when you just sit around, but after you've made a thousand tongue blades, what else can you do? One day I even filled out checklists. You know, I wrote in all the little labels above the columns. They have to be done, but you like to feel like you could do something a little more useful. (1:1B:16)

> I'm bored. I'm stagnant. There are no new experiences, and I'm as good as anyone else up there as far as nursing care goes. Just doing things in view of the medical treatment is boring. And I think I'm going to transfer real soon. (6:4B:24)

> I keep busy all the time. But I just don't find that the work is that challenging. (5:1A:19)

> I finally talked to the charge nurse and told her, "I'm bored. I'm getting a bilateral ear infection from taking so many vital signs." After that she let me have the whole show. I'm really busy now. It's an amazing experience. (2:5A:16)

> I set one year as the time I wanted to work on this floor. Pretty soon I'm going to start making plans for what I want to do after this. Because I can see already by that time my growth here will stop. (9:2C:11)

For the new graduates the constant repetition of menial tasks created a situation in which they could not learn new things, develop their own abilities, or feel challenged to use the abilities which they possessed. Even taking care of the same type of patient sometimes became too routine. To curb the feelings of boredom or uselessness, the new graduates search for outlets and for better opportunities, and if unable to find them within the organization, they may be forced to look elsewhere.

### Suggestions

To maintain the nurse's interest in the work being done and to allow her to use her full capacities are the goals of any action to be taken. Job enlargement and enrichment discussed earlier are one way to stop boredom.

As noted earlier, comments on boredom were most common among new graduates in the most prolonged orientation program. While new graduates need an adequate orientation to learn their functions, prolonged orientations can create a bored and unchallenged employee. There is no magic formula for amount of time allotted to orientation. The key to preventing boredom is to start the new graduate immediately on acquiring the skills and routines that must be mastered to take over her ultimate duties. As soon as the new graduate exhibits understanding and shows some skill, new skills and functions needed at some time in the job can be introduced. As the new graduate acquires mastery, new skills to challenge her abilities must be provided.

When slack times occur on units, it may be useful to catch up on some of the menial tasks which may have been neglected. However, the saturation point for the doing of menial tasks is quite low. Slack time might be put to better use for on-going staff development as well as work on care plans, teaching plans, and other patient care aides and improvements. The doing of menial tasks is not nearly as defeating when interspersed with other more meaningful work.

## COMPETING LIFE INTERESTS

Interrole conflict is the conflict between role pressures associated with membership in one organization and role pressures stemming from membership in other groups[46]. The subject area of competing life interests deals with interrole conflict and accounted for just slightly more than 1 percent of the discussions of the new graduates. The patterning of the subject area was slightly different from the other areas in that the larger number of the themes (43 percent) occurred in the early seminars, with the remaining about equally split between the middle (27 percent) and late (30 percent) seminars. The highest concentration of the subject area frequencies occurred in the three large medical centers located in the large metropolitan areas.

### Theoretical Concepts

The pressures and demands of the job at times spill over into life outside of the organization. The new graduate nurses found that some of their job requirements spilled over and interrupted their private lives. When staying late to complete work, or working night shift, or worrying about their work occupied time outside of work, the new graduates felt as if their own personal needs were unmet. The fact that the new graduates found that their jobs and their social lives at times conflicted is not the fault of the organization. But if the feeling of being consumed by one's work becomes too great, the new graduate will leave the hospital to seek employment in health care facilities which demand less time and have less rigorous work schedules. Therefore, the conflict between work and social roles does at times have a direct consequence for the organization.

New graduates found that the work they did often times consumed more time than they had expected and that it interfered with social plans. Complicating these competing demands further was the factor that new graduates found that they couldn't really talk about their concerns to others who were not in a nursing role.

The range of competing interests talked about went from "It is interfering with my life" to "It just bothers me that I can't get away from it."

> I object to not knowing what my hours are more ahead of time. I can't even
> make plans to go out to dinner with my husband on Monday because I
> don't know if I can. (5:1B:40)

> I don't want to take a lot of work home with me. I try to keep work and
> home separate. But this job gets in the way of my life every day. (7:6B:17)

> The thing that ticks me off is that people say that you can't make it your
> whole life. But how can you not? You can't make appointments for the
> afternoon because you never know whether you'll make it or not. You can't
> say you'll meet people after work because you can't be counted on to be
> there. (3:1A:8)

> Remember the old days when you married your profession? You didn't
> have time for family; you were either a nurse or a wife. I'm sure for some
> the hospital is still their life, and that's where they are wanted and needed.
> But *I* need my life. (3:1A:23)

The new graduates found that the work interfered with their social and
personal lives; there was no discussion of the reverse happening. For the
newcomer the experience of nursing as an all-consuming profession was
upsetting and frustrating, and bad enough in some instances to make the
new graduate think about getting out.

The feelings and frustrations of the new graduate were heightened by
the fact that they took their frustrations home with them but were unable
to talk about their problems with others.

> I find that I can't share my work with people like others do. People love to
> hear my sister tell about her work at school because the stories are funny
> and quaint. There are some funny things, but people don't think they're as
> funny. To be able to tell somebody about what you're doing, they have to
> have a certain amount of understanding about what it is you are doing for it
> to mean anything to them. (1:4B:15)

> It's real hard to tell others who don't understand. Things that get under my
> skin aren't very important to them. It makes me mad when people come up
> with stupid, trite answers like "You ought to be kinder to others."
> (1:6B:21)

### Suggestions

For the most part, the individual must learn to deal with the conflict
between private, social life and nursing demands. Some of the factors
which were identified as work pressures can be attacked by hospital
organizations.

New graduates indicated that there was some difficulty in planning
activities in advance as they did not know their schedules. There is no
reason why hospitals cannot provide their employees with some advance

notice on their upcoming work schedules. As some new graduates indicate, they've "got to get requests in a month in advance." If the employee must plan enough ahead to give the hospital special requests, the employee should be able to expect that on Tuesday of one week she will know what shift she will be working on Monday of the next week.

There are times when particularly heavy days require the newcomer to stay late to manage report or charting. However, if report always lasts beyond the time that is allowed for the report and change of shift, then the sources of difficulty must be identified at the unit level and action taken to correct the problems which prevent nurses from consistently completing work on time.

Although not mentioned in the seminars as a source of difficulty in competing life interests, one problem mentioned by new graduates in the past has been the practice of organizations of calling them in to work on their days off. Other hospitals schedule required inservice programs on the newcomers' days off. The time that the new graduate is off duty is needed for recuperation and restoration. When this time is interrupted, the problem of competing life interests is intensified. Only under emergency situations should the new graduate be called to work on days off duty. If an inservice program is truly necessary for an individual to perform the job in a given organization, then that organization needs to make arrangements to supply the inservice on the employee's tour of duty.

It is easy to say that new graduates must take the time to get away from the overwhelming sense of being consumed by nursing. There is no easy way to turn off the concerns and frustrations that are carried home. New graduates, in talking about their experiences, have expressed that the only way they can maintain their sanity is to force themselves to do other things. "I have to force myself to go to macrame classes or go jogging in the park. But once I get there and get started, I really enjoy myself." Perhaps the best defense newcomers can achieve is to force themselves to do other things which have no relationship to nursing and the care of people, to acquire new habits that can round out their lives and their perspectives and enrich their personalities in the process.

All people who work are apt to experience some pressures resulting from simultaneously engaging in more than one role. The individual who is meeting her own personal needs will be more able to fulfill the requirements of the employee roles. The individual and organization both benefit by minimizing the competing role pressure.

### REFERENCES

1. Kramer, M. *Reality Shock: Why Nurses Leave Nursing.* St. Louis, Mo.: C. V. Mosby, 1974.

2. Alderfer, C. P. "Change Processes in Organizations" in Dunnette, M. (Ed.), *Handbook of Industrial and Organizational Psychology.* Chicago: Rand McNally College Publishing, 1976, p. 1679.
3. Blau, P. and Scott, R. *Formal Organizations: A Comparative Approach.* San Francisco: Chandler, 1962, p. 14.
4. Argyris, C. *Personality and Organization.* New York: Harper and Brothers, 1957, pp. 59–66.
5. Georgopoulos, B. S. "The Hospital as an Organization and Problem-Solving System" in Georgopoulos, B. S. (Ed.), *Organization Research on Health Institutions.* Ann Arbor, Mich.: Institute for Social Research, 1972, p. 16.
6. Krupp, S. *Pattern in Organization Analysis: A Critical Examination.* New York: Holt, Rinehart and Winston, Inc., 1961, p. 98.
7. Katz, D. and Kahn, R. *The Social Psychology of Organizations.* New York: Wiley, 1966, p. 87.
8. Getzels, J. "Conflict and Role Behavior in the Educational Setting" in Charters, W. W. and Gage, W. L. (Eds.), *Readings in the Social Psychology of Education.* Boston: Allyn and Bacon, 1963, p. 311.
9. Getzels, J. 1963, p. 311.
10. Argyris, C. 1957, p. 77.
11. Getzels, J. 1963, p. 314.
12. Argyris, C. *Integrating the Individual and the Organization.* New York: Wiley, 1964, p. 229.
13. Mathews, B. P. Inconsistency: A complex problem in administration. *Hospital Admin.* 7(4): 30, 1962.
14. Mathews, B. P. 1962, p. 34.
15. Johnson, G. V. and Tingey, S. Matrix organization: Blueprint of nursing care organization for the 80's. *Hospital Health Services Admin.* 21(1): 34, 1976.
16. Homans, G. C. "Fundamental Processes of Social Change" in Hollander, E. and Hunt, R. (Eds.), *Current Perspectives in Social Psychology.* New York: Oxford University Press, 1971, p. 462.
17. Homans, G. C. 1971, p. 461.
18. March, J. and Simon, H. "The Theory of Organizational Equilibrium" in Etzioni, A. (Ed.), *Complex Organizations.* New York: Holt, Rinehart and Winston, 1964, p. 61.
19. March, J. and Simon, H. 1964, p. 61.
20. Benton, D. A. and White, H. C. Satisfaction of job factors for registered nurses. *Nursing Admin.*, 2(6): 56, 1972.
21. Kramer, M. Satisfying and Dissatisfying Situations in Nursing. *Proceedings from the Third Annual Research Colloquium.* Northern Illinois University, De Kalb, Ill., Feb. 5, 1975.
22. Homans, G. C. 1971, p. 461.
23. Stevens, B. J. *The Nurse as Executive.* Wakefield, Mass.: Contemporary Publishing, 1975, p. 134.
24. Thomas, B. Job satisfaction and float assignments. *J. Nursing Admin.*, 2(5): 54, 1972.
25. Stevens, B. J. 1975, p. 135.
26. Stevens, B. J. 1975, p. 135.
27. Stevens, B. J. 1975, p. 135.
28. Felton, G. Body rhythm effects on rotating work shifts. *Nursing Admin.*, 5(3): 17, 1975.
29. Matt, P. E. et al. *Shift Work: The Social, Psychological and Physical Consequences.* Ann Arbor, Mich.: University of Michigan Press, 1965, p. 235.
30. Felton, G. 1975, p. 19.
31. Matt, P. E. et al. 1965, p. 235.

32. Felton, G. 1975, p. 18.
33. Matt, P. E. et al. 1965, p. 235.
34. Matt, P. E. et al. 1965, p. 305.
35. Holmes, T. H. and Rake, R. H. The social readjustment rating scale. *J. Psychosom. Res.*, 11: 1967.
36. Jacques, E. *Work, Creativity, and Social Justice.* New York: International Universities Press, 1970, p. 149.
37. Wendt, H. W. and Palmerton, P. R. "Motivation, Values, and Chronobehavioral Aspects of Fatigue" in Simonson, E. and Weiser, P. X. (Eds.), *Psychological Aspects and Physiological Correlates of Work and Fatigue.* Springfield, Ill.: Charles C. Thomas, 1976, p. 299.
38. Locke, E. "The Nature and Causes of Job Satisfaction" in Dunnette, M., 1976, p. 1328.
39. Wendt, H. W. and Palmerton, P. R. 1976.
40. Felton, G. 1975, p. 19.
41. Matt, P. E. et al. 1965, p. 17.
42. Matt, P. E. et al. 1965, p. 312.
43. Matt, P. E. et al. 1965, p. 311.
44. Matt, P. E. et al. 1965, p. 305.
45. Locke, E. 1976, p. 1319.
46. Kahn, R. L. et al. *Organizational Stress: Studies in Role Conflict and Ambiguity.* New York: Wiley, 1964, p. 20.

## BIBLIOGRAPHY

Alexander, E. *Nursing Administration in the Hospital Health Care System.* St. Louis, Mo.: C. V. Mosby, 1972.

Cochran, J. and Derr, D. Patient acuity system for nursing staffing. *Hospital Prog.*, 56(2): 1975.

Fisher, D. W. and Thomas, E. A "premium day" approach to weekend nurse staffing. *J. Nursing Admin.*, 4(5): 1974.

Gahon, K. and Talley, R. A block scheduling system. *J. Nursing Admin.*, 5(9): 1975.

Griffiths, D. E. (Ed.), *Behavioral Science and Educational Administration: The Sixty-Third Yearbook of the National Society for the Study of Education.* Chicago: The University of Chicago Press, 1964.

Johnson, D. W. *Contemporary Social Psychology.* Philadelphia: Lippencott, 1973.

Marrish, A. R. and O'Connor, A. R. Cyclic scheduling. *J. Nursing Admin.*, 1(5): 1971.

Neuhauser, D. The hospital as a matrix organization. *Hospital Admin.*, 17(4): 1972.

Ryan, S. The modified work week for nursing staff of two pediatric units. *J. Nursing Admin.*, 5(6): 1975.

Ryan, T. et al. A system for determining appropriate nurse staffing. *J. Nursing Admin.*, 5(5): 1975.

Stacy, J. RN's tell why they took off their caps. *Modern Hospital*, 108(1): 1967.

Underwood, A. B. What a 12-hour shift offers. *Am. J. Nursing*, 75(7): 1975.

# Chapter 4
# The Individual

The four subject areas in this chapter—self-concept, competency, responsibility, and feedback—all focus on the individual, how she thinks, feels, values and judges herself, and how she seeks confirmation of self and performance. In the section on self-concept, we see the process of building a concept of oneself as a nurse. Also explored is the relation between the self-concept and the value one places on that concept (self-esteem), and how self-confidence is built through confirmation of one's concept and valuation of self.

Competency, one of the major factors affecting the development of self-esteem, is explored in the second section, where we also see the dynamic interrelation of self-esteem, competency, goals, and performance. Competency begets self-esteem. The higher one's valuation of oneself, the higher the goals that one sets for oneself. The higher the goals, the better the performance. Improved performances and increased competency lead to increased positive self-esteem.

In the discussion of competency, we will show that one of the essential requirements of a profession is for each practitioner to build a theory of practice. Such a theory of practice must include diagnosis, which is perception of the issues and problems involved; testing, which is acting upon a theory of action in such a way that hypotheses regarding outcomes are confirmed or disconfirmed; and personal causality, which is the willingness to take responsibility for what one does. This commitment to be responsible is an essential condition for competence and is the subject of the third section in this chapter.

In discussing their concerns relative to responsibility, new graduates on the whole did not indicate abhorrence of responsibility or reluctance to assume it, but rather presented a picture of being quite overwhelmed, and feeling unprepared for the heaviness of the responsibility they encountered.

A major part of the concerns of both responsibility and competency was the vagueness and insecurity created through lack of feedback.

Unless one receives feedback on how one is doing or how one is coming across to others, both the acceptance of responsibility and the development of competence will suffer. This necessary feedback enhances and is acquired through the development of both self-concept and self-esteem, which further feed back into and augment both one's competency and one's sense of responsibility. Feedback therefore is the means by and through which the concerns of competency, self-concept, and responsibility can be met.

## SELF-CONCEPT

> One thing I can really say, is that the first couple of weeks that I was wearing a white uniform and my little staffer pin, I didn't feel like a staff nurse. I felt like I was a student masquerading. I didn't have my student uniform on, but it was all a lie. Now, I feel like I don't belong in school; I feel like I belong here.   (3:5C:7)

As the new graduate nurse moved into the work world, the need to examine concepts of self as nurse became apparent. Who am I? Where do I belong? How do I feel about myself? These were questions asked by many of the new graduates. This section of the chapter on the individual deals with the new nurse's concepts of self. A presentation of the patterning and occurrence of the subject area will be followed by material related to self-concept, with a particular focus on identity, self-esteem, and self-confidence. Then the comments of the new graduates themselves will be used to illustrate the theoretical material. Lastly, suggestions as to how to enhance the self-esteem of the newcomers will be provided.

The self-concept subject area ranked fourth in terms of frequency of discussion. Of the total frequency, 220 themes, 43 percent occurred in the early seminars, 37 percent in the middle seminars, and 20 percent in the late seminars. This pattern was similar to the other major subject areas.

There were more than three times as many negative comments regarding self-concept as positive comments. Of the total 220 comments, 169 (77 percent) were negative while the remaining 51 (23 percent) were positive. There were six subthemes in the self-concept subject area; some were totally negative, others were a mixture of positive and negative comments. The six subthemes were as follows:

I'm not exactly sure what my role is.

I feel inadequate in the use of my skills and abilities.

I am (or I'm not) meeting my own aspirations.

The way others treat me has an effect on me.

My self-confidence is way down (or up).

I see changes in myself as a result of being a nurse.

The themes "I'm not sure what my role is," "I feel inadequate in the use of my skills and abilities," and "I see changes in myself as a result of being a nurse" were totally negative themes, while the other three themes were a mixture of positive and negative comments.

The ranking of the self-concept subject area discussions ranged from three to five in the medical centers. There were no outstanding differences between the medical centers on this subject area.

## Theoretical Concepts

The self can be viewed as a combination of needs, values, and abilities uniquely integrated into an organized pattern that is functionally meaningful for the individual[1]. One's self-concept provides an individual with a basic sense of who and what she is in the world. In addition to the basic image of self, individuals also have socially constructed selves which involve their assumptions and perceptions of the expectations in a given social situation[2]. An individual's occupational role is one such socially constructed self. The socially constructed self of the nurse role will be the major focus of this discussion of self-concept.

The socially constructed self of the nurse is acquired in a school program where one learns the values, norms, and behaviors appropriate to the nurse role. As a result of this socialization, the individual forms a concept of the self as nurse. Just like the more basic underlying self-concept, the nurse self-concept involves a set of integrated and organized needs, values, and abilities. When one chooses to take on the identity of "nurse," one develops this sense of who and what one is and one's place in the social scheme of things. The major part of the socialization process is provided by schools of nursing, although it also continues afterward, particularly in one's initial job as a nurse.

In addition to one's perception of one's actual self, each individual also has an ideal self, an image of what one strives to be but has not yet achieved [3]. In striving to reach the ideal self, one is constantly evaluating that which one is against that which one desires to be. The discrepancy between what one is and what one desires to be provides an individual with a sense of value or worth. The more closely one approximates the ideal self, the greater the value or sense of worth; the further apart the actual and the ideal self, the lower the value or sense of worth attributed to the self. The term self-esteem is used to designate the sense of value or worth which an individual attributes to the self[4].

The process of evaluating oneself goes on in relation to the socially constructed self as well as the more basic self. One evaluates and places a sense of worth on oneself as nurse. The more a nurse approximates her ideal self, the higher the value placed on the nursing self; the more discrepant the actual and the ideal self, the lower the value placed on the nursing self. To determine whether an individual will have a low or high self-esteem, the factors influencing this valuing process must be identified.

The three factors which basically have an effect on one's level of self-esteem are as follows:

1. Living up to one's own values and aspirations
2. Having a history of success and competence in valued areas
3. Receiving respectful, accepting, and concerned treatment from significant others[5, 6]

Individuals who are successfully able to meet their self-set and desired goals and are treated respectfully by others will tend to place a higher value on the self than those who are not successful in meeting their goals and who are not treated respectfully by others.

Obviously, the level of self-esteem is associated with one's conception of the self. For the newly graduated nurse whose conception of nursing practice is centered around total, comprehensive care of patients, the level of self-esteem is derived from successfully living up to and achieving goals related to total care and to being accepted and respected for meeting those goals. If the recent graduate experiences success in this conception of the nurse role and if this role is confirmed by others, her level of self-esteem will be enhanced.

Confirmation of one's view of self and evaluation of self not only enhances self-esteem but also creates a sense of self-confidence. A feeling of confidence or believing in oneself arises from success in undertakings and respect from others[7]. Confirmation by others in essence indicates that an individual has an accurate picture of oneself and one's abilities and can therefore believe in oneself[8]. Likewise, the lack of confirmation by others indicates that an individual has an inaccurate picture of self; one then doubts oneself and one's abilities.

Confirmation from others as to the accuracy of one's perceived identity is particularly important to the newcomer. According to Schein[9], there are basic stages and processes involved in a career. The new graduate as an entrant into a position is tested by both self and others in terms of her capacity to perform and function in the job[10]. It is the process of testing one's competencies, successfully meeting one's level of aspiration, and being confirmed by others that solidifies identity, establishes the level of self-esteem, and creates levels of self-confidence.

The new graduate nurses in this study who talked about their experiences upon entering the work world discussed many difficulties in relationship to identity, self-esteem, and self-confidence. The new graduates' identity of self as a nurse was very strongly associated with the psychosocial aspects of nursing care such as emotional support and preoperative teaching and not strongly enough with the technical aspects of care such as competent skill performance and organization of work. For many of the new graduates, disconfirmation by others of their identity as nurse resulted in decreased levels of success as a result of their not being able to meet successfully the additional role requirements and lacking the time to strive toward what they considered to be appropriate aspirations. Thus the new graduates tended to have very low levels of self-esteem. As the levels of self-esteem went down or remained down, and others did not accept or treat the newcomer respectfully, the levels of self-confidence of the new graduates dwindled further.

The self-concept subject area will explore the effects of the new graduate's initial entry into the work world. The areas to be explored are the new graduate's 1) identity as a nurse, 2) level of self-esteem in relationship to the three factors which affect self-esteem—meeting of aspirations, successful and competent use of abilities, and treatment from others, and 3) levels of self-confidence. Let us begin by looking at the newcomer's identity as a nurse.

*I'm not exactly sure what my role is.* As the new graduate began her new job, one of the first things experienced was difficulty in identifying with the role of registered nurse.

> As a student working on the unit, you eyed the graduate nurses. You had some expectations of them and their roles. Now three months later, you're the graduate. I mean it has been hard to make that identification. "Hey, I'm not one of them, I'm still a student." I've had to adjust and I get confused sometimes as to what to write down at the end of my name. (1:3C:22)

> It's another whole month before we get State Board Results. That's a problem. You've got this permit that says you can function as an RN but you are not allowed to use the title "graduate nurse" or "registered nurse" or "professional nurse." So how do you answer the telephone? They have to know how you are functioning. It's one of those technicalities. And how do you feel functioning as a technicality—really! (2:2A:12)

> I still have days or evenings when I get confused about what my role is. I'm doing two jobs, the nurse and the nursing assistant. I find I do a lot of running and fetching sometimes. (1:2B:25)

At times the newcomers still felt like students and at other times they slipped into a nurse's aide role. New graduates also indicated confusion because they did not know what was expected of them in their new jobs in the role of nurse.

> There were a lot of things that I don't understand and I've had to pick up on my own. Like whether a new graduate nurse is actually supposed to do verbal orders or not and things like that. There was nobody standing there telling me. I feel like my role as a graduate in this hospital hasn't really been outlined to me. It hasn't been outlined at all. (3:1A:6)

I felt terrible. I felt so alone and confused not knowing what I was supposed to do. I kind of fidgeted around, going and offering help here and there. And feeling very self-conscious because I didn't know what was expected of me. Was I supposed to be there as one of the staff, or follow the team leader, or take hold, or what? I was so confused.   (9:1B:6)

The new graduates' identity difficulties stemmed primarily from not knowing exactly who they were yet and what was expected of them. As the new graduates discussed their role expectations and associated functions, the discussions often moved into the area of self-esteem, the second area to be explored.

*Inadequacy in the use of my skills and abilities.*   Even when the new graduate was clear about her role expectations, a sense of insecurity and inadequacy grew out of her inability to perform competently or a fear that she would be unable to handle the role functions competently.

When I first started I felt so inadequate. I just felt horrible. I felt so dumb. I never thought I'd catch on or get used to it. I'm still not used to it.   (3:1C:22)

After my month of orientation, they were going to put me on nights. I was really nervous about that because a lot of times you're the only RN on the floor. I was really nervous because I didn't think that I would be able to handle it.   (9:3A:17)

I had a patient back from surgery. I had a feeling that something was going to go wrong, and basically it didn't. But this feeling stuck with me and it kind of made me anxious to the point where I couldn't think straight. I was having a very hard time and then I got more anxious. I felt very inadequate and frustrated because I knew I should know and I have to know but I was getting into such a state.   (4:3:2)

I was in charge for three nights and I didn't know anything. It worked out really good—no one died. But most of my decisions I made with the other nurse taking care of patients. I didn't know the stuff or how the people worked.   (7:5B:14)

I really did a horrible job. I had suctioning to do and I had a real problem with that. I finally had to go to recovery and ask somebody to come help me suction because I couldn't get it done.   (4:4:13)

The new graduates' evaluations of self in the performance of role functions give the overall impression that they feel unable to use their abilities competently. The negative comments of the newcomers imply that the level of self-esteem in the use of abilities required to perform role functions was quite low.

The new nurses also found that there were times they could not use the skills and abilities which they felt they had, thus further contributing to a low self-esteem.

> There just aren't enough skills to do on the floor. You can't develop as a nurse.  (5:1B:9)

> I think I have a lot of education that I don't get the opportunity to use. At least where I am I don't. Maybe it's because I don't have enough variety in patients or something. I mean I'm on an adolescent floor and most of the cases are accidents. They're in with broken knees, broken wrists, broken legs, or something like that. I just don't get to use the skills that I learned. I hate the thought of losing all those skills.  (2:6A:28)

Because the new graduates were not able to use all of their skills and abilities, the potential for enhancing self-esteem was decreased. When an individual can use all that is hers, the chance for success is increased. Likewise, as a result of perceived success, the meeting of one's aspirations and values enhances an individual's level of self-esteem.

## Meeting Aspirations

Fulfillment of one's own aspirations and values was a mixed bag for the new graduates. Some newcomers found that they could meet their aspirations while others found they could not. Let's begin by examining the area of unmet aspirations as this will provide insight into the self-esteem enhancing potential of meeting aspirations.

> I know that I'm not doing a very good job. I'm not doing the job the way I'd expect a year from now or even two months from now. I can see things that aren't done. You can see when a referral wasn't written and it should have been written. It's obvious when teaching isn't done. And why didn't you have time to do it? Part of it is because you didn't get your time organized.  (3:1C:13)

> Whenever I feel the hospital or anybody is inefficient, it always ends up "If I were only faster or smarter or this or that it would be better." I always end up, no matter whom I'd love to blame it on, feeling really bad. I wish I were doing better and I wish I were faster and more efficient.  (5:2B:15)

> When I get this feeling of having all these pressures from everywhere, I become afraid that I'm not going to get everything done. Often I'll jump on myself and say, "But there's only a few of us on and it's impossible to get this amount of work done in this amount of time." Frequently, I'll start feeling bad about myself. I'm not good enough.  (5:2B:15)

> I think I kind of set my expectations a little higher than they should have been. I took everything very personally. When I made a mistake I felt really bad. I was trying really hard. The first month has been nothing but frustration. I've never cried so much.  (9:1B:4)

For the new graduates, not meeting their aspirations meant disappointment, frustration, and feeling bad. When the aspirations went unmet, the self-esteem of the newcomers remained low.

Another group of new graduates reported success in achieving their aspirations as nurses.

> I haven't had over three patients and so I'm able to give specialized care to the patients I have. And a lot of the patients I've had required specialized care. I've been busy all day, but I knew I was doing a good job.    (4:2:23)

> We just wrote standards of care that are going to be printed up and put in a book for the nursing orders. It was really exciting because when I got done I really felt good because I knew I had done a good job.    (9:2C:12)

> I had a patient who was super apprehensive post-surgery. I had the time to talk to her and support her. It was very satisfying.    (5:4B:9)

The major area in which the nurses met their aspirations was in the psychosocial and teaching aspects of nursing care. When the new graduates were able to provide the kind of care they felt the patients should have and they were capable of providing, they felt good so that meeting their aspirations enhanced their level of self-esteem as nurses.

*Others' effect on me.*    The other staff on the unit became "significant others" for the new graduate nurse. She desired acceptance and acknowledgment from those with whom she worked. Therefore, the unit group had the potential for either enhancing or inhibiting the new graduate's self-esteem. When coworkers treat an individual with respect and concern, then the level of self-esteem increases. But for the newcomers, the treatment from others was heavily weighted toward the negative and thus operated as a force inhibiting development of high self-esteem.

> Every time I turned around she was sending me off to look at a book or something. I felt like "You're really making me feel insecure." As far as checking signing of orders, she really had me rattled saying, "Leave that and I'll double-check it."    (1:3B:5)

> Over the weekend I wanted to change a dressing and I had to go to the charge nurse. She didn't have time to show me so she said she would next time. Today, I was supposed to get a culture and sensitivity from a colostomy loop. The charge nurse asked me if I'd done it, and I said no. I said, "I presume you do this and this and this." She said, "Yes." So I said, "OK, fine, I'll do it." And she said, "No you can't until someone checks you out." It's frustrating because you wonder how much progress you're making.    (3:4A:14)

> When I first came here I had to ask this nurse a question about the IV set-up because it was different from what I had done before. She made me feel like a real dummy because I wasn't sure how to put the stuff together. (1:4C:21)

> I was working the desk Friday night and I heard this day nurse talking about all the mistakes I'd made afterwards. So I let one of the other nurses take the desk. As the night went on, I realized that I should have done it

again to work harder and learn more. If it comes up again, I will do it. I think I was just so nervous that somebody was going to say something again that I didn't do it. (9:3B:36)

Saturday I was functioning fairly well, I guess because I had to. Yesterday, I was helping two of the people who had to stay until 5:30 because they are on ten-hour shifts. I sort of had visions of them saying "Well she didn't really do much today." They probably don't even think enough of you to talk about you behind your back. I had visions of them saying things and I just wanted the other person to say, "You should have seen her Saturday." Anything to make me feel better. I just felt so bad. (6:3A:19)

In addition to the comments made by the staff, one new graduate had this to say about a patient's comment:

I'm sure there are a lot of things to learn. But I'm feeling like I'm not progressing and I'm not feeling responsible. It really kind of topped it off this weekend when two of my patients referred to me as the "helper." "Send in the helper." And there is nothing wrong with nursing assistants, but here is my job and I'm not even doing it. (1:4B:15)

The tenor of the input which the new graduates received from others was that they were not properly performing their role functions. This information had the effect of creating frustration, insecurity, and bad feelings in the newcomer. The overall result was a decrease in the value and worthiness experienced by the new graduate in her functions as a nurse.

One comment reported by a new graduate indicated that the treatment from a coworker enhanced her feelings of self-worth.

We got these new girls about two or three weeks ago. Last week one of the girls wanted to know something and the nurse said, "Well, Anne here will show you how to do it." That's the first time that she asked me, and I guess I felt like one of the staff now. I mean, you know, that she had that much confidence in me. (1:2C:9)

The coworker's action made the new graduate feel like an accepted part of the staff and hence acted to enhance her feelings of self-esteem.

### Level of Self-confidence

Some new graduates indicated a low level of self-confidence, while others indicated they felt more confident. Although feelings of confidence stem from successful undertakings and acceptance by others, the new nurses' comments indicated a much heavier emphasis on successful undertakings than on acceptance by others. This was particularly true for the new graduates who indicated a low level of confidence. The major focus of the comments regarding a low level of self-confidence was associated with a perceived lack of success in undertakings related to the nurse role.

Well, how do you decide on priorities? And then how do you feel when you've left something else undone? I don't have a sense of confidence when I can't make those decisions.   (5:2B:6)

When I pass meds, I just concentrate on that one thing. I can't see the other things going on or do anything else. I wish I could give them a little faster so I could have more time to help, but it takes so long. And I still don't feel that I've absolutely not made a mistake. Today I checked the book three times before I left to be sure. It hasn't become an automatic thing yet. (3:5C:9)

It's hard to be assertive at this point in the game. I guess I feel like my reasons for doing things are still shaky. Takes away a lot of initiative because you are constantly double-checking to make sure you are right. (7:3B:15)

The reason I was thinking about transferring is that I wasn't feeling as confident as I thought I should be. I'm really insecure and when people are on your back it doesn't really help your security at all. And you waste all this energy because you are running around checking everything three times so you finally get yourself so worked up that whatever you are doing is not coming out efficiently.   (1:3C:17)

Understandably, the new graduates indicate two factors which create a sense of no confidence: not being able to make the necessary decisions and having constantly to check and recheck the work completed to make sure it is correct.

The new graduates who indicated a sense of self-confidence referred to both success in undertakings and acceptance by others on the staff.

I can't think of any real turning point. It was sort of a gradual thing. I became more confident and knew the routines of the floor. When you get new people, you can't help but feel like an old hen because no matter how new you are, they're newer.   (3:5C:7)

The best thing is having confidence—doing patient care, working with your own team, and being able to talk to the doctors, being accepted by the staff as a nurse and seeing your patients get well, and having one of the patients say, "Gee, you are a good nurse."   (9:1A:16)

Now that I've gotten three or four IV's started and a few bloods drawn, I've developed confidence in myself. Especially now that I've had to work a few nights. I'm a little more sure of myself.   (6:2A:1)

My self-confidence is building up and that's really nice. I really feel a part of the unit, part of the staff. To be responsible and to finally reach a goal that has been there since second grade.   (8:4:12)

Since self-confidence arises from success and acceptance, it can be expected that those newcomers who reported a sense of confidence also held rather high levels of self-esteem.

The factors which have been explored up to this point which affected the new graduate's self-esteem have been: 1) the degree to which one successfully and competently uses one's abilities; 2) the degree to which one is meeting one's aspirations and values; and 3) one's treatment by significant others. A sense of confidence as a rule is reflective of a high level of self-esteem, not a cause of it. One other area which the new graduates discussed is not directly related either to their sense of identity or to their level of self-esteem—changes in their character traits.

*Changes in myself as a result of being a nurse.*   There were two aspects to the changes the new graduates saw in their socially constructed selves as nurses: "I'm afraid that I'll change and be like the others" and "There are changes in me that I don't like." In the new graduates' comments about the attitudes or behaviors of the other nurses, the other nurses were frequently seen as closed or callous by the newcomers, who hoped they themselves would never be that way.

> Basically my unit is a speciality area. Some of the nurses have gotten so set in their ways that they just about die when we have a boarder. They fly off and say, "What am I going to do?" or "We can only admit one kind of patient." They really panic because they have become so secure in their area and have forgotten so much else. That's kind of frightening to me. I hope I don't become this way.   (5:2B:19)

> To me it's callousness. It's something which I can't understand at this point. I hope I never get like that because right now I'm so involved with my patients.   (2:2B:31)

> I don't just want to find out what someone else wants and do it that way. It rubs me the wrong way. I think you have to figure out what you are going to do and stick to your own plan. I don't want to turn into the kind of nurse who always does what the head nurse thinks is right.   (7:5B:3)

The second aspect of discussion was changes in the self that the new graduates experienced as a result of being a nurse.

> I can see myself getting more cynical, through no fault of my own. It just seems to be that way; I can't do anything about it. The situation is making me be this way.   (1:4B:16)

> I get mad at myself sometimes because I feel I'm not as motivated as I used to be. I feel like lying at home and relaxing and there are things I should be doing.   (3:3C:16)

> My biggest frustration is that we are taught not to make mistakes. That means ask the doctors everything. I'm being taught not to think, not to use my head, to feel like a robot. It really bothers me.   (7:3C:26)

> How do you stay sweet? I can see myself getting very gruff and that's not me. I don't like it.   (7:6:14)

> Sometimes, I see myself slipping onto the edge of being mediocre. It's easy to do and that's also frustrating. If you don't keep up on things, pretty soon you're one of those nurses who doesn't know something.   (9:2A:32)

I stop and say, "What am I doing?" If I'm running into the bathroom so that she has to take the patient then I'm just as bad as she is because that's her trick. I'm finding myself doing it just to get her to do something and I don't like that in myself. It makes me mad. It's just kind of contagious, you know.  (2:3B:21)

The new graduates found that they did not like the changes they perceived occurring in themselves as a result of being nurses.

Whereas the other factors such as meeting aspirations, receiving respect from others were related primarily to the socially constructed self of nurse, this area of changes in the self seems to relate more to the stable image of the underlying personality. Any of the areas discussed could potentially affect the more stable self, depending upon the degree of integration between one's nursing identity and the chronic, persistent images of self, but this area seems to have a very direct and primary effect. The new graduates do not really indicate how far-reaching are the effects of their initial job on their more stable selves except in this area of changes in the self traits. The fact that research failed to indicate a change in overall self-esteem would seem to suggest that the first job did not bring about drastic changes in the long-term levels of self-esteem of the new graduates.

The new graduates experienced a mixture of consequences as a result of entering their first work experience. The consequences were identity confusion, a sense of low esteem in respect to using their abilities, a mix of low and high self-esteem in relationship to their aspirations and levels of self-confidence, and predominantly a decrease in esteem because of the quality of their interactions with others. The fact that 77 percent of the new graduate discussions indicated negative consequences is evidence that there is a marked need to improve the entry experience for newcomers so that self-esteem can be enhanced.

### Suggestions for Enhancing Self-esteem

Although some transition time in the new graduate's identification with her new role is inevitable, providing her with clear-cut role expectations and descriptions of role functions will help to increase the speed with which the new nurse makes the switch in identity from a student to a staff nurse role. Once the role functions are clearly known, then preparation for the meeting of these functions competently and successfully is needed. Although the new graduates experienced some difficulty with specific skills such as suctioning and IV use, there was an indication that more difficulty was experienced in assignment-making and catching on to the routines and duties for the different shifts worked. Some help from others is required to learn some of the skills that the new graduates found difficult. Perhaps the most useful help would be to determine the new graduate's theoretical understanding of the skills at the outset and thereafter to provide the opportunity to practice those skills whenever the chance arises. This may mean having new graduates practice skills on patients other than those they are caring for on the unit. Faculty can be of assistance by ensuring that the new graduates have mastered a basic compendium of skills prior to their entrance into the work world. Additionally, practice is required in the area of managing work through others.

It is not enough just to describe and then allow practice in the necessary role functions. If the new graduate is to meet the demands of the work world successfully in terms of her skills and abilities, then feedback and suggestions as to how to do the job more effectively are required. Assigning someone to be primarily responsible for this feedback activity while the individual is new will enhance future role performance. The more successful the newcomer is, the greater her self-esteem and the more able she will be to meet new experiences with confidence in herself.

Although new graduates will probably never need the total range of skills and abilities learned in school, the more abilities one can use, the greater is one's sense of growing and developing to be all that one can be. The work performed by the newcomers, as well as by the veterans, must use and challenge the abilities possessed. New graduates also must become aware that all of nursing is not as critical and crisis-oriented as it appeared to be or was presented to them when they were students. While the tasks and skills are being learned, they are highly active with variable and unpredictable resistance requiring a lot of decision making. Once skills are mastered, many become rather routine. When the major emphasis at work is on the tasks to be done within a relatively short period of time, the new graduate feels the work does not require all that she has to give. Hence her abilities are not challenged by the job. So a combination of less emphasis on the emergency or crisis nature of nursing by schools of nursing and a stronger emphasis on aspects of care other than tasks by the work world, is needed. This will provide the newcomer with a more realistic picture of nursing and a greater use of a wider range of abilities in the job.

Broadening the view of care in the work world will not only increase the abilities used but will also increase the probability of the new graduates' meeting their own aspirations. If the met and unmet aspirations of the newcomers are examined, one finds that the new graduates felt they were unable to do discharge referrals, or talk to patients, or really have the time to understand the interrelations of disease and drugs. The aspirations which the new graduates indicated were met were such things as having supported a patient after surgery and doing a good job with preoperative teaching. A change in the view of the nurses' work will increase the meeting of these aspirations. However, this change will not come about until nursing administration and nurses themselves hold nurses accountable for the performance of more of the psychosocial and teaching aspects of care. In conjunction with accountability, the resources needed to meet the new expectations must be provided, resources such as an adequate staff and assistance in the reorganization of work at the unit level. For example, for years the question "Do all patients need a bath every day?" had been posed and answered in the negative. However, staff need help to introduce patients and relatives to a system of care based on individual patient needs rather than ward routine. Nurses themselves must also break out of the task-oriented mold. It is only when support is forthcoming for meeting the aspirations of discharge planning, emotional support, and preoperative teaching that nurses will be able to strive to meet those aspirations and feel successful in their attainment. With the meeting of these aspirations, a higher level of self-esteem for the nurses can be achieved.

Confirmation of one's concept of self and level of self-esteem by others leads to increased self-confidence. The treatment of the new graduates by those with whom she works is critical. The new graduates indicated that the treatment they received from others made them feel "nervous," "like dummies," or "incompetent to do the work." Preparation of the staff to work with new graduates is necessary. The staff needs to know what to expect of the newcomers, how they are being oriented, the effects of such statements as "Didn't you learn anything in school?" and how to work most effectively with the new graduate. Training of the staff in the provision of constructive feedback will also allow them to give information to the new graduate in a way that will be more constructive in producing an effective worker. (Feedback principles and additional suggestions regarding building self-esteem can be found in [11].) A change in the type of treatment that the new graduate receives will do much to enhance her self-esteem and self-confidence in her job as a registered nurse.

The suggestions thus far have focused on what others might do to enhance the self-esteem of the newcomer. The new graduate must also take steps to increase her own esteem and self-confidence. It is up to her to seek a clear description of her duties and functions. If the newcomer finds that she lacks skills, either technical or skills for management of people, then she should seek out resources to improve these skills. Regarding unused abilities and aspirations, if the new graduate is good at and believes preoperative teaching or emotional support to be valuable and important, then she must make the time to do these activities at least once a day. If the new graduate does something which she does well each and every day, she can leave the job each day feeling good about herself. In addition, these activities will soon become habit and will then continue to be a part of her working career. As the new graduate becomes more able to do all aspects of the job, additional activities which are important can be added to the work day. This will increase the sense of using one's abilities, performing aspired-to activities, and doing those activities competently. All of these factors will help to enhance the newcomer's level of self-esteem and self-confidence.

## SUMMARY

Self-esteem and self-confidence of the recently graduated nurse in her first job is at a relatively low level. The sense of self-esteem and confidence is related to three factors: meeting the individual's aspirations, using one's abilities successfully and competently, and respectful treatment from others. The expressions of the voices regarding these areas have been presented. Suggestions and ideas as to what might be done to increase the level of self-esteem and self-confidence were given. If there is to be an increase in these areas, each person and organization must look at the degree to which the newcomer is able to achieve these three factors and thereby increase the probability of enhancing self-esteem and one's productivity as a person and as a worker.

## COMPETENCY

> I feel so incompetent. I should know more; it's not others—it's me. I expected myself to know more and I find I don't. I'm incompetent. (5:4B:18)

The concern in this subject area was the possession of the skills, knowledge, and understandings needed to do the job of nurse. The focus in the discussions classified under competency was not on a person's comparison of herself and her abilities with others, or on how she felt in having or not having needed competencies, or on how she thought she would be prepared and found she wasn't, or on how one finds out if one is competent or not. Rather, the central concern was the sheer realization and statement of fact: "I've either got it or I don't. I'm either competent or I'm not." Subthemes mainly concerned the different kinds or types of knowledge and skills in which one possessed competency or not. In this area, the new graduates definitely tended to see things in an all or none fashion; furthermore, as indicated in the opening excerpt, the basis for judging one's competency is one's goals—either those set by the individual or those set by others in the environment.

In looking at this major concern of new graduate nurses, we'll first look at the frequency and patterning of occurrence of competency discussions in the seminars. Then the whole issue of competency will be put into perspective, first in terms of nursing and then with respect to education for professional practice in general. The question of what is compe-

BELMONT COLLEGE LIBRARY

tent professional practice will be raised and discussed. This will be followed by a consideration of some ways in which competence can be increased—specifically social testing. Excerpts from the new graduate seminars will be used to illustrate different aspects of competency. This section will close with some suggestions regarding the development and acquisition of competence in the education and practice of nursing.

### Frequency and Patterning of Occurrence

The subject area of competency ranked second in terms of frequency of discussion, accounting for almost 12 percent of the total 2,163 themes. The patterning of occurrence followed the predominant trend of the major subject areas with 46 percent of the discussions occurring in the early seminars, 32 percent in the middle and 22 percent in the late.

Although competency was a major area of concern, occurring with high frequency in all medical centers, the dispersion in terms of frequency of discussion in the various medical centers was wide. The rankings by medical center ranged from first, second, or third in five of the medical centers, to fourth or fifth in three others, to eighth in the final one. Why this variability of importance of the topic? One of the first possibilities that suggests itself is that competency is differentially affected by type of educational program. Perhaps nurses in diploma programs are less concerned with the issue of competency than are those receiving baccalaureate or associate degrees. The frequency of discussion did not bear this out. Medical center C had the highest proportion and concentration of diploma graduates; here competency ranked first in frequency of occurrence in the seminar discussions. It also ranked first in medical center F, which had a high concentration of baccalaureate nurses. So, looking at the frequency of occurrence in relation to educational program of the seminar participants does not provide us with the answer.

Upon further inspection of the rankings in terms of where the deviant medical centers are located and what was unusual about these medical centers, a possible answer to the wide range suggests itself. In looking at the centers as a whole, we see that competency ranked from first to fourth in frequency of occurrence in all medical centers except two: medical center E where it ranked fifth and medical center G where it ranked eighth. What was different about these two?

Medical center E was located in a very large cosmopolitan city and had the widest mixture of baccalaureate, diploma, and associate degree nurses. This was also the medical center in which the newcomers were advanced the fastest up the hospital bureaucratic ranks. Many of the new graduates were working under head nurses who had been new graduates the year before. The dominant concerns of the new graduates in the seminar discussions in this medical center were role expectations, feedback, and the system. Perhaps there wasn't as much discrepancy between the newcomer's view of her competence and her perception of the competence of those around her. Thus, competency discussions would not be of such a great concern.

The reason for the low emphasis on competence in medical center G is much more evident: that center had the largest number of new graduate nurses working in special care units such as ICU, CCU, and so on. For the most part these units function more on the whole-task system approach to which the new graduate is oriented and accustomed from school. In these units, it is typical that the nurses give direct patient care to one or two patients. Nurses are not required to manage patient care through others, or to work through others to the same extent as is required on the general units. Therefore, although there are speciality skills to be learned in a special care unit, there is a large amount of supervision available, and the skills to be learned are highly valued by the nurse. Hence, it is not surprising that new graduates feel more competent and able to handle themselves in such situations, and hence would have less need to discuss their incompetencies.

The reader will probably notice that in the previous discussion the link was made between frequency of discussion and the fact that these discussions were expressions of concern over incompetency, not competency. Out of the 261 discussions in which competency was the theme in some way, only 24 (9 percent) were expressions of positive themes, such as the following:

I have the skills and knowledge I need.

I was prepared for the job.

My job is an exciting place to learn new things, to become competent.

The most common concern in the competency area was actually neither positive nor negative, but centered around what might be called the proving ground theme, "I have to prove myself to others, or to myself," or "Others are testing me to see whether I can make it." This theme accounted for 24 percent ($N = 62$) of the total discussions. All of the other themes in the competence subject area ($N = 75$; 67 percent) concerned lacks, deficiences, or incompetencies. They were as follows:

I don't have the skills I need to do the job.

I don't have the knowledge I need.

I lack the interpersonal competence to deal
with the staff or to get work done through others.

I am lacking in organizational skills.

I'm incompetent in making the judgments and
decisions I have to make.

Some combination of the above incompetencies.

This list paints a rather gloomy picture for the new graduate, the organization that employs her, and the school that has prepared her. When a
group of new graduate nurses from almost 100 nursing programs all over
the country are so concerned about their incompetencies that the subject
ranks second on the list of their concerns, then it is wise to listen to them
to find out what might be done about this problem. First, it is necessary
to put this problem and concern into perspective. How great a concern is
competency in nursing, and is nursing alone in its concern about the
competency of its practitioners?

## Competency in Perspective

Are the new graduate nurses of today competent? Do they perceive themselves as being so? Do others perceive them as competent? A number of
studies have been done on various aspects of this problem. When all are
considered, the weight of their findings seems to be tipped toward a
negative response to these questions.

Some of the discrepancy in answering questions about competency
seems to be due to the following variables. Who is answering the question? What areas of competency are you talking about? When is the
question being asked? And what kind of educational program did the
graduate come from? Whether a nurse is perceived to be competent or
not definitely seems to be related to whether one asks the nurse for a
report on herself, or whether one asks the employer of the nurse. Generally speaking, supervisors rank new graduate nurses lower in competency
than do the graduates themselves. This is particularly true in the area of
leadership, decision making, and organizational skills. A study by
Brandt et al.[12] of the on-the-job performance of baccalaureate nurses
showed that differences existed between the graduate and her employers
in perception of competence in the area of decision making; the graduates thought they were more capable in this aspect than did their immediate supervisors. In a study of five classes of baccalaureate nurses
graduating from a university program, Hayter[13] found a marked difference of opinion between the graduates and their employers with
respect to the leadership ability of the graduates. This competence was
identified by the employers as being the second greatest weakness of the
new graduates; the nurses themselves thought that it ranked fifth in
terms of their academic preparation. Large's study[14] of baccalaureate
nurse graduates also suggests this same kind of discrepancy between the
graduate and the employer in terms of competency. In the study,
although most of the graduates reported that they felt prepared to prac-

tice the nursing functions selected for the study, they expressed much negativism both toward the educational program and toward the employing agency for their inability to function effectively with technical and managerial skills. These graduates apparently perceived differences in actual and expected competencies, and tended to put the blame on the school and the employer for the problem.

This was not the case not too long ago when a group of new graduate nurses got caught in the cross fire between a school and the local community of nurse employers who refused to hire nurse graduates from the school because they perceived them as being incompetent[15]. In that instance, the finger of blame was pointed at the school, rather than at the individual or the employer.

In our own work, we have found marked differences in the responses of new graduate nurses to the question of competency depending upon when the question was asked[16]. If presented with a list of fairly common skills and functions, including technical, communicative, and management (or leadership), we have found that senior students about to graduate and brand new graduate nurses rank themselves as more competent than do they after they have been employed for about six weeks to two months. At that time, they rank themselves very low. This perception of competency goes up again after about three months. These data would seem to fit and to explain the high concentration of concern about incompetency expressed in the new graduate seminars reported on in this book. Brand new graduates just entering the employment situation don't know enough yet to know what they don't know; hence they assess themselves as being fairly competent. After even a brief exposure on the units, they discover the wealth of knowledge and skills that they lack and hence rate themselves as low in competency.

Although the literature suggests that there really should be a difference in competency between nurses prepared in the different kinds of programs, research evidence does not consistently bear this out. In a panel study which compared the self-reports of diploma and baccalaureate nurses before graduation and after their first job experiences, Smoyak[17] found that nurses from different programs looked more alike than different. Clinical bedside nursing was ranked lowest in perceived competence by both groups. Waters et al.[18] in their study of baccalaureate and associate degree nurses' ability to solve problems and make judgments and decisions based on knowledge found no differences between the two groups. Fair or a little better than fair was the evaluation given to their preparation by both diploma and generic graduates in another study in the East[19]. In this study, there was concurrence between the graduates' and supervisors' evaluations.

One study which does seem to indicate a difference between the competency level of baccalaureate, diploma, and associate degree graduates was conducted by Nelson[20] on the graduates of nine nursing programs in North Dakota. She found that the baccalaureate nurses rated themselves as higher in overall competence, and that there was closer agreement between them and their supervisors on this rating than was true for graduates from the two other kinds of programs. Diploma graduates, on the other hand, rated themselves higher in technical and administrative skills than did the graduates from the other two types of programs. Baccalaureate nurses rated themselves higher in communication competencies. Unfortunately, this study does not tell us how competent the various graduates were, either as perceived by themselves or their employers, only that there were differences between them.

Another issue of importance in placing the question of competency in perspective is to ask whether there is any relationship between academic performance and on-the-job performance. Does a good student nurse make a good staff nurse? Here the evidence is much more consistent, and the answer seems to be a definite "No." In a study of the academic and performance records of a group of diploma nurse graduates, Saffer and Saffer[21] found that the academic records did not predict in any way the quality of the on-the-job performance. There was no correlation between grades for theory and later evaluations of performance. A positive correlation was found, however, between clinical grades and performance. This study verified what Brandt and Metheny[22] had found earlier in their study of baccalaureate graduates, namely, that there was only a very small correlation between measures of academic performance and assessment of on-the-job performance, and between state board scores and job performance. They did, however, find some relationship between clinical grades and job performance. Brandt and Metheny state that their results support earlier findings in the literature of the slight relationship between measures of academic performance and job performance[23].

In summary then, the evidence is mounting that we in nursing have a problem with respect to preparing professional nurses who see themselves as competent, and whom others perceive as competent. Furthermore, it appears that competency in the school subculture of nursing is not directly related to success in the work subculture of nursing. How do we in nursing compare to other professions? Is competency a problem in other professions as well?

*Other professions.* Although issues and attitudes differ from one profession to another, the recent work of the Carnegie Commission on Higher Education[24] provides extensive evidence that there is general discontent in both the oldest, well-established professions such as law and the relative newcomers such as engineering, business management, and urban planning. Five central issues have been identified as being of concern for professional practice and education: whom professionals serve, whether professional schools prepare competent practitioners, whether professionals benefit from cumulative learning, whether reform is possible, and whether self-actualization is possible in professional practice.

For our purpose, we will focus only on the concern of competence for professional practice. Much of what follows here is abstracted from Argyris and Schon[25], with concepts and examples introduced to make the message more explicit. Argyris and Schon argue that it is not surprising that professional schools are criticized for failing to help students become competent practitioners. There are two major reasons why they fail. First, for reasons peculiar to the various professions, professional schools do not help students acquire the skills essential to practice competently in the real world. In many professional schools, students are provided with a common bond, a sense of common professional identity, a common culture, but they are not taught how to practice skills learned in their purity in the school world, in the real, but imperfect, world of life. An example from legal education illustrates this point. In criminal law courses, students prepare for courtroom battles utilizing an adversary process. In real life, however, the actual process of practicing criminal law consists mainly of working and negotiating in a bureaucracy that processes people, like other bureaucracies.

The second argument in support of the argument that professional schools do not produce competent practitioners is based on the premise that professional roles are undergoing such radical change that the skills of yesterday and today will not suffice for tomorrow. Yet professional schools are so preoccupied with the old that they exclude the teaching of emerging competencies. Professions need innovators to improve practice and to clarify issues such as: who is the legitimate client, who should initiate contact, what is the nature of the contract between client and professional, and what are the boundaries of the profession. Friedman argues that professionals need courses that teach skill in managing interpersonal relationships in a way that develops self-knowledge, capacity to learn, capacity for empathy, and ability to live with conflict[26]. In very few, if any, professional schools, be they law, medicine, urban planning, or nursing, will such courses be found.

If, then, competency in professional practice is a primary concern and deficiency, what can be done? What is needed to acquire competence in professional practice?

Schein answers this question very clearly. The foundation for future professional competence is in the capacity to learn how to learn. "This requires developing one's own continuing theory of practice under real-time conditions. It means that the professional must learn to develop microtheories of action, that when organized into a pattern, represent an effective theory of practice"[27]. Such a theory of practice would have certain criteria as follows. 1) The theory should permit detection of and response to its own faults and inconsistencies. 2) It should make the interaction between the client and the professional a mutual learning experience. 3) The theory should enable the professional to seek out new clients, new kinds of clients, and different people who require his services. 4) The theory should include a process for reforming the profession. Such a process would describe the methods by which transition from present to desired behavior could be made. 5) The theory should be conducive to creating a sense of community among the professionals. Such a community must be responsible for carrying out explicit public learning programs. 6) The theory should make it increasingly possible for its members to become self-actualized, capable of using their skills and abilities to meet self-set goals, and capable of setting realistic yet challenging levels of aspiration to promote growth.

An effective theory of practice having the criteria described thus far must include the processes of diagnosis, testing, and accepting personal causality. Diagnosis involves the process of immersing the self in a network of behavioral worlds of the client. A good diagnostician gets inside the world of the client and comprehends that culture so that she can make effective diagnoses of how she, the professional, can best meet the needs of the client. The professional, in the diagnostic phase, must take the unstructured information presented to her in the form of human behavior, must sense which pieces of information are central and which are peripheral, and must attempt to see the perspective of those she encounters. In varying degrees and in different ways, all professionals must interact with individuals, although each can choose the degree to which she wants to respond to the cultures she is working with. If, for example, she chooses the stance of an expert, she may want to learn only as much about the culture as she needs in order to impose her own concept of what needs doing. Or the professional may wish to get much more in tune with her client and be more responsive to the client's culture. In any event, the development of an effective theory of practice requires the professional to build her own diagnostic theory from unstructured information gained, not from reading or theorizing about other cultures, but from her own interaction with clients or perspective clients.

Professional practitioners who have built an effective theory of practice have learned to test their theories and assumptions, both those that are confirmable by direct observation, and those that are not. A hypothesis must be formed that links the observable and unobservable and an action which is thought to follow. Practice or clinical situations are viewed as an opportunity for testing some element of one's theory of action.

There are two major obstacles to testing in professional practice. The first is the difference between the real and the laboratory environment. As any nursing student knows, there is a lot of difference between giving an injection to a plastic buttocks in the lab and giving an injection to a real person who is sick. There is even more difference involved in the testing of the interpersonal aspects of one's theory of practice.

> I know what was wrong with our team leading experience; it was only four days long. That's not nearly enough.
>
> Ours was a little longer than that—nine days. It wasn't good enough but it was better than nothing.
>
> Yeah, but it was sort of a joke, wasn't it? You were really play-like. Felt like you were pretending, huh?
>
> Yeah, and everybody knew you were pretending, so they would play along with you, when actually they were leading you on! [general laughter]
>
> But when I turned grad, I was the team leader and the team! [general laughter]
>
> You really get good cooperation that way! You say: "Self, what do I do now?" (1:1A:15)

Since nursing is a profession in which there is heavy involvement of an interpersonal nature—with patients, coworkers, fellow professionals, and the public, to mention a few—there is need for a large component of interpersonal theory in one's theory of practice. If student nurses are to develop an effective theory of practice, they must have correspondingly large opportunities to test out the interpersonal component of theory in real situations. As many of them discover, the relatively small amounts of time spent in testing the management or leadership process leaves them far short of what is needed for them to develop an effective theory of practice.

A second obstacle impeding the development of the testing aspect of an effective theory of practice is the somewhat artificial nature of the theories of action that students are taught under. Many of the existent theories of action tend to be self-sealing. Often, assumptions about the behavioral world lead us to act in ways that induce or confirm in others behavior that supports our assumptions. Instead of observing and testing what really is there, we see only what our theory leads us to expect to be there. We cut ourselves off from valid information that would discon-firm our theory and assumptions. If a patient is supposed to get relief from 100 mg of Demerol, he'd better behave as though he got relief. Signs indicating that no relief was obtained are often ignored. The same is true of some of the self-sealing theories that students are taught in psychiatric nursing. See for example, the following excerpt:

We had so much psych and so much of this and that appropriate responses, but I don't know. I thought I would be prepared in that area at least, but I found I was never prepared to come into contact with a situation where I just didn't even know what to say. Because there wasn't much to say, you know. In school, no one ever said that there might be a time when you would be sitting by the bedside of a patient and there just wasn't anything you could say. We learned so many of those communication techniques, but he didn't come under any of those standard headings.    (3:2A:11).

The third aspect of an effective theory of practice is the understanding of the process of personal causation. Accepting personal causality means performing responsibly under conditions of the real world—stress, under pressure of deadlines, constrained by time and money. A professional practitioner must be willing to take responsibility for what he does. Such commitment to be responsible is a condition for competence. Without it, theories of action cannot be put into effective practice.

A professional practitioner cannot generate an effective theory of action without commitment to responsibility. Such a commitment requires that one focus on one's own values in a situation and that one take these values seriously. Typically, in our first encounters with real situations, such as a new graduate's first job, we encounter more information than we can handle. This leads to the feeling of being overwhelmed. One cannot generate a perspective on the data unless one can figure out which information to ignore, which to pursue, and so on. Values are the instruments through which we select from more information than we can handle, that which we need in order to act, to test out, and to be responsible for our actions in a given situation.

However, it is not enough only to have values for a situation, and to have these values help us to form a point of view. (We may value a dignified death, which value helps us to hold the view that the human body should not be unnecessarily exposed and invaded.) Unless we are committed to those values, and to the point of view they indicate so that they become a basis for action, consistent action, the practitioner will quickly find that she depends upon the values of those around her, or simply is unable to function in the situation at all. We can observe this process going on in the following excerpt:

And she was wandering all over the floor crying, and then she asked if she could sit in one of the wheelchairs. I had come walking up the hallway, and one of the LPNs was talking with her and so I asked, "What are you doing here?" And she said something about being all upset, and that she was from another floor. And I said, "Well, what are you doing walking around? You're not allowed to go to other floors." And in the meantime, the LPN's getting *mad* at me because I'm questioning her and I'm asking her all the same questions she just asked her. And she's upset. And the LPN goes, "Well, just leave her alone." And, so I left, because, you know, I didn't know how to handle myself when the LPN told me to leave her alone. I didn't think I should have left her, but I didn't know how to handle it. So I said, "Well, all right, just let her sit in the chair, I don't care . . ." I can see myself in that situation as a student nurse. You know, it's strange, but the way you look at things is so different now from then. I would have stayed with her at all costs, and I never would have said the rule thing about not going to other floors. Although now, I know that's true and you'd get yelled at for not enforcing it. But as a student, I never would have said that or left her alone.   (2:5A:46)

Because this new nurse was not truly committed to the values she had learned in school, they did not become a basis for action, and the newcomer quickly succumbed to the press of environmental values.

The aspect of responsibility and personal causality in the building of an effective theory of practice is also related to self-concept and to change agent activity, which will be discussed in the next chapter. Taking one's own values seriously requires a person to have a strong commitment to self. This strong commitment will enable the professional to perform according to her own ideals and values in the face of resistance and disapproval from others. Taking one's own values seriously is therefore essential to innovation in practice, as well as to the building of a personal theory of practice.

Not only does an effective theory of practice contain the three processes of diagnosis, testing, and personal causality, it must also include both technical and interpersonal theories. The former state the techniques which the practitioner will use in the substantive tasks of his practice—for example, monitoring the biological status of the patient, administering medications, doing a dressing, and so on. Interpersonal theories are those which state how the professional will interact with clients and others in the course of practice—for example, how to work most effectively with a dying patient, how to give fluids to a resisting child, how to make out an effective work assignment, how to get a physician to respond appropriately to your concerns.

The overlapping and interconnection of these two kinds of theory vary with different professions. Teaching and nursing have a great deal of overlap, whereas the professions of architecture, engineering, and surgery have areas or zones in which it might be possible to employ techniques without any human interaction. The more that the professional requires interaction with the client in order to perform the professional task, the more interdependent the profession is. In this context, it is easy to see that ICU nursing is less interdependent than, for example, psychiatric nursing.

Now, not only does an effective theory of practice contain both technical and interpersonal theories (in various amounts depending upon the interdependency of the profession), but the practitioner's dependence upon the technical or interpersonal theory will vary during the diagnostic, testing, and implementation phases. The following example might well illustrate this variable relationship in nursing a patient in pain.

|  | Diagnostic | Testing | Implementation |
|---|---|---|---|
| Technical | 20 | 50 | 90 |
| Interpersonal | 80 | 50 | 10 |

The nurse may depend very heavily on interpersonal theory of action in diagnosing and testing a patient's problem of pain due to tension (and not to trauma), but use less of the interpersonal dimension and depend more on the technical dimension in the administration of a pain injection. So also a city planner may need both technical and interpersonal skills during the diagnostic phase, technical skills while drawing up the plans, but then technical and interpersonal skills during the implementation phase. Each profession has a certain and different ratio of technical to interpersonal theories, and a different pattern of dominance in the three different phases of its practice. However, it is inevitable that each dimension of theory building has not only a technical, but also an interpersonal component.

In summary then, professional competence is a major concern of professions in general, as well as of nursing in particular. Professional competence requires the development of one's own theory of practice. To be effective, this practice theory must have both a technical and interpersonal theory; the interpersonal zones of practice, and hence the need for interpersonal theories, are probably much larger than is often supposed. An effective theory of practice must include special competencies related to diagnosis, testing, and to the experience of personal causality in the implementation of solutions. In each of these areas, one needs both technical and interpersonal theories.

## How Competent are New Graduates for Professional Practice?

With the preceding overview as a perspective, we can now raise the question, to what extent did the new graduates perceive themselves as being competent practitioners? Did they feel they possessed the needed technical and interpersonal theories? We will take a look first at skill competence, which is the closest we come to technical theories. In no instance did the new graduates speak of a theory per se; rather they spoke about skills, the tools of theories.

*Skill competence.* As might be expected from the literature and from frequently heard comments from new graduates and older nurses alike, the participants in the seminars expressed a great deal of concern about skill incompetence ($N = 52$; 20 percent of the discussions were in this area). It was not, however, the largest area of concern, nor did the concern over skills persist into the fifth and sixth seminars. Most of the discussions in the skill areas occurred during the very early seminars. Some of the voices in the seminars told of their technical incompetence:

> I found it very difficult being put in the position of team leader when I didn't feel as if I knew what I was really doing as far as technical skills went and always had to ask someone else, say an LVN or a nurse's aide, to do something and then to have them ask me *how* to do it, and I didn't know. I found that very uncomfortable and embarrassing.   (9:2A:5)

> It's awful. Patients look at you because you can't get the IV to run, and then you'd have someone else come in to look at it. They'd touch it and it would run 100 miles a minute. Yeah, or trying to do a dressing when you're uncomfortable. You're a little nervous about doing the dressing, and you go in to do it, but then you forget a hundred things. And you've got to go back and get them and then the patient is looking at you like, "Oh, no, does she know what she's doing?"   (3:1A:30)

> There's a lot I don't know. There's a lot more that I'd like to be proficient at. Still, every time I have to help them draw blood on the kids, I get very nervous. I'm just not comfortable with skills at all. And that interferes with the rest of my care. I worry so about that that I don't have a mental care plan drawn up for going in and working with the kids. And then I question the care that I'm giving them.   (8:4:14)

> I didn't know anything about IV's or passing NG tubes or anything like that. And you're expected to know those things. [many agreeing comments] You just don't know what you're doing; you're totally inadequate and it causes a lot of frustration to the staff and just right off the bat starts a lot of conflicts. I had to add medications to IV's and I didn't know the first thing about it. It was very frustrating. I cried a lot and still do.   (9:2A:2)

The dominant message is: "I don't know the skills; I'm incompetent." Looking closer, one can begin to get a better understanding of why skill incompetence is so troublesome to the new graduates. Telling others what to do when you don't know yourself, embarrassment in front of a patient, conflicts with the staff—these are some of the reasons why the skill incompetence is so bothersome. It does not appear to be the skill performance alone, but rather the effect that the incompetent skill performance has on the self and self-esteem or on one's working relationships with others that creates most of the problem. Notice the feelings of low self-esteem that emerged when the new graduate in the following excerpt was confronted with a blank skill assessment sheet:

> When I started here and had to fill out that skill sheet, I left most of the lines blank because I had just never done any of those things. I know the techniques and the philosophy and that stuff, but I had just never handled it. Boy, filling out that sheet really confirms how incompetent you are!   (3:1A:14)

Other detrimental effects stemming from a low self-perceived competency and low self-esteem were also evident. In the following four excerpts the graduates tell of these effects: feeling highly anxious, feeling stupid, not being able to remember what one does know, avoiding asking questions so as to protect one's already low self-esteem.

> It's really a problem. When I do something for the first time, I ask "Did I do this? Did I do that?" When I first started, for about the first two months, I'd be asking myself, "Did I chart this?" and the next day I'd go back and look and I did chart it, but I couldn't remember charting it. I still have that problem, particularly when I face new things. I'm so incompetent that my anxiety goes way up, and then I get all flustered and can't remember a thing, and then I'm more incompetent.    (9:3B:35)

> This is really stupid and I felt like such an idiot afterwards. We had to have this clean catch specimen on this lady who had a catheter in. When I talked to the nurse about doing it, I said something about having to get a sterile basin to catch the urine in, and she just shook her head and looked at me and said: "What's a catheter? It's already sterile!" You know, just stupid things like that I don't quite remember until I talk to someone. There's so much I don't know that I get so uptight and then I forget what I already really do know.    (6:2B:10)

> I avoid asking questions because the staff thinks I already know. I'm incompetent enough; no point in letting them know more than they have to.    (7:1B:7)

> I don't ask because I don't want them to think I'm incompetent.    (4:6A:16)

One new graduate clearly captured the relation between skills, self-esteem, self-presentation, and relationships with others when she said:

> You know, all through school our instructors said that they weren't going to pound skills into our heads because there was more to nursing than just skills, and they didn't want us to be technicians. I was never sure what a technician was or why it was so awful to be one. I always had the feeling that they knew something that we didn't know and that we would eventually need to know, but I didn't know how else to ask for it except to say that I wanted more skill practice. But, you see, the thing is, the thing I know now that I didn't know then, is that it isn't the skill alone, it's the other things that being competent in starting an IV means, that's important. That's the thing I missed out on by never having really learned the skills until I got out. I had no pride in myself as a nurse[28].

In many ways the whole issue of the importance or unimportance of skills has become so distorted and is so out of perspective that we in nursing have created for the student and new graduate what Laing calls a knot.

There is something I don't know
   that I am supposed to know.
I don't know what it is I don't know,
   and yet am supposed to know,
And I feel I look stupid
   If I seem both not to know it
   and not know what it is I don't know.
Therefore, I pretend I know it.
   This is nerve-wracking
   since I don't know what I must pretend to know.
Therefore I pretend to know everything.
I feel you know what I am supposed to know
   but you can't tell me what it is
   because you don't know what I don't know what it is[29].

What the new graduates seem to be saying is that competence in technical skills is important, not so much for the sake of the skill itself, but because not knowing the skill has reverberating effects in many areas. It causes them to lose face with their coworkers, is an embarrassment to them in front of patient and physician, and prevents building self-esteem and self-confidence. One new graduate handled the knotty problem by pretending:

I've learned to lie a lot. I mean, usually my lies end up OK, like you gotta pretend you know what you're talking about. I found that out very fast. Usually, based on something I've learned from school and from my experience, I would say I'm 90 percent right in my lies. But when I'm not able to consult with someone, I lie. Like answering a patient's question, "Why are my feet swollen?" And if the patient does *not* have an obvious diagnosis that goes with swollen feet, you make it up, and usually you're right. If you can get it together, it certainly is better than getting those funny looks from the patient when you have to say you don't know.    (9:3B:38)

A special form of technical skill is organizational skill. New graduates were not as concerned about this as about more manual-technical skills ($N = 14$; 5 percent), probably because, as one of them put it, "The others don't expect us to be too well organized yet; but you're expected to know the basic skills of being a nurse!"    (6:1:4). Others commented:

Last week, I started orientation to charge, on days. And I've been doing it, but it's rough, because the first month was adjusting to the floor and being staff and settling in. And I was just beginning to feel comfortable and all of a sudden, they said, "Well, you're going to start charge now." And it was all over again—the anxiety attack!    (3:3A:14)

But if you haven't been team leading it's a completely different thing to be responsible for 14 patients and to make *sure* that everything on those patients gets done and that you *know* everything what's going on with those patients. And it's different. And it made me feel really badly that I had so much trouble with it, sort of like: "Boy—I waited all this time and thought I could do it and here I am, and I'm flopping." (1:4B:24)

The last excerpt also indicates the same kind of cumulative effect of organizational incompetence as was observed in skill incompetence. It is not only that one is not organized, but it is what that incompetence does to one's self-esteem and confidence that is particularly disturbing to the neophyte.

Although the development of an effective theory of practice does not speak directly to knowledge, possession of needed knowledge underlies both technical and interpersonal competence. Incompetence due to lack of knowledge was a major concern of the new graduates, ranking third after interpersonal and skill incompetence ($N = 30$; 11 percent).

> The thing that really keeps me from giving better patient care is the lack of knowledge about all the diseases we deal with. (2:2A:3)

> Reading charts and lab values and trying to figure out whether somebody is about to fall into acidosis or alkalosis and how it relates to everything else that's going on—that's really frustrating to me, to not have that information right at my fingertips. At least that's how it is for me. I have to think back to the class and I don't have that information right there on the floor, or right there in my head and I find it frustrating. (9:2A:29)

> I'd like to be able to better prepare patients for tests. But some of them, I just don't know what they are. Someone went down for a hypotonic-duodenography, you know, and I *guessed* what it was. I told the patient what I could about what I *thought* it might be. You just don't know what they are so there's no way to tell people. (3:2A:28)

> I don't know; I'm learning a lot, but I think I'm functioning at a level lower than the other RN's on the floor. I still have a lot to learn. Even passing meds. I always save the covers off them, so I can go home and look them up because I don't get a chance to on the floor. There are a lot of meds I don't know. And I don't like passing them if I don't know what they are, and the patients ask. And when I don't know, I honestly say: "I'm sorry, but I don't know." And they look at you like, "You sure this is for me then?" (4:2:21)

In the foregoing excerpts, again we see that it is not the absence of knowledge per se that is troubling, but rather how this deleted incompetence looks to the patient or to one's coworkers. Perhaps the reason the effects of knowledge incompetence were not mentioned more frequently is that knowledge is less observable than manual-technical or organizational skills. Hence it is a little easier to disguise one's incompetence in this area than in others. Only the individual herself knows that she does not know.

I feel like it's all a front. There's a lot of stuff that I simply do not know, but if I keep my mouth shut no one else knows that I don't know. But it still makes me feel guilty. I feel I should know what's going on with the patient, the disease process, the drugs, the tests. I'd be a better nurse if I knew, but the truth of the matter is that I really can get by not knowing.   (8:4:12)

Another area of professional competence that was of concern to the new graduate nurses regards decision-making and judgment skills. Although many of them recognized that competence in this area does require a certain amount of experience, they were still quite unhappy with their abilities in this area.

I don't feel equipped to handle things that happen. I mean, the organization is one thing, but if something happens, you have to make decisions that are based on a certain amount of experience and knowledge which I don't feel that I have. I still go up to the person in charge and say, "Well, you know, this kid's temp is 102 and I put him on a full liquid diet, and now I'm going to start sponges or whatever. Is that right?"   (3:5A:2)

This is an area in which even the most experienced nurses have some difficulty. Undoubtedly, with an increase in skill, knowledge, and organization techniques and skills, the areas of judgment and decision making, which are in fact a combination of knowledge, skill, and organization, will improve markedly.


*Interpersonal incompetence.*   The last and most prevalent area of incompetence in practice for the new graduate nurses was interpersonal skills and theories ($N = 57$; 22 percent). This probably could have been predicted because, to a large extent, students receive instruction in interpersonal theories, but have very limited opportunities to utilize them in real practice situations. Unquestionably, as we saw earlier, many professions and particularly highly interdependent professions such as nursing, need practitioners schooled with an effective theory of practice that incorporates interpersonal theory as well as technical theory. The newcomers to nursing felt they were severely lacking in interpersonal theories and competence.

Before listening to some of the new graduates describe their experiences in the interpersonal area, let us ask what does interpersonal competence mean? What are its essential ingredients? Interpersonal competence means having the ability to cope effectively with interpersonal relationships[30]. It means being able to accomplish interpersonal tasks—being able to get others to do what you want them to do. Some readers will immediately recoil at this definition and say that this is manipulation. Interpersonal competence can indeed encompass both influence behavior and manipulation. We distinguish between these two on the basis that manipulation is the altering or control of another's responses to achieve one's own personal ends; influence is doing so for purposes of enhancing the development of the other, or for the common good, such as improving patient care. As the terms are used here, influence behavior and interpersonal competence are relative to the individual's purposes.

There are three criteria which can be used both to describe and to evaluate the effectiveness of one's interpersonal competence.

1. The individual perceives the interpersonal situation accurately. He is able to identify the relevant variables plus their interrelationships.

2. The individual is able to solve the problems in such a way that they remain solved. If, for example, interpersonal trust is low between A and B, they may not have been said to solve the problem competently unless and until it no longer recurs (assuming the problem is under control).

3. The solution is achieved in such a way that A and B are still able to work with each other at least as effectively as when they began to solve their problems.*

An individual must be able to identify accurately both her own role, feelings, and functioning in a given situation, and the role, feelings, and functioning of others involved. Having done this, she is then in a position to solve relationship problems competently in such a way that interdependence and work productivity can proceed, and that new problems and challenges are faced, rather than the old constantly rehashed.

Pivotal to being interpersonally competent is development of the skill of establishing and maintaining desired identities, both for the self and for others[31]. Skill in establishing one's own identity or in presenting desired images of oneself will be discussed in the section of Chapter 5 entitled "Management of Backstage Reality." Here we will concern ourselves with the needed skill of identifying the other that one desires to portray. This skill is dependent upon three factors. To perceive the interpersonal situation accurately:

1. The person must be able to accurately take the role of the other and to be able to predict the impact that his own behavior will have on the other person's view of the situation.

2. The person must have a large and varied repertoire of interpersonal behaviors, strategies, things that one can do.

3. The person must have within himself the resources and abilities needed to be able to decide which behaviors and tactics to use at which times[32].

---

* Reproduced by special permission from *The Journal of Applied Behavioral Science.* "Conditions for Competence Acquisition and Therapy" by Chris Argyris, Volume 4, Number 2, p. 148. © by NTL Institute, 1968.

Of these three factors, the first is most crucial. If stripped of its affective overtones, the first factor is what is meant by empathy. It is so important to the development of interpersonal competence because true empathy serves as a self-motivating factor in the development (factor 2) and judicious utilization (factor 3) of tactics and behaviors needed to be competently influential. In other words, if you have a clear and accurate picture of what's going on, this will motivate you to seek alternative ways of working out an effective solution to an interpersonal problem.

What is involved in getting this clear and accurate picture? How is empathy developed? There are numerous writings on this subject; some of the more important ones will be summarized here[33]. First of all, it is generally agreed that empathy has two components: an affective component, i.e., the recognition and sharing with the feelings of another; and a cognitive component, i.e., the ability to structure and view as a logical, integrated whole the value and conceptual world of another. Furthermore, to be truly empathic, it is not enough just to sense or identify the other's world; we must also communicate that feeling or identification with the other. Both affective and cognitive components of empathy are essential for the development of interpersonal competence.

Results of research have indicated that there are wide differences among people in their ability to be empathetic. We know that this ability depends to some extent upon intact senses (so that one can accurately take in stimuli), intelligence (so that one can map meanings out of incoming stimuli), cue sensitivity (so that one can pick out the relevant stimuli from the large amounts coming in), and perceptual vigilance (so that one can constantly listen for and monitor changes in feelings, moods, words, and behavior). We also know that empathy is related to physiological responses[34] and that it is one of the critical variables affecting the outcome of the helping process[35]. In spite of all this, we also know that nurses are not particularly empathetic. In fact, in a study measuring the relative degrees of empathy manifested by workers in twelve different occupational-professional groups, the 112 registered nurses in the sample scored lower on the measure of empathy than all the groups tested, save one. The only group less empathetic than nurses was manufacturing plant supervisors[36]. This same lack of empathy was noted by Duff and Hollingshead, who reported that 71 percent of the nurses studied showed no evidence of empathy[37]. More recently La Monica reported that there was no difference in the amount of empathy reported in a group of senior student nurses before and after their psychiatric nursing experience, the rotation wherein it was expected that students would particularly learn to become empathetic[38]. Lest one think that this deficiency is readily overcome through work experience, such is not the case. In a recent study in which practicing nurses employed in a large hospital were tested for empathy, all were found to score "exceptionally low"[39]. It is therefore not surprising to find that the new graduate nurses in the seminars reported a considerable amount of interpersonal incompetency, and that there was evidence that much of it was due to a lack of empathy.

In the following, rather lengthy excerpt, we can see the kinds of difficulties and dilemmas that new graduates got themselves into when they lacked interpersonal competence.

I was in my second week of being the only RN on, and just right after I had come on, I was down at the end of the hall in this one room. These two guys, patients, obviously had been drinking. It was *so* obvious. So, I just kind of went back to the desk and said to myself, "Now, what do I do?" You know, "We didn't learn about this in school. What do you do?" So I thought about it a bit and decided, "Well, I'll just go down and ask them about it." And so I did and they said, "Well, we had alcohol rubdowns from the previous shift." And I said, "Oh, OK." I thought, "I can't tell them I don't believe them!" But it was really obvious. So I put a note on the chart, on both their charts. I told both their doctors about it, and I told the day shift about it. And that particular morning I wasn't able to tape because it was so busy, so I told them verbally. And the day shift is kind of, well some of them are really funny and they *do* have a good sense of humor but they carried it too far. They laughed at me and said, "What's the matter with you? Aren't you going to let your patients have a good time? They weren't hurting anybody, were they? Why don't you go down and have a little snort with them?" and it kind of really griped me because, then during the whole report they didn't even listen to the rest of what I had to say. And they were always teasing me about it. And I said, "Well, OK, if that's the way you want to be," and we kind of laughed about it but, yet I took it seriously. Well, what they did—they thought it was so funny—was they went down to the two patients and told them that they had scared that poor little night nurse that was brand new half to death with their drinking. And then the patients thought it was funny and they said, "Oh, just wait and see what a hard time we're going to give her tonight!" In a joking way, I guess, but anyway, one of the wives came in and her husband told her about it and she absolutely flipped her lid. She was furious! She was going to sue the hospital for accusing her husband of drinking and she insisted that the doctor be called and the doctor had to come down right away. And I guess the doctor went into another patient's room and the wife followed him in and I guess really created a scene. And then the doctor gets on my back for causing such a fuss in the first place, and the patients jump on my aide, so then she's got it in for me. And through all of this, I don't get not even one kind word from the supervisor! And it was the hospital I thought I was protecting. I mean, although they weren't drunk, drunk, they had been drinking, and drinking isn't permitted in the hospital. Boy, what a mess. (2:3B:8–9)

We can see from this excerpt that the new graduate was indeed temporarily incompetent. She demonstrated a lack of empathy by being unable to define the situation as the nurses, patients, physician, relatives were defining it. But empathy and interpersonal competence are a two-way street. The older staff nurses could certainly have displayed some empathy for the newcomer, and assisted her in her dilemma. Lacking empathy, the new graduate was in no position, nor was she motivated, to find or employ interpersonal strategies that would have enabled her competently to handle the situation in such a way that it would be resolved, and in such a way that she could continue to work effectively with others.

The following excerpt is another very clear-cut example of a lack of empathy on the new graduate's part.

> I'm afraid to just go sit, just take a break, you know. So I always ask everybody else to make sure they don't need any help, and then I'll go and sit down for a few minutes. But I never just go and sit down when I know that somebody else is still busy. But there're other girls who do it all the time. They just take care of the patients they're assigned to and then they sit . . . There's one LPN on my floor that I asked a couple of times one day if she needed help. And by the end of the day, she was really mad at me 'cause I had asked her if she needed help. She thought that I thought she wasn't capable of handling it. She didn't know where I was coming from. I didn't know that she was getting mad. At the end of the day she asked me if I liked her . . . she had the feeling that I didn't like her. And I didn't give her that impression, you know, consciously. And I told her that "there's nothing about you that I don't like." (4:4:21)

The newcomer shows some awareness of the fact that she lacked empathy when she says, "She didn't know where I was coming from," and of course, the counterpart to that is: "I didn't know where she was coming from." This newcomer was quite vigilant for cues—she was picking up information—but she didn't quite seem to know how to put it together into a meaningful pattern.

The new graduates described numerous examples of interpersonal incompetency. Although logically, of course, such incompetency could involve interpersonal relationships with any number of people—coworkers, physicians, other professional colleagues, patients, relatives, to mention a few—it is noteworthy that in only one instance, the excerpt involving patients' drinking, did the new graduates mention any interpersonal problems they had with patients. Fellow coworkers were predominantly the people with whom the new graduates experienced interpersonal incompetency. Some examples of general interpersonal competence difficulties are as follows:

> That feeling that you are a villain if you ask people to do something! Somebody will make a comment or give you that kind of look and I really feel badly . . . They sent me down to ask the blood drawer to draw some blood for a glucose on this lady. And she'd already drawn the blood from the lady for the other tests so she said, "I've already drawn the blood from her!"

And I said, "Yes, I know, but we need one of these." And she really lights into me and tells me I should have told her earlier and all that. Well, it was 20 after 7:00 and there was no way I could've gotten to her earlier. You know, it was like she was trying to assert her authority. And all I was trying to do was to get this patient's blood drawn so she could have breakfast. And then they were taking in the tray but she hadn't had her insulin yet, so I asked one of the nurses to take the tray back to the kitchen to keep it warm because the lady hadn't had her insulin yet. And then, they didn't have the right kind of insulin up there so it took the pharmacy 45 minutes to get the insulin. And then I had to call down for a new tray because I didn't want the person to have a cold tray. Then I had to take the gaff: "What do you think we have here, a restaurant?" You know, so just one thing and it snowballs . . . Oh I wish I could get everybody to be sweet and cooperate with me and not make a federal issue out of things. Others can get people to do that, but I can't.   (6:5A:29)

On 3-11, we got things pretty much set up so that everyone knows what they're supposed to be doing. Like the aides do the I-and-O's and turning. They know they are going to do that when they come on. It's not something that you decide to give them. I notice that some of the attendants are good workers and some aren't. Some you just have to go in and do everything yourself. They just sit there and I suppose I could, when I get to know them a little better, go up and tell them what has to be done. But I really don't know how to do that—to get others to do their work, what you want them to do. I notice that they do more work for the other nurses than for me, but I don't know how to do it except to just sort of suggest it to them. But still they sit in the conference room, smoking and reading. They don't do much to help me. I sort of do their work and mine too.   (6:2A:22)

New graduates often recognize their interpersonal competence problem, but are stymied in doing anything about it and do the work themselves. This kind of situation was noted in about half of the discussions. In others, there was evidence that the new graduates had a general awareness that they would need to develop and pay attention to interpersonal theories and skills; in still others, there was evidence that they were helping themselves to solve their interpersonal incompetency problems. The following excerpts deal with general awareness:

It was really a matter of working through the basics with all of the clinics, with the people, all the interpersonal relations on a different basis. People humor you when you're a student; they really do. There are a lot of things that they'll say: "Well she's a student"—that kind of thing—rather than just telling you directly: "If you were an RN, this would not be acceptable." I think if you got that kind of feedback right away and all along, it would not be nearly so difficult.   (9:1A:31)

When I started I sort of set up some objectives for myself, things that I wanted to work on. My main concern was getting to know the other people that I was going to be working on staff with. But in my orientation of the unit, we were so protected and we were with the clinician all the time, that we walked in for about a week or ten days of five-minute kinds of contact with the rest of the staff, and I didn't even get to know their names. Then when we finally got out on the floor, I was shoved into team leading and I didn't know the people that I was working with, yet I was so anxious I had tremendous tunnel vision. I could barely take in what was happening with the other people I was working with. I didn't know if I was making reasonable demands on them or not, or if some of the things that were said were to be taken personally, or if people were just sounding off because they were having a bad day, or what. I was just walking around with blinders on for several weeks.   (1:1B:9-10)

Increasingly I have found that in nursing, the nurse has to be the one to reach out to others—the doctor, the aide, the patient, to everyone. She has to reach out to everybody on the floor and keep them together, pulling together.   (4:6:3)

In the following four excerpts we see some evidence of this reaching out to others. The new graduates are still telling us of their interpersonal difficulties, but in all four, there is some indication that the newcomer has developed some kind of strategy, some kind of interpersonal theory to her theory of practice that is enabling her to handle the all-important interpersonal aspects of nursing practice.

I think it would depend on the coworkers; how they're going to take it. If you feel that you can talk to them as adults and they're not on any ego trip, then, maybe OK. I work with a male LVN who really wants to be an RN. When he was in another hospital, he was given more responsibility than LVN's here, so he feels kind of trapped here. And anything that kind of puts down his intelligence as a nurse is one strike against the person that is telling him. Therefore in telling this man anything, you've got to really work around him and get into where he's coming from in order to work with him and that's really hard.   (9:1C:14)

I've also found that one way to break the barrier of the age difference is by putting them, so to speak, on the pedestal, putting them in the limelight— For instance, if we're working with traction and it's kind of lopsided, and they come over and help do something, by saying, "Gee, you're the experienced person." Giving them credit where credit's due. They just beam and accept you better. And you work on a more personal level. That's not only with RN's; it's with nursing assistants and LVN's as well. Oh, when you let them know that they can really show you how to do something, or a different way to do something, they feel really good. And you get a lot more cooperation. You just have to show people that you appreciate them and have consideration for them.   (9:1B:30)

It really is a hard kind of a relationship. Like the aides on our floor have been there for a long time and they might know a lot, but you really have to earn their respect before they'll help you out . . . But when they realize that you're working just as hard as they are and that you're not trying to be their boss, that you're just their coworker, then they'll be really nice, but you really have to cross the barrier to them, I've found. And part of crossing that barrier is to be seen doing the kind of work that is tasky, you know what I mean? Talking with or teaching patients doesn't look like work to the aides. They think you are goofing off when they see you doing that.   (4:6:3)

As the new graduates begin to develop empathy they may begin to act upon an interpersonal theory in which they see that different people— aides, other nurses, the patients, relatives of the patients—define situations differently. What is appropriate interpersonal action for one, may not be for the others.

## Social Testing as a Way of Increasing Competence

Thus far in our discussion we have focused on five major kinds of incompetency reported by new graduate nurses in their seminar discussions: skill, organization, knowledge, judgment/decision making, and interpersonal incompetency. In this section we will begin to look at ways in which the new graduates increased their scope of competency. Once one recognizes that one is incompetent, what can one do about it? In discussing this question, very little, if any, differentiation was made as to the type of competency one wanted to increase; all kinds of incompetency were treated together.

One of the first ways in which a newcomer can increase her competency is by passing the tests that she constructs for herself, and that others construct for newcomers. It is in this sense that the first job as a graduate nurse is a proving ground—a place, context, or milieu in which one proves that one is a nurse, both to oneself and to others. Besides proving one's competence, the passing of such tests enables one to be treated by others as if more competent, which is extremely important in raising one's self-esteem. The new graduates discovered that in fact, others were out to test them, and that they would have to prove their competency.

We have five people on the staff and the pace is so fast, and everybody's trying to prove what efficient and super nurses they are . . . I guess that's what a lot of people shoot for. It's your goal. You want to get everything done; you want to treat the patients with respect, and you want to be considered hard-working by the rest of the staff. And that entails, you know, opinions from other people, from patients and doctors, about the work you're doing, the care you're giving. So you have to prove to others that you can do it and are doing it. It goes on all the time.   (6:4A:22)

Where we work, there's a large turnover and the RN's don't last that long. And the LVN's and the orderlies have been there a long time. So it's really like they know a lot more than you do when you're first there, and they're not that helpful! It's really like they'd almost like to trip you up.   (9:2B:3)

Given the realization that others were going to put them to the test, how did the new graduates make out? The following excerpt provides an example of a constructed test taken and passed.

> Oh, it was terrible! But I was really lucky that I had two people working with me, an LPN and an aide who knew things cold and had everything ingrained in his head so he would just walk in and do everything he was supposed to do, and I didn't even have to say anything. I remember when I first started, I remember walking around to both of them and saying, "Now what do you usually do when you work down here?" And they said, "Don't worry, we'll do our jobs." And that was a help, but of course, everything broke loose that day. People had to go down to X-ray, and here and there for lung scans and there were a thousand doctors around, and this never happens at night. And people called in sick, and admissions, and blood ran out—just crazy, but somehow I managed to get through it. But I was a wreck you know, at 3:00. And the next day, the head nurse came back and I said to her, "Did you know that I was going to have to do charge on East?" And she says, "I knew that that was going to happen. I tried to orient you before you'd get thrown into it, but sooner or later you just have to do it." It didn't work though; she knew that it was going to happen and let it happen. But somehow I managed to get through it and afterward, I have to admit, it felt good to just kind of sit back and think "I did it! That's great," you know, it really felt good.   (3:5A:2)

The new nurse who passes the test may not always feel as good about it as in this example, for she may see the test as unfair. In the following example, the newcomer describes a more formal testing situation which she failed. She did not feel good about the test, but it seems as though the cause of the bad feeling was not so much the test as the conditions under which it was done.

> We were in the conference room and I was reading a chart or something and the head nurse started asking me if I knew my emergency drugs. "Well," I said, "it's been awhile since I had ER, ICU and inservice classes." So she starts throwing out these drugs to me, asking what this does and that and what the action is . . . I wouldn't have minded it had I been alone, but an intern was sitting there and I felt like a dummy as it was. And she kept throwing them at me, even when I didn't know them—I would say at least 20. I didn't appreciate that at all under those circumstances.   (6:2B:16)

The new nurses really felt good when they passed tests constructed by others providing they could get a handle on the criteria for passing, and providing that they saw the tests as being fair. In the following two excerpts, we see examples of what was considered to be unfair testing. In the first, the newcomer felt that the test was too difficult; in the second, she felt that the criteria were unfair.

> So it's like you're saying to yourself, "OK, you're new, you need the experience, so get in there and do it all." But the thing is they hand me things

that are over my head, and then won't help. And when you need to know something and ask a question, they're never around [laughter] . . . I feel secure in taking a difficult patient as long as there's a doctor there, or somebody else that *knows* what's going on and can help. But when they give me somebody that is super over my head, and I'm the only one there and no one ever comes in to say, "Hi, how's it going?" or "Is your patient still alive? Are you still alive? Do you need to go to the bathroom?" You know, you feel like, "What is this?" Because you know darn well what they're doing, because you can hear them sitting out at the desk talking and carrying on, and you begin to wonder if they're just trying to see if you can do it or not.   (2:2B:18)

Then my husband said to me, "Maybe they're trying to tell you that you just can't do as thorough a job when things are in a rush and you have to hurry. The other staff know how that is, but they don't know how else to tell you except that you're just going to have to pick up your speed and the only way that can be done is if you don't do as thorough a job." I don't know. The whole thing is the epitome of what this idealism versus realism is all about . . . Idealistically, you shouldn't have to hurry . . . When a patient is expelling her enema, you shouldn't be standing there asking her questions. You should, you know, let her have her privacy. And I could be doing things—interviewing her and so forth while she's doing this. But it shouldn't be that way. It's just really, instead of trying to hurry putting in an IV, you should take your time until you're good enough at it. Then you pick up your speed, you know, by yourself instead of really practicing rushing at it and blowing several of the veins.   (6:4A:4)

The following excerpt describing a testing situation is of particular interest for several reasons. First, it shows a mixture of both self-testing and testing by others. Second, it describes a testing situation that is currently in progress; the test isn't really over yet. And third, it clearly indicates that the new graduate is aware of the criteria for passing the test— the kinds of things she must do to show competence in the test situation.

It's not that I'm utterly dedicated, but I'm thinking of myself now. If I don't show myself to be a trooper now, then they're not going to think too much of me. You know, in some ways it's ridiculous. You can't do only your regular work and be thought of as a real good worker. You have to do *more* to show that you're a trooper. But I feel like when I'm there, I'm still not functioning even up to regular. I'm not as good as at least I hope I will be sometime. So no way can I pass the test of being a trooper . . . So I feel like if I don't at least put in the time, lots of time, then they won't even think I'm trying to be a trooper. And *I* won't think I'm trying. I still can't function very well, but just the fact that I'm there, I guess, shows something.   (6:3A:20-21)

This nurse's knowledge of the criteria for passing the test will undoubtedly help her to pass it if she chooses to do so. In the following example we see evidence of an other-constructed test in which it is evident that the new graduate felt that the testing was creating jeopardy for the patient:

> I figure that since the doctors aren't complaining and the patients are reacting the way they are to me, that I'm doing something right. But you'd never know it by what the other staff members have said. There are people who will say why it was good, but most don't say anything. When I first went on nights, all they did was pick me apart. They actually once stood at the door of the delivery room when I was having a very difficult delivery and the doctor was hinting that he'd really like another nurse in there because we were very busy. We were planning on a bad baby and that sort of thing. The other nurse just stood there and took notes on the things that I wasn't doing quickly enough. I was taking blood pressures while he was giving funnel pressure and she said, "You should have been giving the funnel pressure." I said, "And who was going to take the blood pressure?" "You know," I said, "didn't it ever occur to you that you could have walked in and done one or the other for us?" But she was taking notes. It flabbergasted me! When I got back down from upstairs and I was cleaning out the baby warmer and putting it back in the delivery room she pulls these notes out of her pocket and starts reading them, and I thought, "OK, that's really not putting the patient first. The least you can do is put the patient first, and then yell at me later. But help when help's needed." (2:2B:13-17)

Here we see that the new graduate was aware that she was being tested, that she was aware that she had not passed the test, yet was very angry at the whole idea of being tested under these circumstances. It is important for newcomers to learn how to ask the questions that need to be asked in order to ascertain the content, criteria, and circumstances of testing situations. For further elaboration and specific information on this process, the reader is referred to the "proving ground" module in the book, *Path to Biculturalism* [40].

Although we saw in the last excerpt that the new graduate did not know the criteria for passing an other-constructed test, it is also very apparent that she could articulate the criteria she was using to judge her own performance: no complaints from the doctors and the patients reacting in some kind of positive manner to her. So it would seem as though the nurse was passing her own self-constructed tests. Now let us examine some examples of nurses discussing self-constructed tests.

> It's great just to find out how well you can function. Last Saturday, there was this lady who was having twins. And I never saw twins born before; it was really exciting . . . I wanted to be a part of it. And you know, every medical student in the place that was within call was in there. God, it was just really exciting with everybody standing around. And there was one other circulator and myself. And you know, I really felt like I was adding, contributing, helping out by getting the little things ready that have to be gotten ready for delivery. And I looked around for a second and saw all those people standing there and gazing. And I said, "That's me!" As a stu-

dent nurse, you know and I know just how they feel, and I really know I've come a long way when I can come into a situation like this and function instead of just standing there. Golly, it was such a nice feeling. (6:6A:21–22)

When I stopped saying "I don't know" when doctors or nurses asked me questions, and started saying, "I'll do it"—that's when I knew I had made it to myself, for myself.

For me, it was going on nights by myself. I could see how good or how bad I am. The responsibility was there and there was no one else around except me. (5:5A:27–28)

Passing one's own tests and the tests of others and thereby proving one's competency is contingent not only upon the fairness of the test and the fairness of the criteria for passing the test but also upon the goals of performance. Competency is intimately tied up with goals and performance, and there are a number of things we know about this relationship through research.

First, we know that performance is a function of the goals a person is trying to reach; the higher the goals, the higher the performance. The level of self-set goals (goals a person sets for herself) in a specific task situation defines what is meant by competency in that situation; how competent a person considers herself to be in any given situation is a function of the level of her goals. Self-set goals that are higher than current level of performance will lead one to label oneself as incompetent. See for example the following excerpt:

Do you know how you can know something when you really sit down and think about it, but at the time you don't know it? Most of the time I feel generally pretty frustrated and incompetent because I feel like I'm just really working hard, you know, and I'm learning a lot, more and more every day, but I'm still not at the level yet that I want to be at. (3:5C:16)

Self-perceived competence for a task will generally facilitate one's performance on a task, particularly if there is some way of getting feedback which tells one how close one is getting to one's goals[41]. Self-perceived incompetency can motivate improved performance, providing that the distance between goal and performance is not too wide.

The research findings in relation to externally set goals (other-constructed tests) are somewhat different. It has been shown that the higher the goals someone sets for us[42], the higher is their opinion of our competency; this high opinion in turn results in one's perceiving oneself as being more competent, and hence should lead to higher performance. In some ways, we see this principle operating when a head nurse assigns the new graduate to increasingly more difficult patient care assignments. The message is that she sees the new graduate as competent. If the new graduate understands this message (instead of thinking it means something else, like, "She doesn't like me; she's trying to kill me with work"), the result should be higher performance. In the following excerpt, a new graduate explains that mastery of technical skills is the goal she perceives has been set for her but does not give us any indication as to whether this goal motivated her to high performance.

> All I can hear are the words ringing, "You'll pick it up." [general laughter] "Give yourself six months and you'll pick it up. Granted, you'll fumble a little bit." And I did; I really did stumble. These first couple of months are really, really hard because you just don't have the dexterity and the basic technical skills. That is a real need for you to have because a lot of times that's how you're recognized as being successful before anything else. Your acceptance and your rate of success, how people judge you as being successful, are all dependent upon that.   (9:3B:10–11)

Investigation has shown that there is a maximum tolerance level between a goal for future performance and one's current performance. If the gap between goals and present performance is too great, the individual becomes too discouraged to proceed, or else engages in self-defeating frenzied activity[43] as in the following excerpt:

> I was on by myself and had four admissions and it was absolutely chaotic. I asked for help but got none. I was on the brink of tears all night, and just kept working faster and faster, but nothing seemed to help. I finally made such a big mistake, I thought I would just die, absolutely die. I went to start this IV on a patient—I'd seen it in the cardex. Well I went back and I stuck this lady four times trying to get it. Finally I called the doctor and he got it in after three trys. And so then I went to go back at 9:00 P.M. with an antibiotic, and I look at the label and it says Kelly, and I look at the name on the wall card and it says McCarthy. And I said to myself, "Oh God, I put the IV in the wrong person." Yes, I did. I got the IV set up, stuck it into the other patient, called the doctor so he wouldn't get alarmed the next morning, called the supervisor and filled out an incident report, and then hung my head. I was scared to death! I thought I would die. That's my whole career—down the drain.   (6:5B:23–24)

Obviously, neither utter discouragement nor frenzied activity is going to result in improved performance. A happy medium must be reached with respect to externally set goals for the new graduate. They've got to be high enough to challenge the development of her competence, but not so high as to be unattainable.

*Other ways of improving competence.*   Two very common solutions to the problem of incompetency used by the new graduates are to shelve the idealism of school temporarily and to become better organized. Many expect that by following these courses of action, they will develop the competencies rewarded in the workplace and have the time to perform the competencies valued in their academic training. The second plan generally meets with a little more success than the first, providing one does not become enamored with organization for the sake of organization. The first plan generally fails, as predicted by the maxim, "Use it [the school ideal] or lose it."

The new graduates were very free in sharing and in asking for help as to what to do about specific interpersonal relationship problems. They probably asked for more direct help in this area than in any other. An example of sharing the solution to an interpersonal problem was given by the new nurse who said,

> I finally went to this girl and told her, "Look, I really feel threatened by you. I think you're really aggressive and I think you probably feel overwhelmed like I do a lot of the time." And, you know, that one came out great! I think it's better to get those feelings out. That was one way to approach it, and I don't think she was ever really aware of the way she was coming across to others.   (1:4C:20)

The following, rather lengthy excerpt is presented not only because it illustrates the direct asking for help in this area, but because it typifies some of the interaction frequently observed in the new graduate seminars.

> Sometimes you have a run-in with one person, when you've asked her to do something, and that's really bad. And even if you try to be nice later on, or something like that, still, that person is defensive. And you're defensive, and you never really iron it out. I don't know how to handle that; I'm having trouble with that, and she still won't do anything for me, or that I ask her to do.

> I've run into that too. I had one aide say to me that a patient noticed that the two of us just don't get along. And I said, "You know, I'm sorry if it's so obvious." I really felt bad about that. I don't know what to do. I admit that I don't really get along with her, but it's come out very defensive. Like I would try to be helpful to her, and try to come out helpful. But she got very upset. She misreads it but I don't know how she reads it. And then the aftermath was bad too. I'm really quite a calm person so if someone's upset, I just say, "OK, fine," but this person just blew up in front of the patient, and I couldn't stand that, so I said, "OK, let's just go out and talk about it." And then the patient asked me, "Why did she have to say that in front of me?" And I can see the problem of that, too . . . I don't know what to do. I have to work with her; it's not like school where it would have been only temporary.

> I think the best way to handle that would be a confrontation. I know that's hard to do. You can sit and talk about it in theory, but going in and saying, "Hey, we've got a real problem. We both hate each other but we've got to work together, and so we should go talk about it." You know, that's hard to do. I don't know if I'm that big a person; in fact, I know I'm not. But that's what I think should be done.

Yeah, well maybe it's not that big a deal. Maybe I'm making more out of it than I should. Cause, you know, looking back on it now, I know it was a horrible day for her. And we haven't worked together alone since then, so maybe it won't be a problem. Maybe she'll have forgotten about it by the time we work alone again.

I doubt it.

Me, too.

Did you ever involve your head nurse in this?

Oh, no. That's not the best thing to do because some head nurses will really hold it against both of you, but especially against the new RN. It depends on the kind of head nurse you have, but some of them can be so petty.

Yeah, you're right. They expect you to be able to get along with everyone and not stir up the waters. Sometimes, I think it's just better to forget it and start over. Try to be amiable and act like nothing happened.

Yes, be nice and help 'em and please 'em.

Yeah, but how do I get her to do her job and be nice to the patients? She doesn't do it automatically, and if I say something to her, then that's when we got into it . . . And it really bugs the rest of the staff. They're uptight and unhappy because she was uptight. And they could feel the friction. And that's hard to be in a team leader situation in a case like that.

When I have that kind of problem, I kind of work around it. You know, delegate more to others who will take it, or do more of the work myself. I just work around the way the others want to do it. As long as it's not harmful to the patient.

I don't think you can always work around a situation like that. Or that it's particularly effective to do it that way. I think you have to bring it out into the open.

Granted, I do too. But what do you say after the opening line? I don't think I'll have trouble saying, "We've got a problem." But what about after that? (8:5:22-24)

The foregoing conversation illustrates an interpersonal relationship problem that many new graduates felt incompetent to handle. They asked for help, and received various advice. What is very clear is that even though they wanted it desperately, there was no indication that these new graduates possessed or were using any kind of interpersonal theory upon which to construct an effective theory of practice.

*Suggestions for improvement of competency.* The voices of experience have been very clear in their message: "We feel incompetent." Let's address ourselves now to a consideration of what might be done to help them to improve their competency and, of course, subsequently, their performance. These suggestions will be organized around three major areas: effective theory of practice, preservice or inservice orientation, and appropriate goals.

## Effective Theory of Practice

Students and practicing nurses alike must develop effective theories of professional practice. Not until all nurses look at professional practice as a process of diagnosing, testing, and assuming personal causality for the actions taken will the practice of nursing be all that it can be. In developing these theories of practice, attention must be given to both the technical and the interpersonal components. In nursing, we need both. Ultimately, nurses need to be steered or guided into those specializations in practice that are most consonant with their personality needs. A nurse who is very technique-oriented will not be an effective practitioner in a rehabilitation unit; one who is not will be markedly uncomfortable in an intensive care unit. Be that as it may, because nursing is such a highly interdependent profession, all nurses must have some techniques, some interpersonal skills—the latter, for use not only with patients but, in some respects even more so, with coworkers and others with whom nurses work.

One of the most critical needs in nursing education is for an understanding of the interrelation among skill mastery, self-confidence, and self-esteem. There is no question that high self-esteem leads to high performance. A large measure of the low self-esteem of new graduates is caused by their feelings of incompetency, particularly in using manual-technical skills. This incompetency and the low self-esteem it spawns can be overcome by *skill mastery*. Once-over-lightly exposure is not the same as skill mastery. Skill mastery is the breeding ground of self-confidence.

For years nursing educators have been loathe to place much emphasis on the mastery of skills. They gave many reasons: there is too much else to teach; a skill will be outdated by the time it is used; the training is not necessary because a nurse is supposed to use her head, not her hands. Regardless of what reason is given, the plain and simple truth is that the deemphasis has had bad results. Something was lost when skill practice was eliminated from generic nursing programs.

> My instructors always said that the skills would come with practice. Well, that might be so, but you have to have a place to practice. And you have to know that somehow you'll really be able to learn them.   (5:5A:7)

As we have shown in this chapter, it's not the skill per se that is so important. It's what mastery of that skill does for one's feelings of self-esteem, self-confidence, and ability to get along, to relate competently with others, that is so important. What is being suggested here is not to go overboard and reinstitute the checklists whereby each student had to be shown to have 400 skills before graduation. Rather, what is being proposed is for a faculty (preferably in conjunction with local nursing service hospital and community health personnel) to agree on perhaps 20 basic, highly used skills. And then to teach these to students to the point of mastery, not one-over-lightly. These skills must include some complex and fairly technical skills, like administering IM injections, suctioning, monitoring or starting of IV fluids, and inserting Levine tubes. These are skills used fairly extensively in nursing service, and their mastery by the student will do much to provide her with sufficient technical competence so that she has grounds for the development of a healthy self-esteem and self-confidence.

There is another factor in skill mastery that must be recognized. Early saturation and concomitant mastery of selected skills by students will enable students to learn that skills are a means to an end, not an end in themselves. If manual-technical skills are learned and incorporated into the student's conception of whole-task care, she will learn that they are simply a means to achieve whole-task care. Rather, when students graduate, they discover that they are lacking so many skills that the learning of them becomes an end in itself.

Research[44,45] has confirmed the observation that individuals need a sense of competence and that they need to try to become more effective in their human interactions. Interpersonal theories must be taught and practiced so that they can become an integral part of each student's theory of practice. The practice of these theories must include the opportunity to test them out, not in ideal, hand-picked situations where everyone is set to cooperate with the student, but in real, imperfect situations. Faculty may also wish to consider having the unit personnel make out the assignments for students during the clinical rotation in which students are focusing on the testing of management and interpersonal skills. In this way the student will get a much more realistic view of the work situation, feel more a part of the staff, and will have real opportunities to test interpersonal competency skills on less than cooperative staff. Testing means being allowed to fail and to pick up the pieces after one has failed. Hand-picked situations do not permit this freedom to fail.

Nursing service needs to recognize that the further testing and mastery of interpersonal skills will have to become an integral part of inservice staff development. Theories for management and conflict resolution strategies can be taught in schools of nursing, but actual practice to the point of mastery will be difficult because of the short, spaced, and interrupted periods of time the student spends on the unit, and because of the mutual noninvolvement and noncommitment between student and unit staff. Involvement will not occur until an interdependency is created between the staff and the student nurse—a condition not likely to occur.

An essential component of developing interpersonal competence that must be learned by students and practitioners alike is empathy. Cognitive methods alone, such as lectures and reading, have little effect on helping one to achieve ability in social skills such as empathy[46]. Probably the most effective way of practicing empathic skills is through role-playing with feedback. Immediate playback of a videotape recording is one of the most effective methods of feedback[47]. It is highly doubtful whether one can train oneself in empathy. There is strong evidence to indicate that groups and social interactions are necessary to learn this skill[48]. It is hoped that before long empathy training programs will be set up in preservice and inservice programs alike.

### Preservice or Inservice Education

Increasingly, nurse-employing organizations have been accepting responsibility to be sort of a middle training ground where entering new graduates can acquire on-the-job classroom training to supplement voids in their occupational preparation. But how long can we expect this to go on? Can nurse-employing organizations afford to continue or to augment this practice? Conover indicates that business organizations are becoming increasingly reluctant to do this[49]. As the supply catches up with the demand in nursing, nurse-employing organizations will probably also be unwilling to do this. Where then will this leave the new graduate?

There are really two sides to this issue. Educators must understand that by abdicating their responsibility for fully preparing students to be nurses, they are losing a magnificent opportunity to mold the profession and to affect its ongoing development. By graduating what one of the new graduates called a "half-baked" product and leaving the rest of the baking up to the service organization, educators are not only shirking their responsibility, but also are limiting their potential influence. It's like leaving half of the socialization process to chance.

The other side of the issue is the extent to which nursing service should become enmeshed in the educational process—the cost of which must ultimately be passed along to the patient. It is understandable that nursing service wants a competent, effective professional worker. The question that must be asked is whether such workers can be produced by establishing lengthy educational programs, or by rotating new employees to and through various units and services, a practice used in internship programs. It is our suggestion that the most effective type of unit orientation is to place the new graduate on the unit where she will be working—preferably, if at all possible, a unit of her choice. Then orient her immediately on the shift and to the place where she will be working. Rotating her around to various shifts and services will give her a broad understanding of what's going on, but it will do nothing for her competence. As one new graduate explained it:

> We had a guy who was real bad off and we were expecting him to go at any minute. I was working back in the unit and the girl I was working with had to get off to lunch, so I went out and asked the clinician if she could send

someone to relieve the girl because, with that guy, I really needed someone back there with me. And she said, "Well, you know, we have a meeting at eleven," and she added, "You don't feel comfortable back in the unit by yourself? You wanted to get there and now you don't feel comfortable?" And I said, "Well, I'm sorry, but no, I wouldn't feel comfortable." And she answers, "That's why our orientation out here on the floor is so long. So you'll feel comfortable back in the unit when you go back there." I just can't make her understand. What good is that going to do? You know? You have to get experience, and you have to have some time to orient in the place where *you're going to be.* I'm still not going to know anything until I get into the situation, the particular situation.   (1:3B:3)

For the most part, the newcomers have had enough of the general; they need the particulars in order to function competently and effectively.

Another factor that will help the newcomer in developing competence in the work situation is to hold the number of extraneous variables to a minimum. Keep new situations tough and challenging, but simple. In working with neophytes, help them to sort out the relevant from the irrelevant. Ask them questions like, "What are all the things you are considering in making that decision?" If the newcomer mentions interesting but irrelevant information, tell her so quite clearly. The newcomer must learn to differentiate between the "need to know" kind of information and the "nice to know."

### Appropriate Goals

The last, but not by any means the least important, area in which the new graduate might be helped or might help herself to improve her competency is in the choice of goals. Self-set goals must be realistic of attainment. Newcomers would be wise to set overall long-term goals; for each long-term goal, they need to establish small stepping stones. There is a movement under way in nursing services to help the newcomer to set goals for her practice. This is important and should be continued as there is a tendency for most new graduates not to set specific goals in terms of practice. Accomplishment and progress toward meeting specific goals is much easier to assess than is progress toward grandiose goals. By meeting these short-term goals, the individual's self-perceived competency and correspondingly her self-esteem and self-confidence will be enhanced. Future goals can be set higher. With higher goals, higher performance is likely to result.

Service organizations can be extremely helpful to new graduates by providing the ample feedback that is so necessary to the building of competence in performance. The "No news is good news" method of reinforcement or reassurance is not very helpful to the newcomer.

Whoever is responsible for setting goals for the newcomer would do well to remember that goals should be high enough to be stimulating and challenging, but not so high as to be overwhelming. There is often a tendency to reset goals too low when a neophyte fails on the first time around. Doing so is devastating to any newcomer, because not only do such low goals no longer motivate and challenge, but most importantly, they clearly communicate the message that the goal-setter no longer perceives that person as being competent. It is well to remember a firm and all encompassing principle: "No matter what is being learned substantively, it should be learned in such a way that it is accomplished by feelings of psychological success and confidence in self and others, and in the group"[50].

Confidence in others is at times destroyed by their imposition of unfair or dangerous tasks such as the tests some graduates described which potentially were harmful to the patients. Service organizations need to exert some control in the testing process so that criteria for evaluating newcomers are more clearly defined and known dangerous tests discouraged through negative sanctions.

## SUMMARY

This section of this chapter began with a presentation of the patterning and occurrence of the second ranked concern of new graduates: competency. First, competency was placed into perspective in terms of nursing, and then it was looked at in professional education as a whole. The question of how competent new graduate nurses were for professional practice was raised, and some of the ways in which competency can be increased were presented. The section ended with suggestions for improving competency acquisition, the last of which is here now presented.

### A Word of Caution

It is well to remember Galsworthy's challenge: "Idealism increases in direct proportion to one's distance from the problem." With graduation, the idealistic new graduate nurse gets very close to the problem. There is a tendency for her to give up her ideals in favor of speed, efficiency, and competent performance. This does not have to be. One does not need to give up one's ideals, but to make it possible to attain them. This can be done by developing an effective theory of practice which theory includes both technical and interpersonal theories. Mastery of a small number of skills will build not only technical competence but, most importantly, one's self-esteem and self-confidence. Develop empathy so that you can develop interpersonal competence and can be effective in working through and with others. Set high but realistic and challenging goals for yourself. In this way, your idealism will not be lost as you tackle the problem of competence.

## RESPONSIBILITY

In filling a registered nurse position, a new graduate takes on certain duties of that position. Although these duties will differ somewhat according to place, every organization has some required duties which go with the position of registered nurse. According to Webster, duty means having the responsibility for certain assigned tasks and functions. Responsibility means being trustworthy and accountable in the performance of assigned tasks and functions. The responsibility subject area of the new graduate seminars dealt with the trustworthiness and accountability aspects of duties. The discussion here will commence with a presentation of the patterning and occurrence of the subject area in the seminars, and then will focus heavily on some theoretical notions regarding the components and aspects of responsibility. Excerpts from the new graduate seminars will be used liberally to illustrate different points in the theory. The section will conclude with ideas and suggestions as to how the responsibility components might be dealt with.

Responsibility was discussed in seminars in all medical centers, ranking seventh in terms of frequency of occurrence. It was definitely of more concern to the new graduates earlier in their employment than later. Over half (55 percent) of the 112 discussions of responsibility occurred during the early seminar sessions, 30 percent in the middle seminars, with only 15 percent during the late seminars.

The topic ranged in rank at the various medical centers from second to eleventh, with most clustering in the sixth to eleventh ranks. Two medical centers, A and D, stood apart from the others with their high ranking of the theme at 2 and 2.5. Medical center A had the longest on-the-unit orientation of all the medical centers, which probably accounts for the high concentration of concern with lack of responsibility felt by the new graduates there. Medical center D was the only center in the study with a decentralized administration. There, new graduates experienced more uncertainty and sensed greater responsibility than did new graduates in the other medical centers. The fact that the organizational structure places more responsibility and accountability at the unit level most likely accounts for this difference.

The responsibility subject area contained two overall categories of themes. The categories and the themes within each category are as follows:

Amount of responsibility

I've got too much responsibility.

I'v got too little responsibility.

Responsibility and uncertainty

The nature of the field and job create uncertainty.

I don't have enough experience.

The change in supervision puts a lot of pressure on me.

I'm responsible for the care others give too.

The amount of responsibility category accounted for 55 percent of the themes while responsibility and uncertainty made up the remaining 45 percent of themes in the subject area.

## Theoretical Considerations

In the performance of one's work, there are prescribed and discretionary activities. Prescribed activities are assigned tasks, particular routines, and policy-guided actions. Some prescribed activities have to do with what slip to fill out to get a certain lab test or x-ray done; what time of the day certain activities such as reordering of supplies or filling out 24-hour reports for the supervisor must be done; what to do when a patient returns from surgery. Some prescribed activities call for the use of discretion and others do not. For example, no discretion may be applied to decide what slip to use to order a test. If the proper slip is not used, no test. However, whether the prescribed treatment of a postoperative patient has been carried out long enough can be and is determined by the nurse.

For the new graduate, one of the difficulties is that some prescribed activities are discretionary for her, although not for oldtimers. For example, the new graduate has to think about and decide which of myriad slips to fill out for a certain test, or what the routine is.

Although some are prescribed, a large portion of the tasks of a nurse are discretionary. In the exercise of discretion, "The person doing the job must exercise his own control and judgment from within himself. He himself must decide, choose, judge . . . conclude just what would be the best thing to do in the circumstance, the best way to go about doing what he is doing"[51]. What to do with any given patient at any point in time for the eight hours that a nurse is on duty calls for many decisions and judgments. The evaluation and assessment of patients requires discretionary activity. Is this postoperative patient stable? Are the patient's symptoms indicative of a drug reaction? Which staff member is appropriate to care for *this* patient? A pair of excerpts from the seminars illustrate some of the decisions and judgments new graduates feel need to be made:

> You feel responsible for evaluating the patient, his progress, and letting the doctor know what is going on and trying to communicate about what's happening to the patient.   (2:1A:4)

> I function as a team leader, but I don't feel like I'm looking enough. I made sure everything is done, but is the patient doing all right? Are there any

changes that the doctor should be notified of? You know, it's hard to sit down and look at all these laboratory things that—does the doctor know about it? Does he need to be notified? Is something abnormally wrong that I should give a report?    (2:2A:19)

The need to decide, to judge, to exercise discretion is seen and felt by the new graduate in the performance of her role functions.

While the new graduate was still a student, the need to decide, to exercise discretion was not fully felt. When one is a nursing student, time is spent prior to clinical experience reading and preparing to care for one or two particular patients so that the decisions are often made ahead of time and merely acted upon the next day. In addition, the student can at all times call upon the instructor to assist with the decision, thus obviating the need for the student to make the judgment. Not only is the instructor present, but the staff are also available. Many times the student needs only to report to the staff what is happening and the decision or judgment as to what is required is made by the staff nurses. Some areas of decision making—which patient to see first, or setting priorities when all patients' needs cannot be met because of lack of time—the student never deals with at all. Although the student may feel as though she can attempt to decide what to do, the pressure to do it alone and in a wide range of areas is not present.

### Amount of Responsibility

What effect does the need to exercise discretion in a job or role have upon the new graduate? "We appear to derive our sensation of level of work or responsibility from the discretion we are called upon to exercise . . ."[52]. Thus the more one is called upon to use discretion, the greater is the amount of responsibility felt; the less one needs to use one's discretion, the smaller is the amount of responsibility felt.

*I've got too much responsibility.*

It's been six weeks and I'm working on a surgical floor. And I'm definitely feeling a lot better about myself. The first thing that overwhelmed me was the responsibility. Especially working nights. There would be two nurses alternating between wards and I thought "You've got to be kidding!" But, you know, I've learned—hopefully I've learned how to pick priorities.    (4:1:4)

I think [one of the biggest adjustments] is the responsibility of, you know, someone's life in your hands, so to speak. Needing to know how, what to do and having it help.    (8:4:3)

The common threads through the new graduates' discussions of the amount of responsibility were their sense of being overwhelmed at first and the need to choose priorities. The impression given is that there is a lot of responsibility that goes with making the decisions and judgments that need to be made. So the more the deciding, judging, and choosing required, the more the responsibility felt. Moreover, since some of the routine, prescribed activities have not yet become routine for the new graduate, they require decision making, thereby increasing the sense of responsibility further.

*I've got too little responsibility.*    Comments about too limited responsibility were made but were less overt than those about too great responsibility.

> I think on our unit, the full implication of being a nurse hasn't hit us yet because we've done nothing yet. None of us have. None of us have done team leading yet. You know, we're still like students working overtime.   (3:1C:11)

> I don't mind doing patient care, but I'd like to team lead once in a while. And I'd like to be treated like an RN or even a GN instead of an aide. You've got five patients, and you've got an aide to help you and the two of you do it. But you don't pass your own meds and you don't do your IV's. What do you do? You're making beds and giving baths and seeing that they get to therapy and all that stuff.   (7:2B:10)

> I'm the third RN on my shift. We have one LPN, three RN's, and sometimes an aide on there. So actually most of the time, I feel like a highly paid nursing assistant because the people that team lead do all the RN activities. Let's say they give me six of the hardest patients who are complicated with dressings or whatever. But then they go ahead and do all the IV stuff and all the dressing changes. So actually, you're only putting people on bedpans and taking the vital signs!   (2:3A:16)

The total lack of any mention of responsibility or decision making is strikingly different from the previous examples. The sense of the examples is that the activities engaged in require very little, if any judgment. There may be considerable disagreement among nurses as to how prescribed these activities really are, and if they should be prescribed, but from the perspective of these new graduates, the tasks are prescribed. They do not require the exercise of discretion. In the absence of the use of discretion, a smaller amount of responsibility is felt.

The perception that causes the feeling of no responsibility or insufficient responsibility is important in understanding the emotional reaction to that feeling. When one believes that it is possible to fulfill one's wish or desire (for example, to accept more responsibility) but that someone is preventing it, frustration results[53]. A number of the new graduates indicated that they perceived that others were preventing them from assuming responsibility.

> I haven't been given the opportunity to use my resources, my education. I don't have a lot of responsibility. I can't think of anything that I have done to make them think I can't take responsibility.   (1:4B:5)

I think you've hit on another key word—stereotype. Here we are, all new graduates. They all think we're a bunch of clods and fools who don't know a damn thing. And they have to watch you.   (9:1B:29)

New graduates' perception that they are not being given responsibility, for what reason, creates a sensation of frustration. This frustration is much more apparent in the second excerpt than in the first. The source of that frustration is important because what one is able to do is influenced by what one thinks[54]. If a new graduate such as the one in the first excerpt picks up cues from head nurse or others that she cannot handle responsibility or must be watched at all times, later on she may not take responsibility when the opportunity is given. What one "can do" is often influenced by what one thinks she can do, which in turn is affected by the opinion, suggestions, and stereotypes of others[55].

### Responsibility and Uncertainty

A second important factor in one's perception of the amount of responsibility in one's job is uncertainty—making decisions and carrying out actions without really knowing how good or bad the decision was until sometime later or perhaps never[56]. The longer one has to tolerate uncertainty and yet continue with the work, the greater is the sense or feeling of responsibility[57].

You've got to learn to make a lot of decisions on your own and that can be a real heavy trip for a lot of people. All of a sudden to be thrown out and not have anybody that you can run to and say, "Is this right? Is this right? Is this right?" Decision making is a big thing that is involved.   (9:3B:4)

Supervision of the individual nurse therapists has been taken away because of the financial crunch. So here I am, running my own groups without any supervision besides what I can sneak from talking with the head nurse. I really feel like I was given so much responsibility—running my own groups . . . Even though I had some training, that's different. Besides, actually doing it, I felt like I needed ongoing support and more feedback every time I'd come out of group. What did I do wrong? How could I get that silent person to talk?   (9:2C:15)

The uncertainty—about which action to take about the rightness or wrongness of action taken—makes the responsibility seem like a heavy burden.

Uncertainty can have even more dramatic consequences than those expressed in the foregoing excerpts. "When the individual believes that his cause/effect resources are inadequate to the uncertainty, he will seek to evade discretion"[58]. When one believes that for whatever reason one cannot control or overcome the uncertainty, one will seek *not* to make decisions or judgments.

The more things I find that the team leader has to do, the longer I can wait.   (2:3A:30)

The blood was done—all these things. You think, "OK now, when you have all those other responsibilities, and the phone ringing, and everybody piling on top of you at the desk and asking questions, you know, "I don't want to be charge nurse! Just give me ten beds to make and I'll make them." (6:5A:30)

I felt in such chaos because it was the first time I was in charge without the head nurse being there . . . No serious problems came up but just a couple of crazy things. Like, we had two people with CVP lines and the lines just stopped. We were afraid they were clogging and so we were taking them apart and constantly fixing them. And then one of our graft patient's blood pressure flew up and we thought for sure he was going to blow his grafts. It was just absolutely crazy and I'm thinking "My God, why do they do this? I don't want to handle all this responsibility by myself." (3:5C:11)

In these examples, we see three possible responses to uncertainty by the new graduate:

1. Avoid the taking of responsibility as long as possible.

2. Get away from responsibility.

3. Attempt to find some way to have less responsibility by not having the responsibility alone.

Although they represent varying degrees of avoidance, all three responses are attempts to avoid full responsibility.

Since uncertainty seems to have a rather substantial effect upon the amount of responsibility felt and accepted, perhaps it would be of value to examine the factors which create or contribute to the uncertainty felt by the new graduate. There are primarily four such factors: 1) the nature of the field and the job, 2) lack of experience, 3) change in type of supervision, and 4) dependence on others to do some of the work.

*The nature of the field and job.*    The first factor affecting uncertainty is the nature of the field or the work itself. Within the field of nursing, different ideas as to how to handle nursing care exist. For example:

There is a question of whether if the kid hasn't cried at all but is fairly pink to leave him or stimulate him. One shift said to stimulate him because you have to make him cry, and the other shift says if he's pink, he's breathing, just leave him. And I've noticed that between nurses, some will just leave the kid and just let him pink up gradually and others will stimulate and others will put him on oxygen. That was one of those things where I had to decide what worked best for me and that the consensus could be wrong. I tried to decide what I felt was best. (2:2B:2)

Different ideas and thoughts exist. It is hard to say that one is right and one is wrong or that one choice is better than another in any given situation. The differences in ideas and practice are there and they create uncertainty for the new graduate.

The other aspect of this first factor is the uncertainty of the job. As one of the new graduates indicated, "crazy things" happen. Patients' CVP lines stop up and a skin graft patient's blood pressure "flies up." The best that any nurse can do is to be aware that anything can happen with a CVP line. And the question still remains, will it happen to this one today? Some patients have a rise in blood pressure after surgery; some have a drop; some have neither. So which will it be, and will it happen with the patients who had surgery today? Such unpredictable events contribute to the uncertainty felt by the new graduate.

Compounding the problem of uncertainty is the fact that the practice of nursing is presented to many students as if it is a certainty—as if there are prescribed ways of handling nursing care. Take for example, the following excerpts from a text used in teaching nursing: "The necessity for maintainence of high serum antibiotic levels makes it imperative that medication be administered at the exact time intervals prescribed"[59]. "[If there is] any alteration in rate or rhythm, including a significant decrease in the heart rate (to less than 60/min) . . . the drug should be withheld and the physician notified immediately"[60]. In addition to the message that students read in their texts, faculty tend to give students the impression that there are "right ways" to carry out nursing practice. A student described this situation:

> My clinical instructor tells me to do a procedure one way; my team leader tells me to do it another way; the doctor wants it done his way; and my own instincts tell me my way works best. So, I start a simple task, like a dressing change, and I am almost paralyzed with conflict. In the end, I do it my way and take the risk. Later in the day, the team leader readjusts it. (She doesn't change it to her way, but doesn't leave it my way either.) And after clinical, my instructor tracks me down for an explanation . . . I give her my rationale for my method and add that it was altered by the team leader. My instructor gives me her rationale again and makes some comment concerning the team leader—something like one can suggest change but can't force it . . .

The incident described leaves the student with the impression that there is certainly *a* right way in which the task of a dressing change must be handled. Although the student cannot help but be aware of differences in thought and practice as a result of the situation, the message interpreted by the student is that these differences result from poor practice on the part of some nurses, and not because of a legitimate difference in ideas inherent in the nature of the field. Thus when the new graduate encounters differences, they create problems for her because she was not previously prepared for them and did not expect them.

*I don't have the experience.* Another factor contributing to the uncertainty felt by the new graduate is her lack of experience with uncertainty and responsibility. As two of the new graduates so aptly expressed,

At first, when I had the authority and I was the one that was called upon to make judgments, it kind of shocked me. A few weeks before, I was running to everyone else. And I think that's been really hard, but a change to realize that.   (8:2:2)

There was one nurse and me. She was saying that she was scared to death. It's the fact that I'm new and inexperienced. She says, "Oh, the responsibility is just overwhelming me." Well, that's how a new graduate nurse feels when she comes on and she's faced with a situation that isn't really frightening but to her it is because she doesn't really know what she's doing yet.   (6:4A:14)

Thus some new graduates find themselves in a role of authority, called upon to make judgments, when just a short time ago they were running to others to get help in making such judgments. Others find that they are faced with situations they really do not know how to handle yet. The kinds of decision, judgment, and uncertainty that arise when one is on a unit as a student are quite different from those that come up when one is working eight hours a day, forty hours a week. As a result of limited time on the units, recent graduates lack experience in predicting what will happen to patients and what to do if and when things do happen. Students write care plans hypothetically predicting a patient's course and appropriate nursing action, and yet seldom do they have the opportunity to validate the plans. The validation may be missing as a result of lack of experience with patients having the problem being considered, or such short exposure to the patients that the chance to see progression is absent. When the unpredicted events occur, the new graduate is left with the sense of tremendous responsibility because she doesn't have previous knowledge to draw upon and doesn't know exactly what to do. Perhaps another part of the explanation of these differences between being a student and being a registered nurse is given by the new graduate who said,

I felt, even though I was very pleased with my education, both the clinical and the academic part, I always felt that you're always protected. You have that protective coating where you never have the full responsibility—the instructor's always there. You're never really totally responsible. A lot of the patients know that you are a student and you're not looked upon the same way as if you were a registered nurse. I felt like I never really had the chance to find out what my capacity was until now when I'm working.   (3:2A:15)

"You never have the full responsibility." The protective coating prevents the new graduate from feeling the full weight of the responsibility and uncertainties of the registered nurse role. This lack of experience with uncertainty as a student makes it difficult for the new graduate to deal with uncertainty and with the corresponding feeling of full responsibility.

*Change in supervision puts a lot of pressure on me.*    The ever-present instructor is the basis for the third factor affecting uncertainty—a change in the type of supervision for the new graduate. As a nursing student, one can always count on an instructor to be no more than a phone call away. In the early parts of clinical work, the instructor is usually physically present on the unit. In later portions of training, the instructor may not be on the unit, but her presence is felt. When there is any question or need, the student need only pick up the phone. If there is no response from the instructor, the student can always fall back on the real team leader or other staff nurses. Then the student graduates and becomes a staff nurse.

> There is tremendous pressure to think ahead, anticipate problems, and alone—no instructor there.    (7:1B:6)

> My biggest adjustment? Being on the unit and not having an instructor to fall back on.    (6:2B:4)

There is no instructor, no one to fall back on. Who takes her place?

> Yes, there's a lot of difference in not having a protective instructor watching you to make sure that you're not doing anything too wrong. They catch your mistakes before you make them. Now there's nobody!    (1:1B:9)

> I think the hardest thing about nights is getting used to the responsibility that *you are it.* I mean, you know, if something goes wrong there's no head nurse you can ask. There's always the nurse on the other side, but she usually doesn't know too much about your patients.    (1:2C:13)

The replacement for the instructor is no one or someone who "doesn't know too much about your patients." As the new graduates indicate, this is a difficult adjustment and it involves a lot of responsibility. It also increases the duration or time-span of uncertainty.

The time-span of uncertainty is the length of time that one must make decisions and judgments in a role without the results of those decisions coming to the attention of the immediate supervisor[61]. For students there is a very short time-span between action or intended action and attention (or feedback) from the immediate supervisor. The instructor is always there—she even catches mistakes before they are made. For new graduates there is no one to fall back on—no one there to ask for help.

*I'm responsible for the care others give too.*    In the movement from the student nurse role to the staff nurse role, the new graduate comes face to face with another factor which contributes to increased uncertainty—having to depend upon others to do portions of her work. As a student with two or three patients, the student could do everything that needed to be done for those patients by herself. As a staff nurse, there is no way that she can do all of the work for her patients herself. She must depend on others to help with the work.

You're responsible for the care of the patients . . . You just can't do it all. You can't play aide, team leader, and head nurse, and play it all at the same time. I think that I found that there are different areas. The staff on my floor is really beautiful, and we all really work together. But there are some that leave people set up for baths and they come an hour later and the people are still waiting. It's disgusting. I get so upset because I hear of this stuff . . .    (2:1A:5)

In having to depend upon others, the new graduate loses some control over the care the patients are receiving. Will the patient get his bath? How long will he wait? Will all the care that is to be done for the patient get done? Contrast this uncertainty with the words of new graduates who feel that they have as much control as they had in school:

I got to work in the ICU a couple of times and that was kind of neat. I just had one patient. You are responsible for them. They are really dependent on you and you really have got to be on the ball and know what you are doing and do the whole job yourself. I liked that kind of job.   (6:2A:11)

I think a lot of satisfaction comes from primary nursing. The satisfaction of being responsible for the things you do and accountable. And you have fewer people to depend on and fewer people that are responsible to you. It's more like you take on more of it yourself and at the end of the day you're able to say, "I did these things."   (9:2B:18)

Having fewer people to depend on so that you, yourself, are responsible for and do the care of the patient is satisfying. The more the new graduate can do herself, the more control she has, and hence the more satisfying the job. Conversely, the more the new graduate has to depend upon others, the more uncertainty in the job.

Whether they have control over the care activities themselves or must depend upon others for care activities, the new graduates talk about having and feeling responsibility for the care. Where does the responsibility for an action lie? There is support in the literature for the fact that ultimate responsibility remains with the individual who delegates activity[62,63]. The new nurses provided some interesting insights into responsibility and its delegation:

Again I sit here thinking that all of us are in charge-like positions and we're always saying, "OK, we're responsible for this team" and we're not only responsible for all the clients on that team but then we've got all the people and they may be auxiliary staff, student nurses, or whatever. And in the interim, although these people all have licenses or certificates or whatever, we're still responsible for all these people too. If they do something, in the final analysis, whoever gets blamed, it'll be you.   (9:1C:17)

In fact, when I think of that night, you know, she [the head nurse] must have had some things going on that were really bugging her. That didn't help *my* feelings that night. I felt more incompetent than I have ever felt . . . it was my error, and I knew that. And I tried to explain to her we had a hell of a night and it was something that I thought had been done because I had given the responsibility to someone else. They said, "Yes, I'll do it" and it wasn't done. Well, it was done, but the girl was in such a panic that she couldn't find it. It was *there* and it *had* been done. My error was not checking to find out, but it *was* there.   (1:4C:11)

So the responsibility remains with the new graduate for those who work under her. Of course this principle works to her benefit when others delegate responsibility to the new graduate.

No, she didn't make me. She said "I think it would really be a good idea if you could be in charge tonight." And I am not the type to go and say "Hey! Can I be in charge?" But I like to be asked to do stuff. Because if I just go ahead and ask, it's more of a risk, because I asked to do it. Whereas, if I'm assigned somehow I feel like I won't be blamed as much if I do something wrong if I was asked to do it. If I went ahead and volunteered, then I should have known what I was getting into.   (6:5A:16)

"Somehow, if I'm assigned or asked, I won't be blamed as much." Although this was a rare statement, it does indicate that the new graduate is aware that just as she retains responsibility for those activities she assigns to others, others retain responsibility for activities assigned to her. Whenever an individual assigns or commands another to perform some activity, the ultimate responsibility remains with the individual doing the commanding or assigning.

### Relief for the New Graduate

The new graduate does feel a strong sense of a lot of responsibility that must be dealt with in her new position. With some insight into what might be behind this sense of responsibility, it is now appropriate to examine what might be done about this concern. As with most problems there is no one simple solution. The major objective must be to help the new graduate move into a position of responsibility as quickly as she is capable of doing so. Looking at factors such as discretionary activities, prescribed activities, and uncertainty can help to decrease the feeling of responsibility for the new graduate as well as assist her to assume her new responsibilities more easily.

The first task in dealing constructively with responsibility is to determine the amount of discretionary activity involved in the job. Does the job require many decisions and judgments to be made? Or is the job composed mostly of prescribed and routine activities? In jobs which are a mixture of discretionary and prescribed actions, which tasks require judgments and decisions and which do not? Making this determination between discretionary and prescribed activities allows one to determine how complex the job will be. The more discretionary the activity, the more complex the job and the more skill will be required. The more prescribed the tasks, the simpler the job and the less skill required. The more complex the job, the longer will be the time required to prepare an individual to do the job. Not only does this determination tell us how long it will take to prepare an individual to do the job, but it also tells us the kind of help an individual must be given in order to perform the task.

The two different types of activities, discretionary and prescribed, require different types of intellectual activity and thus different kinds of preparation. Discretionary activities require observation, analysis, and interpretation, whereas most prescribed activities require attention to detail and concentration on the task. Take, for example, the task of giving medications. The discretionary aspect of this task involves the determination of the response of the patient to the drug. Is the patient having therapeutic or adverse reactions to the drug? Depending upon the patient's response to the drug, what action should the nurse take? For a new graduate to perform this aspect of the task properly she needs to know what to look for, how to interpret her observations, and what to do based on her interpretation of the data. The prescribed aspect of the task involves using the "right steps" of giving medications: check the med card with the order, check the drug with the card, check the patient with the card, hand the patient the correct drug, and record the drug in the proper place. The procedural steps do not require judgment, only attention to detail, to the task at hand. The different aspects of the job require different assistance in preparing the individual to do the job. Perhaps the worst disservice we do both to students and to new graduates is to mix the two aspects of a task. While expecting the nurse to pour medications, the helper is questioning her to determine if she has at her fingertips the necessary information to make the observation and interpretation as to the effect of the drug. This distracts the nurse and interrupts the concentration and attention needed to perform the task. We would do better to teach students and nurses how to deal with breaks in concentration for those tasks which require it so that both the discretionary and prescribed aspects of the task can be done correctly and safely. Distinguishing discretionary and prescribed aspects of tasks and separating them from the overall job can help those who are charged with orienting new graduates or teaching students to provide the right kind of assistance.

Another reason for determining and separating the kinds of activity involved in a task is to reduce the amount of discretionary activity required by any newcomer in an organization. Whenever a newcomer enters a new institution, prescribed activities for a time require the newcomer to make decisions. For example, what slip should be used to get an x-ray or where does one go for a certain supply or how does one get maintenance to replace a light bulb? Obviously the energy required to completely eliminate this problem by having *all* organizations use the same procedures and forms is not worth the result. However, the additional sense of responsibility placed on a newcomer who must exercise discretion in the performance of these activities is counterproductive. Introducing the individual to a plethora of policies and procedures during an initial two-week orientation program when the individual is not using the procedures and is inundated with a wealth of information is the type of practice which contributes to a sense of unproductive responsibility. Something needs to be done at the unit level to help the newcomer quickly convert these seemingly discretionary activities into prescribed ones. Whether this is done by storing slips in such a way that they clearly say what they are used for, or by instituting a quick card reference which indicates the procedure for changing light bulbs, doesn't matter. The point is that organizations must, in some practical way, standardize and routinize those prescribed activities that use up unnecessary energy, so that energy utilized in making decisions where no decision is called for can be channeled into more productive avenues. In the long run, this will benefit not only the newcomer but the patient and organization as well, since the newcomer will feel more in control of the situation and thus more able to handle the responsibilities of the job.

Perhaps one of the major reasons that responsibility weighs heavily for the new graduate is her limited or untested ability to make judgments and decisions. If the new graduate is unsure of her decisions and judgments or doesn't know exactly how to make them, the heaviness of the responsibility in the job will remain despite efforts to reduce it. Thus, one of the tasks confronting educators and service people alike is the development of the decision-making ability of the nurse.

At the preservice educational level, students are taught how to make plans of care for patients based on assessment. This, in essence, is teaching students to decide how to proceed based upon sound rational judgments and deliberative thought processes. Many new graduates come to work well prepared to make decisions as to the best plan of care to enact for a particular patient if they are given sufficient time (at least 12 hours), energy, and resources to develop such a plan.

When entering the service settings as new graduates, nurses are not only required to decide what care to give each patient, but what to do when they can't possibly do everything for every one of 20 patients, what to do in situations they never encountered as students, and what to do without sufficient time to marshal all of their resources. Interestingly enough, we have developed inventories to determine what a new graduate knows about medications and their administration, and inventories to check out the new graduates' repertoire of manual-technical skills and their levels of mastery, but we have no way of knowing or determining their ability to make clinical decisions and judgments under varying circumstances. Perhaps it would be useful to determine an entering employee's decision-making ability as well as her technical skill. Whether decision making is assessed or not, it is necessary to devote more time and attention to the development of this ability, since so much of the work of nursing is based upon the nurse's ability to observe, analyze, and interpret what she sees so that the appropriate line of action can be taken. How can the ability of a nurse to decide and act be determined and then increased if need be?

One strategy that has been used in nursing to help individuals take on a role is that of role modeling by way of the buddy system. The reasoning behind this strategy is that if a new graduate is paired with an experienced registered nurse, she will learn the duties and functions of the role by observing the experienced nurse. This strategy usually works well in helping the newcomer learn what to do and when to do it, but it actually does little to assist the person in making decisions. A strategy of role modeling linked with participant observation offers much greater potential in accomplishing the learning both of role functions and of the process of decision making.

Participant observation is a research strategy associated with field research. The fieldworker makes observations of behavior in its natural settings rather than in artificially established settings. The methodology involves not only observing and recording what people do and say, but, equally important, discovering who the people in a situation are, how they fit into the ongoing action and setting, and what meanings the observed persons themselves give to their behavior. It is the latter aspect of participant observation that is so crucial in the combined participant observation/role modeling strategy that is being proposed here. We are not proposing that new graduates come onto a clinical unit and do research on the other staff nurses. Rather, what we are proposing is that some opportunity be provided for the newcomer to observe another staff nurse, specifically selected because she exhibited the ability to make sound judgments and decisions. The new graduate would be paired with the model for a stipulated period of time. She would not *work with* the model, but rather would observe the model in the performance of her clinical tasks, and as is typical with the participant observation method, would query and abstract from the model her rationale for actions, meanings to her behavior, and the logic of her decision-making processes. For example, a new graduate might observe that the nurse model makes rounds to only some of her patients and then immediately goes and pours her morning medications before seeing the rest of the patients. The new graduate formulates questions to ask of the nurse whom she is observing. She may notice that all the patients that the nurse saw first are going to surgery that day and may conclude this is probably the motivation for seeing these patients first; she will want to verify this with the nurse model. But since medications are not due until nine o'clock, why not see all the patients before pouring the meds? Why does this nurse order her day this way? In another instance, the new graduate may notice that the nurse goes into a room to check an IV and for some reason goes instead to the other patient in the room, then leaves the room to get a blood pressure cuff, returns to check that patient's vitals, goes to the patient's chart, and then telephones the physician. As soon as the nurse concludes these activities, the new graduate might well ask, "What did you see that caused you to do those things in that order?" Further benefit can be gained from this strategy by using more than one nurse as a role model. In this way, the new graduate sees that nurses may make the same observation and arrive at slightly different interpretations or even the same interpretation and take different actions. It is vitally important that the new graduate achieve this learning. Everyone must understand that it is the process that the new graduate is concerned with learning and not the specific actions of the nurse. By learning from the model how the nurse hooked the pieces together to arrive at her decision and how the nurse chose what to do, it is hoped, the new graduate will be helped to apply all of her knowledge and information to make her own decisions and will not merely imitate the decisions of others. Through the use of this strategy, the new graduate sees the duties and functions of the nurse in practice and comes to understand the process by which the nurse makes decisions which guide action.

Several factors are needed in using a combined role model/participant-observation strategy. First, it is imperative that role models for the new graduates be carefully selected so that the new graduates learn sound decision making. Second, the role models need to understand the process and the strategy, so that questions raised are accepted as a means to help the new graduates' understanding and not as a challenge to the way the nurse performs her duties. Third, both the new graduate and the role model require preparation for the observer role so that observation, formulation of questions, and asking questions will be productive. Many students are now learning participant observation methodology as part of their preservice research courses. Nurses can be taught this methodology through inservice programs. Although the initial setting up of this strategy may require some time and effort, once a system is operational, the investment pays off handsomely.

The participant observation strategy can be used not only for teaching new graduates the process of decision making, but also as a means of determining what kinds of decisions and judgments the new graduate makes and possibly where she is having difficulty in making decisions or in making appropriate decisions. By reversing roles after the time period allotted for the new graduate to observe, and placing the newcomer in the position of the observee, participant observations can be performed on the new graduate. Although at first the reversed observation may seem a bit threatening, if conducted in a gentle manner and with every-one understanding the purpose and process, it can be both productive and well received.

These strategies enable the new graduate to take on responsibility without feeling overwhelmed by it. Learning how to make decisions and judgments necessary for action reduces the new graduate's uncertainty and hence her anxiety and frustration. Other means of reducing that uncertainty are discussed in the remainder of this section.

Students have a tendency to place blame on the faculty for the predica-ment they find themselves in as new graduates, claiming "I wasn't ade-quately prepared." In some instances this statement may be true. Stu-dents generally are not prepared well for the uncertainties of the field. Students rarely see patients for any length of time and thus are unaware of some of the events likely simply because they never see them. Some of this problem is being alleviated by the use of long-term clinical assign-ments while the student progresses through school. Thus the student begins to see some uncertainty through her clinical experience. Because of the nature of the educational experience it is often difficult to obtain for students the experience of seeing the uncertainties without eight-hour-a-day five-day weeks. But situations do occur in the clinical areas which could be used as potential jumping-off points for a discussion of differences in practice which are uncertainties of the field. The student who described the incident quoted earlier about the dressing change had an excellent opportunity to examine a common uncertainty. What about sterile versus unsterile dressing changes for some wounds? Go one step further, what about sterile suctioning versus nonsterile suctioning? Seminar discussions exploring areas of nursing where legitimate differ-ences exist in schools of thought will enable the new graduate: 1) to meet uncertainty, 2) to make reasonable decisions as to what actions to take, and 3) to determine when poor practice is really in operation.

Many times, the new graduates attribute unpredicted happenings to the failings of the nursing staff. A student described this situation:

> This little old lady had surgery a few days ago. Today when she got up walking, she threw a pulmonary embolism and died. And that shouldn't have happened. I mean if patients get the right activity post-op they don't throw emboli.

Whether the staff did or did not provide adequate care is not the question here. The point is that although the student had no data whether the care was given or not, her conclusion was that it couldn't have been because, if it had, the embolism would not have occurred. The fact is that there are times when everything that a nurse knows to do is done and a patient still gets an embolism. Students need to examine the real possibilities of unpredictable and uncontrollable events. They should be provided with experiences with patients who have had an unpredictable course of treatment and response, or with case history study. Not all that they see is poor practice. Students need to develop a basis for distinguishing between the uncertainties of practice and improper practice.

Another way students can be helped to deal with uncertainty is to encourage consultation with other nurses. Students are taught to ask questions when they do not know what to do or to conduct care conferences to draw up a plan of care for the patient, yet seldom are they encouraged to seek real consultation from peers. Before consulting with peers one should make an assessment, interpret the meaning of the assessment, and hypothesize a line of action. Sometimes nurses are unsure if the proper interpretation has been drawn and if the course of action will be appropriate. Nursing has not formalized the idea of consulting with peers: presenting the assessment, interpretation, and proposed action and seeking the advice and input of other nurses—even to the point of asking another nurse to see the patient and then concurring or disagreeing. Formalizing a consultation process with peers imparts the message that uncertainty in nursing exists; input from others may decrease the uncertainty involved in deciding upon a course of action.

A second area of uncertainty which creates difficulty for the new graduate is lack of experience. New graduates lack experience not only with mastery of basic manual skills but with the total scope of being a working registered nurse. As indicated earlier, lack of skills confounds the picture for the new graduate, as she doesn't know what is a result of her own lack of skill and what is an inherent part of the uncertainty of the field. Because manual-technical skills have not been practiced to the point of mastery, wherein they require little thinking and less concentration on detail, these skills require the new graduate to think and make decisions about how to perform routine procedures. This is an unproductive use of energy. Enough decisions are necessary without making performance of skills matters of decision and thus contributing to the burden of responsibility felt. New graduates need to come to work with a basic number of skills mastered in order to decrease this burden.

An obstacle preventing students from learning the total scope of their upcoming role is the lack of a "total immersion" experience. In the past diploma programs and the early BS programs, the students worked all shifts and full shifts, often carrying the very same functions as the graduate nurses carried. The total immersion experience allowed the students to see the uncertainty present in the field of nursing and forced them to deal with the uncertainties they would have to face when showing up on a unit not knowing who the patients would be and without extensive preparation to care for the patients. Now the total immersion experience occurs after graduation. The new graduate must cope when she has no idea who her patients are. The patients are not always classic examples of the disease process they have, and often the newcomer is required to perform aspects of the job which she has heard about but has never done. Completely restoring the total immersion experience to the nursing school curriculum seems unreasonable, but totally ignoring this exposure to reality seems equally unreasonable. Aspects of total immersion could be captured during a designated segment of a clinical rotation by having students come to the clinical area theoretically prepared to care for patients but without having prepared for specific selected patients in advance. This would force students to make on-the-spot plans and decisions and then proceed to care for the patients. Seminar discussions about the experience and ways and means to cope would provide the students with some understanding of what is to come. Students could have some clinical experience on evenings and nights so that they could see what that experience is like. What is the difference between working days and nights? What is it like to try to recycle one's life to work evenings and still meet other daytime obligations? A taste of what is to come can help students prepare so that they are not devastated by the uncertainty they encounter.

Total immersion experiences for new graduates vary widely. In some organizations, new graduates are plunged into reality and thus rendered incapable of dealing with the uncertainties they meet; in others, the new graduate continues to have an experience much like those of school and finds that there is nothing in the job that is different from what she has already learned, so that some of the job becomes boring because of its prescribed and routine nature. New graduates need to be challenged. Individualized orientation programs after a basic orientation can more adequately meet the needs of the organization as well as of the new graduate. A large portion of the experience of reality for new graduates occurs during the intensive orientation usually conducted on the day shift. Frequently new graduates are then moved to the evening or night shift where they receive very brief orientations to the shift routine and then are in charge. Although the new graduate learns to deal with one set of uncertainties during orientation, these are not the same uncertainties she faces in her work on evenings or nights. To decrease the sense of responsibility resulting from these uncertainties, the new graduate must be helped to deal with the uncertainties that are expected in her day-to-day work. This means that if the new graduate is going to spend the major portion of her working time on nights, then the major portion of her orientation and gaining of reality experience should occur on the night shift.

The third aspect of uncertainty which new graduates are faced with is a change in the type of supervision. The student is accustomed to a very short time span of uncertainty in receiving information as to the soundness of her decisions and actions. In the movement to work, she often finds that the time between action and feedback is much longer and, at times, nonexistent. It is necessary to increase the student's ability to tolerate longer time spans of uncertainty. The "protective coating" of the student days needs to be dissolved. In many schools, as the student progresses through the program, the instructor becomes less immediately available. The student may need to telephone rather than just to go down the hall to find her instructor. However, from the words of the new graduates we can see that the mere physical absence of the instructor from the unit is not doing the job of making students take more upon themselves. Whenever students are in a tough spot they merely send up the distress flag. So the change required in the course of a student's progression is not in the proximity of the instructor but in the function of the instructor. The instructor needs to act more as a consultant to the student. The student must make decisions and act. If the student remains uncertain as to the quality of her decision, she should be expected to present her data and then to defend her decision and plan of action. Input from the faculty member should be elicited on a consultative basis. The faculty member is not there to tease the data, decision, and evaluation out of the student.

The foregoing is particularly true of student-staff interactions. If the student's clinical experience is to be a meeting of the real world with her school learnings, then the student must be the one to deal with the situations encountered and must not call in a faculty member as a troubleshooter when the going gets rough. The instructor needs to be certain that the student will not jeopardize the health and safety of the patients, but, especially in matters where the student is having difficulty with the staff, the student, not the instructor, must learn to handle the problem. Mistakes will be made. Students will get themselves into corners and have less than optimal results from attempts to work with others. But they are there to learn and need to learn while help is available and not when they are truly on their own. Indirect help with problems such as with ruptured interpersonal relationships can be as effective or more effective than the faculty member's simply stepping in and taking over for the student.

The protective coating of school is as detrimental to effective role transformation as is a new graduate's perception of a complete absence of any resources in the work setting. Whether it is one's first experience as a registered nurse, or a head nurse, or a supervisor, resources for questions and validation of proposed actions are needed. To tell a new graduate to call the supervisor when the supervisor is always so busy with her own duties that she couldn't possibly help anyone for lack of time is not providing a resource. The new graduate does need more supervision initially than she will later on. She does need honest feedback as to her performance. Usually by the end of orientation, persons available as resources when needed are usually adequate; these persons need to know what kind of assistance to provide for the new graduate. As in the role model strategy, the kind of help most often needed and of greatest usefulness is assistance in making decisions and taking appropriate action. Many times all that is needed is for the supervisor to validate a new graduate's decision regarding a course of action.

The fourth and final aspect of uncertainty for the new graduate is depending upon others to do some portion of the work. Students, as a rule, are taught theory regarding team management and dealing with auxiliary personnel but rarely do they receive a realistic clinical experience in this area. The lack of experience is partially due to the buffering effect of the faculty, partially due to the buffering effect of regular staff, and partially due to the fact that the staff can manage to go along with just about anything as long as they know it isn't permanent and the student really is trying to learn. In reducing the uncertainty that results from lack of exposure to real situations, a much stronger bond between nursing schools and nursing service is required. For the student to have a strong experience in working with others to achieve a job, the instructor must take a consulting rather than troubleshooting role with the students; regular staff must act less as buffering agents and place the duties in the hands of the students; staff need to be encouraged to be more like themselves rather than adapting to the idiosyncracies of the students for three days a week. This may be the hardest type of preparation to offer at the preservice level. One possible way to do it is for faculty and students actually to take over the running of a public health agency or hospital unit for a period of time. Service agencies should help students and new graduates alike to learn what work can be delegated to others and what they themselves must do to ensure that the work gets done properly. They need to know what to do when others perform poorly and how to give feedback. Helping students and new graduates understand the concepts of active and inert tasks can provide a basis for delegation of tasks. Teaching students how to give feedback in a way that is acceptable to others will help them to feel capable of approaching and working with others to upgrade the care being given.

To recap this section: uncertainties and the use of discretion in a job create a sense of responsibility; either a sense of too much responsibility or a sense of too little responsibility in a job can cause difficulty. Helping new graduates learn to live with responsibility is the concern of both educators and service organizations. Suggestions for how this might be done include training for uncertainty, a realistic immersion experience, and a new strategy for unit orientation.


## FEEDBACK

The inputs into living systems consist not only of energic materials which become transformed or altered in the work that gets done. Inputs are also informative in character and furnish signals to the structure about the environment and about its own functioning in relationship to the environment . . . The simplest type of information input found in all systems is negative feedback. Information feedback of a negative kind enables the system to correct its deviations from course[64].

A feedback loop for a new employee serves the same purpose as feedback in any other living system. The purpose of the information input is to allow for maintenance of appropriate behavioral courses. In their work in the hospitals, the new graduates encountered a variety of information inputs. This last section of the chapter on the individual deals with the feedback which the new graduates did or did not receive. The patterning of occurrence, theoretical concepts, excerpts of the Voices, and suggestions in regard to feedback will be presented.

The feedback subject area had a total frequency count of 196 and ranked fifth overall. Although feedback was a major theme, the pattern of occurrence was more like the minor than the major themes in that 28 percent occurred in the early seminars, 38 percent in the middle seminars, and 34 percent in the late seminars. Perhaps the new graduates became more concerned about feedback as the end of initial three months of employment approached and they expected a preliminary evaluation at that point. There was very wide variation in the frequency of discussion of this theme in the individual medical centers; the rank ranged from first to tenth. There seemed to be no particular pattern in the clustering of medical centers, and no reason for the wide variation could be found.

Five themes constituted this subject area. The overwhelming majority (71 percent) of the comments in regard to feedback were in the themes "I don't get any feedback" and "All I ever hear is negative feedback." There were 42 percent in the "I don't get any feedback" theme and 29 percent in the theme "All I ever hear is negative feedback." "I get positive feedback" accounted for an additional 17 percent of the comments, and the remaining 12 percent encompassed both "I've used this specific approach to get feedback" and "People provide feedback in different ways."

## Theoretical Concepts

When entering a new organization or career, one's ability to evaluate oneself using appropriate criteria may be limited. For the new nurse who enters the work world with a predominantly whole-task orientation towards work, evaluation is based upon the criteria learned while in school. The newcomer is uncertain as to the expectations and demands of the service setting, is exposed to some of the organization's requirements for competency for the first time, and thus has difficulty in evaluating herself. If the new nurse is to improve in meeting the expectations of the work group, input from the environment as to how well the expectations for performance are being met is required.

The input from those working with the newcomer must be recognizable by the newcomer as feedback. For many new graduates the differences between the type of feedback used in the school world and the type of feedback predominating in the work world created a problem in the recognition of input. While in school, the feedback received was marked by five distinctive characteristics. It was planned, particular, balanced, firsthand, and tended to be patient-focused. For example, if the student did a sterile dressing change, a faculty member was there, and both faculty member and student knew that immediately after the procedure there would be a session for the express purpose of providing the student with input as to how well she had done. The student received very specific feedback information as to the nature of her performance. The student often heard comments such as, "You handled the forceps well and did not contaminate the sterile field. You could improve on explaining the procedure to the patient, and your charting indicated an accurate description of the kind but not the amount of drainage found." This feedback was balanced in terms of negative and positive input. The feedback was firsthand: the faculty member was right with the student and watched everything that the student had done. Finally, the feedback was focused on care provided for a particular patient.

At work, the feedback tends to take quite a different form. As the new nurse comes on duty at 3:15 P.M., the head nurse indicates, "I hear things were kind of a mess when you left last night." As a rule, the new graduate never is sure when she will receive feedback from others and when she does, the feedback tends to be very global and negative. She wonders, "What was a mess last evening? The utility room, the patients, or the charts?" Furthermore, "Is this a serious concern or just a passing comment?" It is difficult to take corrective action when the information is so vague. It is also difficult to get more specific information from the head nurse since the head nurse got the information from someone else and did not directly observe that the unit was in a mess. The nature of the feedback is somewhat different as well. Feedback at work is usually focused on the organization of work or the unit as a whole rather than on specific activities performed for an individual patient. As a result of these differences in feedback between school and work, the new graduate often does not recognize work feedback or is unable to use the feedback constructively.

Recognition of feedback is further complicated by the indirectness of feedback in the work world. Grumbling, passing comments, and methods of patient assignment are all possible means of providing feedback. These are in contrast to the grades, formalized conferences, and written comments on paperwork used in school. Thus at times, the feedback given to the new graduate at work is often not recognized by the newcomer as an indication of input about her performance.

The differences which exist in feedback between the two subsystems are related to institution's expectations of its members as well as the duties required. For the head nurse, providing ongoing continuous feedback is not a priority job requirement, whereas for the faculty member, giving feedback is of the highest priority. Whereas the faculty member is primarily responsible for the supervision of her students, the head nurse is charged with the running of an entire unit. Whereas the faculty member is expected to provide continued and ongoing feedback to students, the head nurse is expected to deal with her staff evaluations once a year. Otherwise the emphasis in her role is placed on the adequate caring for the patients on her unit.

Whether or not legitimate reasons exist for the differences in feedback is not the major point of concern here. A newcomer cannot, without input from those around her, be expected to correct and improve her functioning. The input provided must come in a fashion which allows for intake into the system and in such a way that it can be utilized.

The new graduates provided information as to the type of input they received from those around them and the value they found in this input.

*I don't get any feedback.*    The largest percentage of comments (42 percent) by the new graduates indicated that they received no feedback of any kind from those working with them on their units.

> I haven't heard from the charge nurse, the team leader, or the head nurse. It's not that I'm looking for a pat on the back. I just want to get some idea of what I'm doing—if it's right, if it's wrong, if I need to improve, or if I'm doing a terrific job. Just something.    (2:5B:41)

> Well, it's not very comfortable to be picked at on small details, but sometimes there isn't even that kind of feedback. You aren't even told there is something going wrong—just silence. You have no idea how you're doing.    (1:3C:20)

> Don't you feel the same way? If you did something wrong, wouldn't you wish someone would show you? No one tells us on our shift. At least I've never been told.    (2:1A:3)

> I had to try to adjust and I thought I was doing a pretty good job. I guess I wanted to hear that and I never did.    (9:3A:22)

Lack of feedback was disturbing to many new graduates. The newcomers were uncertain as to their performance and desired to have some confirmation as to just how they were doing. The primary reason indicated for the need for feedback was that improvement was difficult if one did not know what to work on and improve. The consequences of no feedback or of feedback stored up and given all at once were best put into words by the new graduate who said:

I like to be told at the time when I'm doing something wrong. If you are in a situation where when they do evaluate you, they tell you, "You didn't do this and this and this," nothing gets done. They wonder why you aren't improving and maybe you don't know what you're doing wrong. So you're hit with it. It's just like saying "This is what you did wrong. Now what have you got to say for yourself?" If you don't know at the time, you can't correct it. And it makes me feel like "What does that person know?"    (9:1C:5)

Thus the consequences of no feedback are not only lack of improvement but in some instances, a loss of respect and credibility for the individual who finally provides the feedback.

An additional consequence of lack of feedback was that the new graduates tended to look for subtle nonverbal clues to give them some kind of a picture of how they were doing. Although at times the new graduates drew inferences based upon behavioral clues, there was no validation of the correctness of the inference.

Sometimes, the absence of poor feedback is good. I mean, I haven't heard anything bad. And nobody has written me up for anything. That makes me feel kind of good.    (3:5C:28)

I'm just counting up the months until my six-month evaluation. That's how bad she makes me feel. I know I can improve through experience, but personally, I think I'm right where I should be at this point. But I don't know what she thinks.    (6:5B:14)

For most of the newcomers, no news was good news. This deduction may or may not be true. The effects of no verbal feedback can be worse for this group than for the group who is distressed because they do not know how they are doing. At least if one does not know and has no expectations as to how one is doing, the actual evaluation and feedback when they eventually do come will not be disconfirming. But for those who assume that everything is all right, the result of disconfirming feedback can be shocking and produce a blow to self-esteem and self-confidence as they discover that they have been unable to accurately perceive their own abilities. For such persons, the lack of feedback creates the potential for difficulty both for them and for the individual providing the feedback.

*All I ever hear is negative feedback.*    The second largest number of feedback discussions reported by the new graduates concerned negative feedback. There was a tendency for the newcomer to hear from others only when something had been done improperly or not done at all.

Do you find that any time they have something to say, it's usually negative? They don't come find you unless you've done something wrong, which doesn't make you feel too good.    (9:3A:21)

I never hear anyone say, "She's a good nurse" or "Hey, she did real good today" or "She handled that well." I never hear anyone say that. Maybe it is just human nature that we always look for the negative aspects and are more critical.    (2:5B:47)

"New graduates don't know anything." They tell you that every day. (5:3B:42)

Every time I get feedback, I'm told that something was wrong: "Well, you dummy, didn't you know . . . ?" The first thing that comes out is that you should have known.    (2:5B:37)

The majority of new graduates indicated that the negative feedback was given directly and verbally. But messages were also conveyed nonverbally.

I had trouble with this aide. I constantly had to check up on her and remind her to put vitals on the chart at the bedside. I have things to do and it takes my time to keep checking on her. When I ask her to do something, she does it—but the looks she gives me! Like "What are you doing?" I mean the looks she gives!    (5:6A:3)

People on our floor look down on some of the graduates. They act like "You didn't go to college. You don't have a college experience so you don't know anything." They don't come up to you and say it but I feel it. (1:3C:14)

At times the feedback the new graduates received was global; that is, they felt they were being told they couldn't do anything right. At other times, the new graduates received feedback for specific activities which were inappropriate. Whether or not it was clear that the feedback was global or specific, many new graduates were certain they would hear when something was wrong or mistakes were made, although when this would happen seemed unpredictable.

The feedback the new graduates received was not always negative. Seventeen percent of the new graduates' discussions indicated that the feedback received was positive.

A couple of times, I've been taken aside by the head nurse and I've gotten some positive feedback. She asked me what I wanted help with and told me that she was pleased with the way that I fit in and how I was doing.    (8:5:4)

The staff will give little suggestions. And they are right there if you need them. And if you do something well, they'll say: "That's really good." (1:3B:9)

I've had a lot of older RN's give me suggestions. They've been pretty good about it. I've never felt put down or anything. I've had little notes left that say, "Good job," or something like that.    (8:5:21)

They gave me positive reinforcement. They said, "Oh, you charted very well; that was really good." And it was a shock. I feel like I'm really making headway.    (2:2B:14)

While negative feedback was solely related to the unit level staff, positive feedback also came from other than nursing sources.

I forgot to give this man his meds when he went home and his wife called. So I called the physician and he complimented me on knowing what to do. (5:1A:32)

I wrote up some histories on some of the patients and some people were duly impressed with them. One of the residents and one of the occupational therapists said they were very helpful and well organized. (9:2C:16)

I was on alone this weekend and a lady from the kitchen came to tell me how well I had done. I felt good. (5:4A:29)

One of the patients had just delivered about three hours before and I decided to check on her. So as I was leaving, one of the nurses said that this lady's husband wanted to see me. As I went out of the door on the way, he was coming down the hall. He had a box of candy for me. It was so nice. I gave everybody a piece of candy—I was so ecstatic. (6:3A:28)

Like negative feedback, the positive feedback tended to be very global; "You're doing fine," or "You're functioning well" were the most common positive messages received by the new graduates. While these comments did not usually give the newcomers any specific information as to what exactly was good, it did serve as a boost to morale and feelings of well-being. The overall reaction to the positive feedback was that it made newcomers feel good about themselves. This is important, although more specific feedback would have accomplished the same thing while letting the newcomers know what behavior should be repeated or corrected.

*Feedback approaches.*    There were two themes which dealt with feedback approaches or methods. The new graduates reported on different ways in which they had obtained feedback from others, and on the methods that others used to provide feedback to them.

When I first started, things got to be kind of a mess so I talked to the head nurse and I told her "If I'm doing anything wrong, please let me know at the time because I'd like to improve and I'm really trying." She opened up, and that brought out a lot of things. So by approaching her, it seemed to help the situation. (9:1C:10)

I just ask for it. I say, "How did I do?" It's very direct and I usually get it. (3:5C:26)

The only way I ever get feedback is when I start cutting myself down. Like when I first started team leading. You know, I apologized to people for things I had done or else I said how awful I had done. Then they'd give me feedback which otherwise I hadn't gotten. (1:3B:11)

A few of the newcomers used more indirect approaches to get feedback. One new graduate found that her approach didn't work.

I've asked my head nurse a couple of times for a critical evaluation of how I was doing, but she is always so busy that she hasn't really sat down with me to talk or anything. (6:2B:17)

The next three excerpts describe ways in which the feedback provided which were unacceptable to the newcomers.

> The main thing we are talking about is poor communication between everybody. They were just talking about people behind their backs. And if you have something to say about somebody, go on and say it to her face. (1:6B:2)

> Some people were saying I was doing well. Others were saying that I was just socializing all the time. If someone is going to talk about me I'd like to hear it directly.   (5:1A:26)

> A nurse was specialing a patient and right in front of the patient, she was told not to proceed as she was doing. It bugged her! And I was so mad!   (5:6A:18)

New graduates could accept negative or neutral feedback given in a tactful manner.

> She doesn't holler at me in front of other people. She lets you know when you've made a mistake, but she uses tact in telling me about mistakes.   (7:4C:22)

> It's kind of funny, but a few weeks ago, we were sitting around the desk talking and the head nurse said, "Don't plan on getting any praise for your job. We'll let you know if you're not doing a good job, but otherwise, you won't hear too much."   (1:2C:20)

While the method described in the second of the foregoing excerpts may not be the most positive way of providing feedback, the new graduate now knows for certain that no news is good news. The newcomer in this situation is much further ahead than those who received no feedback and didn't know for sure what its absence meant.

The lack of feedback in the work world may stem from the desire of those in the system to give the new graduates an opportunity to take hold before they begin to give feedback. There will be errors and mistakes at first and everyone deserves a chance. The message from new graduates is that to receive no feedback is to have no chance at all. Equally devastating is overemphasis on totally negative feedback. Whatever the reason for the type and style of feedback in the work world, a need has been clearly stated by newcomers. We need more feedback and more balanced feedback. Let us proceed to some suggestions for providing feedback constructively and positively.

## Feedback Suggestions

One of the first factors that must be dealt with in the area of feedback is the development of the ability to provide one's own self-evaluation and self-reinforcement. To do this, one must develop criteria for evaluating oneself. Usually, new graduates have developed some kind of criteria for self-evaluation during the socialization process of school. However, criteria the new graduate possesses when she comes to the job need to be broadened and given a slightly different emphasis from those she used during the school years.

The skills of self-evaluation can be acquired through the process of role modeling discussed earlier. This strategy will aid in the development of the necessary evaluation criteria. The sooner the criteria are developed, the sooner newcomers can count on their own abilities for evaluation and reinforcing their own behavior. Therefore, when the skills are developed, the need for external feedback and validation decreases.

As one looks at the reactions of the new graduates to feedback, it is apparent that positive feedback produced a better feeling state than did negative feedback, as might be expected. But which kind of feedback produces the best results in the long run? Operant learning and behavior modification theory provide some insight into the best kind of feedback to provide. As a rule, negative feedback acts to eliminate or extinguish a behavior, because the learner wishes to avoid the negative consequences associated with the enactment of a given behavior. Positive feedback tends to increase the performance of a given behavior because the consequences are usually a reward. The best feedback is a combination of the two types of feedback. Negative feedback should be given to eliminate inappropriate behaviors, with positive feedback given to strengthen desired behaviors. Mixed feedback has been demonstrated to produce the best results[65].

There is also some indication that different personality types respond better to positive or to negative feedback, as in the Hunnicut and Thompson study, for example[66]. Although that study was done on children, the results would seem to be equally applicable for the mature adult. Its findings indicated that extroverts responded better to negative feedback while introverts responded more favorably to positive feedback. While the authors are not suggesting that new graduates be subject to measures of introversion, readily perceived behavioral indicators that cause people to say that an individual is introverted or extroverted can be used. Perhaps if those responsible for feedback to newcomers made the attempt to determine a new graduate's basic personality tendency and then gave the proper feedback type, more improvement would be seen in the new nurse's performance.

The schedule and patterning of feedback also acts as a variable in the effectiveness of the feedback provided. The least effective pattern is the fixed-interval schedule for providing feedback[67]. This type of feedback specifies given times when evaluation will be provided—for example, at three months, six months, or one year of employment. The fixed-interval schedule tends to generate the minimum expected work output with sudden and dramatic increase just before the evaluation is due. The most effective schedule is the variable-ratio schedule[68]. This means that feedback is given at varying times depending upon the amount of the behavior performed. For example, a new graduate might team lead for three days and then receive feedback on how well she had done; another day passes and feedback is given again; a week passes and feedback is provided. Since the feedback is related to the behavior and is not specified in terms of time and since the ratio is not always the same, this kind of schedule results in a higher, more stable, and more consistent level of performance.

If we examine the usual patterns for evaluating and providing feedback to new graduates, we find that the great majority of hospitals employ a fixed-interval schedule. Thus it can be expected that the result will be the minimum expected output of behavior. It would be better to provide feedback based upon behaviors performed and to give feedback at varying intervals.

An additional factor related to the effectiveness of feedback is the completeness of the information given regarding the required response. The more complete information is, the better the response rate[69]. In other words, the clearer the new graduate is about the expected role behaviors and functions, the better her performance will be. Those responsible for the work of the new graduates must be able to provide feedback in a constructive manner, and if feedback is not forthcoming, new graduates must elicit the needed input from others. Detailed information on these two aspects of feedback has been presented elsewhere and will not be repeated here[70].

The work involved in providing useful feedback can at times seem more than the results would warrant. Each individual must decide whether better performance, increased respect for supervisors, decreased misunderstandings, and increased confidence are worth the effort[71]. The more able we are to produce an employee who can use appropriate criteria for evaluating the self, the narrower the gap between self-appraisal and appraisal by others. As Longfellow said, "We judge ourselves by what we feel we are capable of doing; others judge us by what we have done." The less discrepant the evaluations by self and others, the higher the level of self-esteem and the better the overall performance of the new graduate in her first job.

## REFERENCES

1. Argyris, C. *Integrating the Individual and the Organization.* New York: Wiley, 1964, p. 23.
2. Schein, E. The individual, the organization, and the career: A conceptual scheme. *J. Appl. Behavioral Sci.,* 7(4): 470, 1971.
3. Argyris, C. 1964, p. 23.
4. Wells, L. E. and Marwell, G. *Self-esteem: Its Conceptualization and Measurement,* vol. 20. Sage Library of Social Research, Beverly Hills: Sage, 1976, p. 59.

5. Wells, L. E. and Marwell, G. 1976, p. 37.
6. Fitts, W. H. et al. *The Self Concept and Self-actualization.* Nashville, Tenn.: Counselor Recordings and Tests, 1971, p. 13.
7. Bonner, H. *Psychology of Personality.* New York: Ronald Press, 1961, p. 437.
8. Argyris, C. 1964, p. 29.
9. Schein, E. 1971, p. 416.
10. Schein, E. 1971, p. 416.
11. Kramer, M. and Schmalenberg, C. *Path to Biculturalism.* Wakefield, Mass.: Contemporary Publishing, 1977.
12. Brandt, E. M. et al. Comparison of on-the-job performance of graduates with nursing school objectives. *Nursing Res., 6*(4): 50-60, 1967.
13. Hayter, J. Follow-up study of graduates of the University of Kentucky College of Nursing, 1964-1969. *Nursing Res., 20*(1): 55-60, 1971.
14. Large, J. T. Perceptions of Baccalaureate Graduates as Beginning Practitioners. Ph.D. thesis, Teachers College, Columbia University, 1970.
15. On April 2, 1973 the *San Diego Union* reported that health employers in San Diego were not hiring San Diego State University BS graduates. Only 15 of the 165 graduated in the previous six months had been hired. During this same time, the local community colleges reported no particular difficulty in placing their graduates.
16. Kramer, M. Some Effects of Exposure to Employing Bureaucracies on Role Conceptions and Role Deprivation of Neophyte. Ph.D. thesis, Stanford University, 1966; Kramer, M. *Reality Shock: Why Nurses Leave Nursing.* St. Louis, Mo.: C. V. Mosby, 1974.
17. Smoyak, S. A. A Panel Study Comparing Self-reports of Baccalaureate and Diploma Nurses before Graduation and after Their First Work Experience in Hospitals. Ph.D. thesis, Rutgers-The State University, 1970.
18. Waters, V. H. et al. Technical and professional nursing: An exploratory study. *Nursing Res., 21*(2): 124-131, 1972.
19. Wescoe, F. H. Nursing Service Expectations and Nursing Education Goals as Factors in Initial Employment and Nursing Education Goals as Factors in Initial Employment Situations of New Nurse Graduates. Ph.D. thesis, Indiana University, 1972.
20. Nelson, L. F. Competence of nursing graduates in technical, communicative and administrative skills. *Nursing Res., 27*(2): 121-125, 1978.
21. Saffer, J. B. and Saffer, L. D. Academic record as a predictor of future job performance of nurses. *Nursing Res., 21*(4): 457-462, 1972.
22. Brandt, E. M. and Matheny, B. H. Relationships between measures of student and graduate performance. *Nursing Res., 17*(3): 242-246, 1968.
23. Brandt, E. M. and Metheny, B. H. 1968, p. 246.
24. Carnegie Commission on Higher Education. *Higher Education and the Nation's Health.* New York: McGraw-Hill, 1978.
25. Argyris, C. and Schon, D. *Theory in Practice: Increasing Professional Effectiveness.* San Francisco: Jossey-Bass, 1975.
26. Friedman, J. *Retracking America.* Garden City, N. Y.: Doubleday, 1973, p. 143.
27. Schein, E. M. *Professional Education: Some New Directions.* New York: McGraw-Hill, 1972.
28. Pittier, L. Letter of June 14, 1977.
29. Laing, R. D. *Knots.* New York: Pantheon, 1970, p. 56.
30. Argyris, C. Conditions for competence acquisition and therapy. *J. Appl. Behavioral Sci., 4*(2): 148, 1968.
31. Weinstein, E. "The Development of Interpersonal Competence" in Goslin, D. (Ed.), *Handbook of Socialization Theory and Research.* Chicago: Rand McNally, 1969, p. 757.
32. Weinstein, E. 1969, pp. 757-758.

33. For an overall treatment of the subject see: Kramer, M. and Schmalenberg, C. The first job—A proving ground: Basis for empathy development. *J. Nurs. Admin.,* 7(1): 12-22, 1977; Truax, C. and Mitchell, K. "Research on Certain Interpersonal Skills in Relation to Process and Outcome" in Bergin, A. and Garfields, S. (Eds.), *Handbook of Psychotherapy and Behavior Change.* New York: Wiley, 1971, pp. 299-344.

34. Gellen, M. I. Finger blood volume response of counselors, counselor trainees, and non-counselors to stimuli from an empathy test. *Counselor Educ. Supervision,* 10(1): 64-74, 1970.

35. Truax, C. and Corkhuff, R. *Toward Effective Counseling and Psychotherapy: Training and Practice.* Chicago: Aldine, 1967.

36. Truax, C. B. et al. Therapeutic relationships provided by various professionals. *J. Commun. Psych.,* 2(1): 33-36, 1974.

37. Duff, R. S. and Hollingshead, A. B. *Sickness and Society.* New York: Harper and Row, 1968, pp. 225-240.

38. La Monica, E. and Karshmer, J. Empathy: Educating nurses in professional practice. *J. Nursing Educ.,* 17(2): 3-11, 1978.

39. La Monica, E. Empathy Training as the Major Thrust of a Staff Development Program. Ph.D. thesis, University of Massachusetts, 1974.

40. Kramer, M. and Schmalenberg, C. 1977.

41. Korman, A. Toward an hypothesis of work behavior. *J. Appl. Psychology,* 54(1): 39, 1970.

42. Locke, E. Toward a theory of task motivation and incentives. *Organizational Behavior Human Performance,* 3: 157-189, 1968.

43. Stedry, A. and Kay, E. The effects of goal difficulty on performance. *Behavioral Sci.,* 11: 459-470, 1966.

44. White, R. Motivation reconsidered: The concept of competence. *Psychological Rev.,* 66: 297-334, 1956.

45. Argyris, C. and Schon, D. 1975.

46. Argyle, M. and Rendon, A. "The Experimental Analysis of Social Performance" in Berkowitz, L. (Ed.), *Advances in Experimental Social Psychology,* vol. 3. New York: Academic Press, 1967, p. 85.

47. Argyle, M. and Rendon, A. 1967.

48. Cartwright, D. Achieving change in people: Some applications of group dynamics theory. *Human Relations,* 3: 381-393, 1951.

49. Conover, H. H. and Daggett, W. The other half of job competency. *Business Educ. Forum,* Feb. 1976, pp. 8-9.

50. Argyris, C. 1968, p. 153.

51. Jaques, E. *Equitable Payment* (2nd ed.). Carbondale and Edwardsville: Southern Illinois University Press, 1970, p. 81.

52. Jaques, E. 1970, p. 87.

53. Heider, F. *The Psychology of Interpersonal Relations.* New York: Wiley, 1958, pp. 142, 216.

54. Heider, F. 1958, p. 97.

55. Heider, F. 1958, p. 97.

56. Jaques, E. *Measurement of Responsibility.* Cambridge, Mass.: Harvard University Press, 1956, p. 93.

57. Jaques, E. 1956, p. 90.

58. Thompson, J. D. *Organizations in Action.* New York: McGraw-Hill, 1967, p. 119.

59. Moidel, H. et al. *Nursing Care of the Patient with Medical-Surgical Disorders* (2nd ed.). San Francisco: McGraw-Hill, 1976, p. 512.

60. Moidel, H. et al. 1976, p. 252.

61. Jaques, F. 1970, p. 90.

62. Heider, F. 1958, p. 246.

63. Laird, D. A. and Laird, E. *The Techniques of Delegating.* New York: McGraw-Hill, 1958, p. 158.
64. Katz, D. and Kahn, R. *The Social Psychology of Organizations.* New York: Wiley, 1966, p. 22. Reprinted with permission.
65. Bandura, A. *Principles of Behavior Modifications.* New York: Holt, Rinehart and Winston, 1969, p. 316.
66. Thompson, G. and Hunnicutt, C. The effect of repeated praise or blame on the work achievement of "Introverts" and "Extroverts." *J. Educ. Psychology,* 35(5), 1944.
67. Bandura, A. 1969, p. 28.
68. Bandura, A. 1969, p. 28.
69. Bandura, A. 1969, p. 573.
70. Kramer, M. and Schalenberg, C. 1977.
71. Veninga, R. Interpersonal feedback: A cost-benefit analysis. *J. Nursing Admin.,* 5:41, 1975.

## BIBLIOGRAPHY

Cohen, A. "Some Implications of Self-esteem for Social Influence" in Gordon, C. and Gergen, K. (Eds.), *The Self in Social Interaction.* New York: Wiley, 1968.

Cooper Smith, S. *The Antecedents of Self-esteem.* San Francisco: W. H. Freeman, 1967.

Dawis, R. and Lofquist, L. Personality style and the process of work adjustment. *J. Counseling Psychology,* 23(1): 1976.

Dermer, J. D. Interactive effects of uncertainty and self-control on the acceptance of responsibility for, and satisfaction with, performance. *Human Relations,* 27(9): 1974.

Feather, N. T. Attribution of responsibility and valence of success and failure in relation to initial confidence and task performance. *J. Personality Social Psychology,* 31(2): 1969.

Fishbein, M. Attribution of responsibility: A theoretical note. *J. Experimental Social Psychology,* 9(2): 1973.

Flippo, E. *Principles of Personnel Management.* New York: McGraw-Hill, 1961.

Greenhaus, J. and Badin, I. Self-esteem, performance, and satisfaction: Some tests of theory. *J. Appl. Psychology,* 59(6): 1974.

Katz, R. L. *Empathy: Its Nature and Uses.* London: Free Press of Glencoe, 1963.

Keefe, T. Empathy: The critical skill. *Social Work,* 21(1): 1976.

La Monica, E. and Karshmer, J. Empathy: Educating nurses in professional practice. *J. Nursing Educ.,* 17(2): 1978.

Levita, D. *The Concept of Identity.* New York: Basic Books, 1965.

Notter, L. E. and Spalding, E. K. *Professional Nursing: Foundations, Perspectives, and Relationships* (9th ed.). Philadelphia: Lippincott, 1976.

Redman, P. W. Responsibility. *Int. Nursing Rev.,* 7(2): 1960.

Reeder, L. et al. Conceptions of self and others. *Am. J. Sociology,* 66: June 1960–June 1961.

Turner, R. "The Self-conception in Social Interaction" in Gordon, C. and Gergen, K. (Eds.), *The Self in Social Interaction.* New York: Wiley, 1968.

# Chapter 5
# The Ambiguous,
# Tenuous Span

In the last chapter on the individual, much concern was expressed regarding the development of high self-esteem, competence and self-confidence. Why so much concern? It is because high self-esteem is the core characteristic of an individual that enables her to successfully cross the bridge to her environment. It enables her to successfully articulate the meeting of her own needs with the needs of the organization wherein almost one-third of her life is spent. It enables the nurse to begin the journey from the protective environment of the school to her place in the work world as a mature professional practitioner. To make this journey between the system and the individual, one must cross a bridge composed of the tenuous, ambiguous spans of backstage reality, role expectations, change, and friction. Each of these factors are challenges from the environment which, if successfully managed, enable an individual to utilize her environment for optimum need satisfaction of self and the organization.

The link between self-esteem and the topics of this chapter is direct. The higher a person's self-esteem, the more value she places on who and what she is and the more likely it will be that she will use her own values, beliefs, and attitudes in an attempt to influence others toward change. A system needs input to sustain its health, meet its own needs, to replenish itself, and to make contributions to its employees, so that they in turn will want to continue to contribute their services. High self-esteem, competency, responsibility, and the ability to obtain needed feedback are the skills an individual needs in order to articulate happily and productively with the system. This articulation can be seen in the extent to which the individual can perform the four kinds of behavior that are the concerns of this chapter, management of backstage reality, coping with role expectations, inducing change in the system, and handling friction.

Upon entering the work world for the first time, it is highly likely that new graduate nurses will experience reality shock. They will find that the individualistic whole-task approach to nursing care learned in school differs markedly from the segmented part-task functioning of the work world. It is a shock to find that the operating principle for the delivery of nursing services has switched from meeting all the nursing care needs for one or two patients to meeting some of the nursing care needs of everyone according to number of personnel and amount of time available. This shock is magnified when the newcomer discovers some of the "backstage" realities—things that go on behind the scenes in the job. Sooner or later the individual must cope with these two major discrepancies—the differences between the whole-task and part-task systems of work organization and the differences between the front region view of nursing and the back region reality. One common way of coping is reduction of emotion; shock and surprise give way to resignation and acceptance. As noted earlier, accepting the existence of backstage reality is not the same as accepting the practices found in the back region for oneself. When one does accept the practices as legitimate functions of the job, however, one moves those practices into the arena of role expectations, both for oneself and for others. The process of coping seen in the movement from the shock phase to role expectations is illustrated in the following diagram:

|  | Shock Phase of Reality Shock | Acceptance that Backstage Reality Exists | Role Expectations |
|---|---|---|---|
| *Emotion Expressed* | Shock; anger | Resignation; sadness | Certitude; conviction. Righteous anger if expectations not met. |
| *Typical Verbalizations* | "I couldn't believe it!" "I was amazed!" "It shouldn't be that way!" | "That's the way it's done." "Everybody does it that way." "I know it's not the right way (or the way I was taught), but that's how it's done here." | "Everyone should do it that way." "The way it's supposed to be done is . . ." |

In any situation, there will be some backstage reality or some practices, some ideas, that, it is hoped, a newcomer will want to change or will want to see incorporated into the practices of the work group. Modification of all practices or initiation of new practices will require that the individual be an effective agent of change. Even with such abilities, it can be expected that a certain amount of friction will result. Without change and friction both the social system and the individual are dead.

## MANAGEMENT OF BACKSTAGE REALITY

Can I ask how somebody else has handled a particular problem that came up twice today? I do things that are supposed to be done on day shift like changing to new IV bottles and changing tubing all the way down to the needle. And I've had the patient say, "Nobody else ever does that." How do you talk to the patient without really saying, "The other nurses are wrong; they should do it too"? I know they're wrong. I know it's the right thing to do, . . . but I don't want to destroy the patient's confidence in the nurses or in the kind of nursing care he is getting, so I can't really tell him. (4:4:28)

The dilemma described in this excerpt represents a concern commonly voiced by the nurses in the seminars. They ask "How do I constructively and effectively manage the impression that patients receive of me and of the other nurses, and at the same time, how do I cope with my own feelings and attitudes about some of the shocking things that I discover are really going on?"

Management of backstage reality can best be viewed as a series of overlapping steps. The first step is the new graduate's discovery that there is a backstage or back region to nursing. This is where the performance of the work of nursing is prepared for enactment for various audiences—patients, physicians, nursing office supervisors, relatives, other departments, and so on. More often than not, as a student in a school of nursing the new graduate did not see this back region or caught only infrequent, partial glimpses of it. Hence, upon graduation she possessed little knowledge or understanding of it and fewer skills to cope with it or manage the desired impression of it.

After the shock of discovering the back region, the nurse must learn to deal with her feelings about what she has discovered and then with how she is going to fit into the back region. Existing simultaneously is the newcomer's desire to establish her identity as a nurse. To accomplish both of these tasks, the newcomer engages, either consciously or subconsciously, in the art of "impression management." She attempts to manage the impression that others receive of her as an individual, but she discovers that she must also cooperate with other staff members in staging the performance of certain behaviors or routines for various groups of people—patients, doctors, supervisors, relatives. Sometimes, as in the preceding excerpt, the two impression managements conflict.

The discovery that impression management goes on in the work world and that the way things appear to be on the surface is not necessarily the way they really are was a concern universally discussed in the new graduate seminars. This theme came out primarily in the early seminars, although elements of it continued throughout. Of the 112 occasions when this theme was discussed, half (53 percent) occurred during the first two seminars; 30 percent were in the middle two and the remaining 17 percent in the last two seminars in the series of six.

The sequential nature of the theme of coping with backstage reality was evident in the timing of discussions related to this theme during the seminars. In the early seminars specific incidents of backstage reality and shock and amazement at their discovery predominated. In the middle and late seminars, struggles to understand, to rationalize, to probe the meaning of various performances and characteristics of the back region predominated, as well as specific queries on how to cope with the backstage reality through impression management. There were 12 subthemes under the backstage reality theme which covered the types of backstage discoveries made, entrance rights into the group, and reactions and methods of coping with the back region discovered. The predominant subtheme was: "I was taught to give patient care (baths, care plans, etc.) in a certain way, but now I find that's not the way it's done at all." The discovery, "There are rules and policies to follow, but some people either don't have to follow them, or don't follow them all the time," was a subtheme mentioned throughout the seminar series.

Backstage reality ranked eighth in terms of frequency of discussion. In four of the medical centers, the theme ranked between fifth and sixth; in the other four, it ranked between ninth and tenth; and in the remaining one it was eighth. Reasons for these differences in frequency were not apparent and the usual variables of educational program, size of hospital, location, and control did not appear to explain the differences in rank noted.

This chapter will follow the steps in the backstage reality management process. First, a framework for looking at this process will be presented. Then, some differences between the reality of school and the reality of work as perceived by new graduates will be discussed. The process of managing the back region discoveries boils down to the questions whether to accept or not to accept, and to what degree. Examples of how different new graduates handled this all-important process will be presented, as well as some suggestions for managing, clarifying, and working with the impression management process.

## AN IMPRESSION MANAGEMENT FRAMEWORK

All the world is a stage and all the people actors in it.

*Shakespeare*

Impression or image management may be addressed as it concerns individuals (for instance, patients who would mask their symptoms, seeking to keep them from becoming visible to those around them), teams or groups of people (for example, the nurses on a unit who project an image of cheerfulness or hope to a critically ill patient and his family), or organizations (for example, a manufacturing organization that attempts to project an image as a company more concerned about the quality of its product than about profit). Almost two decades ago, Goffman analyzed and described social interaction and particularly social interaction within social establishments in terms of the means used by people to control the impressions others receive of them. He likened this phenomenon to theatrical performance. Although there is no hard research data to support his rather unusual way of looking at interaction, his analogy provides a useful and meaningful framework for tying together bits of experience. It is within Goffman's context of impression management in social interactions as a theatrical performance that some of the initial experiences of new graduates will be examined[1].

As individuals, all of us can probably recognize and tie together the bits of experiences in our personal lives in which we knowingly and deliberately attempted to manage the impression that others received of us—the presentation of self in an employment interview, portraying a knowledge of some subject matter to a person whom we wanted to impress. Our everyday language is filled with phrases that connote this impression management: "Put your best foot forward," "Made a good impression." This kind of individual impression management also goes on in our work as nurses. We each want not only self-respect, but the approval and respect of others. Self-presentation is one way of manipulating social situations to gain approval. That may sound a bit harsh and perhaps Machiavellian, but if we were carefully to observe our own behavior as well as that of others, we would see, in fact, that it is true. Watch, for example, new graduates coming into their first jobs. Unsure of themselves, unsure even of their own identity as nurse, most newcomers will expend considerable time and effort to manage the impression that others receive of them. Some will decide that the best (and perhaps safest) impression they can create is that of a continued learner, eager and willing to glean as much information from others as possible. Others may try a different tack and present themselves as mature and experienced beyond their years, sure of themselves in the new role, poised, and so on. By managing the impression others receive of us, we communicate to others our individual needs, how we want to be treated, and how we expect others to interact with us. Impression management is neither right nor wrong, nor is one kind of impression necessarily the one to be favored. The point is that impression management is a common social reaction; positive self-presentation is a particularly common reaction to a challenging and threatening situation (such as a new job)[2]. Furthermore, self-presentations are means of establishing identity and gaining both self-approval and the approval of others. When the impression management is successful, we establish identity and approval both in our own eyes and in the eyes of others.

The same kind of image management is performed by teams of people. It is learned in our society first in the family team, wherein children are socialized for "company manners." In fact, small children are often left at home when parents go visiting until the parents are reasonably assured that the child can carry off the performance that the family wishes the outside world to have of the family team. The kind of team impression management that will be of concern in this chapter is that which is prevalent in the work or occupational group. Goffman described it as follows:

> Thus, one finds that service personnel, whether in profession, bureaucracy, business, or craft, enliven their manner with movements which express proficiency and integrity, but, whatever this manner conveys about them, often its major purpose is to establish a favorable definition of their service or product . . . We commonly find that the definition of the situation projected by a particular participant is an integral part of a projection that is fostered and sustained by the intimate cooperation of more than one participant, and, moreover, that each member in such a troupe, or cast of players, may be required to appear in a different light if the team's overall effect is to be satisfactory.*

Within the walls of a hospital, for example, there are various teams of performers—nurses, physicians, patients and others. The members of each team cooperate among themselves and sometimes the different teams cooperate to present to audiences (patients, nurses, physicians, and others) a particular definition of the situation. Doctors and nurses cooperate to play out performances of routines in prescribed ways so as to give patients desired views of their condition and prognosis, the efficiency of the staff, and so on. One common image that nurses project for patients is that everyone—doctors and nurses—"really cares" about them and their welfare. Another is the positive image a patient is led to have of his physician even though the individual nurse or team of nurses may privately hold the image that the physician is less than competent. Another example of team impression management is the picture of hope that the nursing staff portrays to a patient about to be operated on for a serious cardiac condition. Or the nursing staff might define a situation as being more serious than it is for a patient with diabetes who is not taking his condition seriously and not taking care of himself properly.

New graduates were very much aware of some of the audiences to which they and their coworkers play. The following two excerpts illustrate impression management to patients and to students, respectively:

---

* From *The Presentation of Self in Everyday Life* by Erving Goffman. Copyright © 1959 by Erving Goffman. Reprinted by permission of Doubleday and Company.

Oh no! I wouldn't tell the patient! It's happened a lot. They [the patients] see you rushing around and so they will say, "Gee, isn't there anyone to help you?" or something like that. And I just don't feel they should be in on that, you know. They might get the feeling they're not getting the care they should because there aren't enough people. Oh no, I would never tell them we were short.   (3:3A:28)

A lot of things have happened, and a lot of mistakes have been made. I don't want the students to know this. I don't want them to see what other RN's are doing, so I deliberately try to steer them out of the way of activity that I don't want them to see.   (7:6B:7)

There are at least three different views of each situation: the view the team thinks the audience holds of the situation, the view the team wants the audience to have, and the view the team projects. These different views are carefully prepared and selected and are, at times, discrepant. These different views of the situation lead to the development or creation of the two divisions—the back region, where the performance of a routine is prepared, and the front region, where the performance is presented. The nursing team presents to the patients (the audience) only those aspects of care and activity that will enable the patients to obtain the definition of the situation or the impression of the nursing and medical staff that is desired. To do this, access to back regions (for example, utility rooms, nurses' stations, and patient charts) is often rigidly controlled. Access is controlled because the real performance often goes on there, and if the audience were to see it, the desired impression could no longer be maintained. Among members of the team, familiarity usually prevails, solidarity is likely to develop, and secrets that could give the show away are shared and kept. For successful impression management to occur, there must often be a tacit agreement among performers to act as if a degree of accord existed among them. Usually, agreement is stressed and opposition is underplayed. The result is certain kinds of carefully controlled communication when the audience (the patient) is present. A new graduate presents an example of a communication in front of a patient-audience which she felt violated the idea of controlled communication and allowed the patient to see the back region of the staff.

Yesterday the person in charge—I was doing something in a patient's room, getting a person on a stretcher—came in and started reordering everything. Then when I was trying to get the stretcher out, she said right in front of the patient and his wife, "I don't think you should do it that way. And I don't think you should be talking while you're working. Just stop talking— you're talking too much." This, right in front of the patient and his wife! I have many feelings about it. I felt like hitting her with a real zinger, something that would shut her up. If someone is going to criticize you, it should be between you and them and nobody else—not in front of patients, or other staff, or housekeeping.   (5:6A:18)

Communication when the audience is present is quite different from that exchanged in the absence of the audience. For example, consider the difference in dialogue and feelings expressed about a patient, his illness trajectory, motivation to get well, and prognosis when nurses talk among themselves in the coffee room, as compared to when they talk directly to the patient and/or his family.

Knowledge of and familiarity with the back region are usually allowed only to loyal members of the team, and their exposure is upsetting. Thus, performers, audiences, and outsiders all utilize techniques for "saving the show" by avoiding likely disruptions or correcting for unavoided ones, or by making it possible for others to do so. A vivid example was experienced by one of the authors [M. K.] when she once was sent in to care for a young terminally ill mother who was not to be told the seriousness of her condition. The author, new to the unit, was assigned to care for this patient because the other nurses had gotten "too close to the patient," and could no longer pull off the show that the physician, family, and they themselves expected.

Organizational impression management, although similar in many ways to team impression management, has some aspects that are unique. However, it is beyond the scope and purpose of this book and will not be discussed here.

With the preceding as a brief overview of individual and team impression management, let us now examine some of the specific aspects of the self- and team-presentations that are so prevalent in our society. First, it is crucial to understand that in these presentations, the audience is not singular. Although there may be similarities in the performances put on for the various audiences—physicians, other nurses, patients, relatives, personnel from other departments, and so on—it is much more likely that the performances will differ. The following scene was recorded in the field notes of an observer on a medical-surgical unit:

> When I [the observer] came in this morning, J. greeted me with a big smile and said she'd have plenty of time to talk with me today as the census was low and they had a full complement of staff. It was therefore quite surprising to me when an hour later I overheard M. (a staff nurse who is frequently in charge when J. is off)—J. was at coffee—telling the nursing supervisor that she really didn't see how she could release any of her staff to float to another unit because, although the census was quite low, the patients were so sick that they almost required special duty care . . . (Same morning as above) I feel quite guilty. I was sitting in the far corner of the T-shaped linen room out of sight of anyone (I was eating a breakfast roll) and overheard K. [LPN] saying to one of the aides on her team, "You'd better save up work for today and do it while the sup and the doc are making rounds so it looks like we're busy. Be sure you're doing treatments and stuff when the docs come around because we like them to see us doing stuff like that. (7/28/76 #1; 10)

The definition of the ward situation presented to the nursing supervisor audience was that the unit was busy; to the physician audience it was that the nurses were occupied doing technical things for their patients. It would seem that the latter definition of the situation was also presented to the supervisor audience.

A second important fact to understand is that a given individual is not a singular performer. In managing impressions for audiences, a person may act or perform in a variety of roles. Let us look more closely at the three most common roles in which an individual might find herself.

### Individual as Performer

The person presenting herself to others may wish others: 1) to think highly of her, 2) to think that she thinks highly of them, 3) to perceive how in fact she really feels toward them, or 4) to obtain no clear impression at all. She may wish to ensure sufficient harmony so that the interaction can be sustained, or to defraud, get rid of, confuse, mislead, antagonize, or insult others. Regardless of the particular objective and the motive for having this objective, it is in the person's best interests to control the conduct of the others, especially their response to her. This control is achieved largely by influencing the definition of the situation which others formulate. The person can express or portray herself in such a way as to give others the kind of impression that will lead them to act voluntarily in accordance with her plans. For example, a common initial impression many new graduates try to present is: "I'm only a learner, a beginner. Teach me."

Newcomers are particularly able to influence the impression others have of them and thus reciprocal roles because others commonly seek to acquire information about the newcomer or to bring into play information already in possession about that person. They will be interested in the newcomer's educational background, her conceptions of self as a nurse, her attitudes toward them, the kind and type of her previous work experience, her competence, her trustworthiness, and so on. Although some of this information seems to be sought almost as an end in itself, there are usually quite practical reasons for acquiring it. Information about the newcomer helps others to define the situation, enabling them to know in advance what they can expect of her and what she may expect of them. Informed in these ways, the others will know how best to act in order to call forth a desired response from the newcomer. The newcomer, on the other hand, by influencing the initial impression that others receive of her, can greatly control subsequent interactions.

New graduates were consciously aware of the kind of impression they were trying to present to various audiences. To patients, new graduates attempted to impart the following image:

Allergy patients are very nervous patients, I've noticed. We have four and they're really panicky . . . That's very typical of them. They have a lot of trouble breathing. . . . And that makes *me* very nervous as a nurse when they can't breathe. And I don't want to come across to them as nervous. I have to appear non-nervous even if I'm shaking inside . . .  (2:6B:6)

In the following excerpt we see evidence of image management going on with members of the same team:

I've figured out that they're going to put me on Thanksgiving and Christmas both!!! because everybody else will want the holidays off. Which if they knew, is really fine with me at this point, that I work both those days, I don't really care; I don't need the exact days off. I won't tell them though. I'll let them think it's really important to me, so if they feel like, you know, they have to give me something, you know, it's the only way it works up there. You can't, you can't say anything straight. That's another thing. I've had my attendants come over and tell me who to talk to and who not to talk to. You know, you don't tell anything to so and so if you don't want it known all over the floor.  (6:6B:32)

Although a number of aspects of the individual impression management performance might be considered, one is of crucial importance for new graduate nurses. Goffman notes that one's initial projection commits one to what one is proposing to be and requires one to drop all pretenses of being other things. As social interaction progresses, additions and modifications in this initial informational state will of course occur, but it is essential that these later developments be related without contradiction to, and even built up from, the initial positions taken by the participants[3]. It would seem that it is easier to choose what line of treatment to demand from and extend to the others present *at the beginning of an encounter* than to alter the line of treatment that is being pursued once the interaction is underway[4]. The latter course is the very kind of dilemma into which the new graduate in the following excerpt got herself:

Boy, I really blew it! When I first came on the unit, I was so scared, I could barely walk down the hall. I look so young, I guess everybody thought I was still a student. And I had tape over the RN on my name tag because I hadn't passed my boards yet. Well anyway, this doctor (I found out later it was the chief resident) asks me something about this patient, and I'm stammering all over the place and finally I managed to get out, "I'm new here," and he smiles and says, "Oh, a student," and then he begins to explain all about the patient and all. Well that was really great and it took me off the spot, so after that whenever I got into a tight spot, I'd let people assume I was a student, and everything was fine. Well, I'm really paying for that comfort now. Now that I'm a little less shaky and have passed my boards and all and really do know something, now I can't convince that doc or some of the patients either that I really *am* a nurse. He still treats me like a student . . . And it just galls me when I go to answer a patient light and the patient asks if I'll go out and get a *real* nurse.  (9:3B:10)

## Individual as a Member of a Team

A team is any set of individuals who cooperate in staging a single routine or performance. We commonly find that the definition of the situation projected by a particular participant is an integral part of a picture that is being fostered and sustained by the cooperation of the group or team. Individuals who are members of the same team will find themselves, by virtue of this fact, in an important relationship to one another. For instance, while a team performance is in progress, any member of the team has the power to give the show away or to disrupt it by inappropriate conduct. Each teammate is forced to rely on the good conduct and behavior of her fellow members, and they in turn are forced to rely on her. This good conduct and behavior may result from a cooperative venture, or positional power, force, or bargaining may be used to maintain solidarity of behavior. Regardless of the underlying means used to achieve the solidarity, there is still the element of drama presentation whereby the performer either increases or decreases the strength of performance and of his relationship with the team. The following seminar excerpt illustrates this effect:

> It really burns me up when no one takes any responsibility for a new patient who has come to the floor from two other services—say, medical and orthopedic. No one will write orders and you can't give nursing care when there are no orders. You really get caught in the middle because the patient wants things, like a sleeping pill or something to eat, and you can't tell the patient that no one wants him. You have to keep up the impression that he is wanted and someone is looking out after him.   (5:3B:8)

To understand how a person performs not only as an individual but also as a member of a team, it must be recalled that the objective of a performer is to sustain a particular definition of the situation, thus representing as it were, his claim as to what reality is. Alone, with no teammates to inform of her decision, a person can quickly decide which of the available stands on a matter to take and then wholeheartedly act as if her choice were the only one she could possibly have taken. And her choice of position may be nicely adjusted to her own particular situation and interests. When we turn from the individual performance to the team performance, we find that the character of the reality that is projected changes.

## Individual as the Audience

A third common role is acted when one person serves as the audience for another person or for another team. This can be seen quite readily when a newcomer enters a preestablished or formed group—say, for example, a unit where the nurses all know one another, having worked with one another. The newcomer will undoubtedly attempt to create or manage some kind of impression of self; it can take various forms: "Poor me,

I'm only a beginner, so teach me"; "I haven't had much experience, but I'm intelligent and really quite competent"; "I've worked lots as a nurse's aide and I really know the ropes"; "I've got a degree; see how smart I am." At the same time, she constitutes the audience for the other nurses. This team of nurses will convey to the newcomer how they define nursing on the unit, the role of the nurse, what constitutes good nursing care, how much work is expected, and so on. When an individual plays the audience part correctly, she enables the actors to play their parts, to gain their own approval. Although this audience role probably serves a useful social function, the reciprocal nature of this simultaneous performer-audience role is not only stressful for many newcomers, but it causes a lot of confusion and uncertainty.

> I'm trying to get them to see me as a person who really knows and who gives good nursing care. And at the same time, they're trying to present me with their picture of what good nursing care is, and it's a picture I don't buy. It's gotten so that I'm not sure what I think anymore. It's sort of like that song in the *King and I* when Yul Brynner says, "I'm not sure what is, and I'm not sure what's not," and stamps his foot.   (8/10/76; #6; 8)

The new graduates in the seminars were somewhat naive about others' impression management. They did not seem to be aware of the process, nor of how to respond to it. Although numerous examples were given in which the newcomer served as an audience for the impression management of others, seldom were the new graduates able to move beyond emotional reaction to a situation. Most new graduates were unable to see that if they refused to play the audience role as expected they would interrupt the performance.

> One thing that really shocked me—I wasn't prepared for this at all—was getting report when I went on nights from the P.M. shift. They give you this lovely report of all the work they did—your IV's and all that kind of stuff. Then you go out and find the IV's are empty; all the fluids have run in; ten patients are wet, and everything is wrong; the oxygen tanks are empty. So, in direct contrast to what you heard five or ten minutes ago . . . it's a total cover-up when they make it sound like they'd done all this work when they had actually done nothing.   (9:2A:18)

Even new graduates who indicated an awareness that they were being played to had no hint of how to handle the situation.

> You can always tell who's going to call in sick. The one charge nurse—what she would do usually is make out the assignments the night before. If she doesn't make out the assignment, it's guaranteed that she's going to call in sick. If there are five RN's on, you can guarantee that another girl is going to call in sick. If there's someone who asked for certain days off, you can guarantee the night before she's on, she's going to call in sick—especially if it's a three-day weekend. Everybody tries to give everyone else a good

impression—make it seem like they're all dedicated, hard workers, but after a while you can see behind it. You learn all the little habits and ways; it took me my first two months that I was on nights to learn all this. (9:1B:11)

## School-based Impression Management

The discovery of the back region and the corresponding frontstage behavior was a dominant concern for many of the new graduate nurses. It might be asked why the new graduates had not learned of the back region while they were students in school. The answer is that new graduate nurses do not discover the backstage of reality until they graduate because in all likelihood their impression of nursing was managed for them by their instructors. This impression management is intricately woven into the whole professional socialization process whereby the student is subtly manipulated into seeing nursing as it *should* be, into seeing the nurse do and perform as she can and ought to perform. Again, it is not germane to the discussion here whether such image management should or should not occur. It simply does. Often, the school management of her impressions is so pervasive and extensive that the student cannot perceive the backstage reality of the work world even if she is in a position to do so. More often than not, however, students are not in a position to perceive the backstage reality of work. In fact, they and their instructors constitute one of the prime audiences for the presentation of the unit staff's image management.

New graduates had varying reactions to the discovery that their impressions had been managed while in school. Some began to gain insight into why instructors may have managed their student impressions; others continued to be shocked and appalled that instructors hid the real world of nursing from them.

> I sometimes wonder if the reason they [instructors] did not really let us get into team leading was because they knew that if they gave us a taste of it, we would say, "Forget it!" and go into something else before we ever really got started in nursing, and they'd have nobody to even make the effort to stay with the nursing program. (1:1B:15)

> I was sitting here thinking about a quote from one of my instructors when I did go back after a couple of months and told her I was pissed off, that they didn't prepare me more strongly. And she made a comment, "We're teaching you the ideal, while helping you deal with the real." That comment really stuck with me—they are teaching us the ideal situation so you have something to strive for, and they say they teach you the real . . . *but they don't.* They don't really teach you the real. What I found is that they don't give you enough of the meat of the reality that you can weigh with the ideal. I knew that what I learned in nursing school was the way that it was supposed to be, but not having worked, I was at a disadvantage. You were

an aide before, but I had never worked anywhere. I knew nothing about a work situation; this was all new. And the school just didn't give me any idea that this was going to happen.   (9:1A:10–11)

I think one of the biggest shocks too was you're just fresh out of school and you have all these great ideals in nursing care and then you go on the job and you're a team leader and you give your report in the morning and people go, "Well, I'm not going to lunch then, I go to lunch at 11:30." "I'm not going to pass the trays; I'm sick of this patient; I'm not taking her." . . . And you're just kind of stunned. You're used to nursing school where you give an assignment and everyone takes it very pleasantly and does a good job, and comes back and reports to you. And here you have all these people refusing assignments and complaining and running out and stealing all the linen. You go out and there's no linen, and they have all their beds made . . . Relationships with ancillary help are a big problem. We got a lot of that in theory in school, a lot of team leadership theory, but we only got to practice it a very few times in a clinical situation . . . It's a problem! Actually being confronted with it day in and day out where you're continually being tested by them, and they're refusing to do things very often and changing your assignments and not always having the support of your head nurse.   (9:2A:7)

The foregoing samples of some of the differences between school and work realities are revealing, not only by their content, but also by the emotions expressed. Besides anger, resentment, and frustration, there was a pervasive tone of sadness, a deep sense of loss. This was one of the areas where the first job could be readily seen as crisis. For some of the new graduates the crisis had already passed and the backstage realities were described with acceptance and resignation.

You don't have time to use psych things at work very much. If you're passing meds and taking patients and team leading or whatever, you know, you just can't use a lot of it. You might use them occasionally, but they're so many things, so much knowledge that you don't use . . . And the doctors don't explain things to you . . . everything is so cut and dried. They look at one aspect of a patient (orthopedics) and that's all, and that's not good for you because you're trying to look at a total patient, all of his needs, and they're not concerned with what you're concerned with. You know, you feel, "like wow, what's the use?" I find I might as well look at it their way.   (2:6A:29)

Anybody could do what I do. I was taught to think, but I don't think here. I'm just a robot; all I do is tasks.   (5:1B:42)

I was taught all the way through nursing school that if you can't handle something, you should just admit it and that people would respect you for that. But that's not the way it is—they respect you more if you just go ahead and do it.   (7:5C:17)

## Quality of the Performance

When a person plays a part she is implicitly requesting others to take seriously the impression that she is trying to foster[5]. The audience is being asked to believe that the person they see actually possesses the qualities she appears to possess, and that whatever procedures that person carries out will have the consequences that she implies they will have. The quality of the performance is affected by the performer's own belief in the reality that she is attempting to portray.

At one extreme, there is the performer who is fully taken in by her own act; she is sincerely convinced that the impression of reality she is staging is valid. At the other extreme, we find the performer who is not at all taken in by her own routine. This possibility is quite understandable, since no one is in quite as good a position to see through an act as the person who puts it on. See, for example, the following excerpt:

> When you feel incompetent, it's hard to come across any other way when you're dealing with people. And I want others to see me as competent . . . Oh, I feel like I can get by, but like somebody mentioned before, it's amazing how you can get by [said angrily and with a tone of disgust]. It's really amazing. Not only me, but other nurses too. A lot of them do things and don't have any idea of why or what they're doing. (9:2B:19)

Moreover, the performer may not be at all interested in the long-range effects of the performance. She may only be trying to achieve an end, that is, impressing the audience as a temporary means to achieve some desirable goal. When a performer has no belief in her own act and has no ultimate concern with what the audience thinks of her, we can label her cynical. This does not mean that cynical people are "bad" people. Not all cynical performers are interested in managing the impression of their audiences for purposes of self-interest or private gain. They may be doing it for what they consider to be the audience's own good, or for the good of the majority or of the community. For example, consider the performances that are often put on by a medical team in an attempt to withhold from dying patients the information that they are dying. (See reference 6 for more examples of this.)

Ordinarily a performer's attitude changes from disbelief to belief in the performance she is giving. Attitudes or beliefs are changed to become congruent with behavior or performance. However, the attitude change can also go in the other direction—from belief to disbelief; from conviction to cynicism. It is not uncommon that in professions which the public holds in awe, recruits are often allowed, encouraged, and socialized to follow the reverse cycle—from belief to cynicism. This was noted in Becker and Geer's study of cynicism in medical students[7]. Goffman proposes that the reason for this is not that the students come to the slow realization that the performances they are putting on are deluding to the audience (the public), but that they use this cynicism as a means of insulating their inner selves from contact with the audience[8]. There was some evidence from the new graduate seminars that this happens for nurses as well.

> When I came into nursing school, I had stars in my eyes and I was all gung-ho. I really *believed* that I had something to give and that I, as a nurse, could really do something to help people. But then I've gradually come to see that some people are going to get well in spite of what you do, and others are going to die no matter what you do. And when this happens, I find that I still put up a front in front of patients and families. I still have to make them believe that what the doctor has prescribed is going to help— even if I know that it's really only sort of temporary. Know what I mean? Yeah . . . I also find that by making a person, say like someone with a terminal problem, by making them believe that there's hope, that they might get better, then I don't have to deal with, you know, with maybe they'll say something to me about dying, and that scares me.    (1:2B:8)

### Admission to the Back Region

The new graduate's discovery of and reaction to the back region is inevitable. If a newcomer is simply around for any period of time, and keeps her eyes and ears open, she will see and hear things that are new, strange, and perplexing. She will uncover the backstage reality. Becoming a member of the team and being let in on the meaning, the rationale of the backstage reality and of the frontstage performance, however, is another story. Sometimes there is a more or less formal passage into the team, as exemplified in the following seminar excerpt:

> I felt really good about charge. It was really exciting and neither one of the two I supervised had any major problems. On Monday, the head nurse came back and she told me that things had gone well; that I had done a good job. I got the keys to the 30 closets where they store the supplies. It's a symbol of trust to get the keys. She gave them to me. It's much better now that I've made it.    (5:5A:12)

Other times, a newcomer may perceive that the staff is united and presents a team front, and that she is not yet part of the team.

> Well, it's a very sad feeling to have to go off into the linen closet and cry because you feel shut out and someone made you cry.    (1:3B:11)

Then suddenly she becomes part of the team, but it is not made clear what she did to earn the membership rights.

> The floor is a closed floor. Whenever anybody's sick or something, they cover for themselves, and they do all their own scheduling and things. And most of the people have been there a long time, at least two years, some

four, five, six, eight years—so they all know each other well—a very closed staff. And I felt really like the outsider coming in. But then one day, one of the girls was talking to me and another came up and said, "Well, we've decided that we will take you in and we won't ostracize you" . . . And I'm thinking, "Here I am, the first week on the floor, and they're telling me that they're going to be nice to me and take me into the fold!" You know, and I just, I didn't know what to say . . . (5:2B:28)

Sometimes, the new graduate discovers that self-deprecating modesty earns admission into the group. In his description of a fundamental dilemma of social life—that between being respected and being liked by our associates—Blau[9] notes that often our efforts to achieve respect hurt our chances of being liked. A person who is motivated to become an integral part of a group will not simply wait until the others discover her good qualities; she will try to manage the impression others receive by proving herself an attractive associate, by revealing characteristics of herself that she assumes the group will value positively. Paradoxically, the more attractive a person appears to others in a group, the more reluctant they will be, at least initially, to approach her freely. This is because the attractiveness of another makes us vulnerable and creates a need for defenses. We are most impressed by qualities that are superior to our own; the possibility of rejection of us by the attractive person creates the need for us to protect ourselves through defense mechanisms. Thus results the situation that if the newcomer is successful in impression management—seeming highly attractive—she may find herself unapproachable. One important method of increasing approachability and penetrating the defenses of other group members is for a person to demonstrate that, even though she has attractive qualities, she is also quite easily approachable. She does this through the process of self-deprecating modesty. By completely reversing her earlier strategy of presenting only the most impressive parts of herself, she now flaunts her weaknesses. Often this is done by pointing out mistakes or by relating incidents that make us laugh at, as well as with, the person. Such a process shows one to be a person willing to admit to one's shortcomings. Such self-deprecating modesty is disarming since it obviates the need for defenses. One of the new graduates relates how such a process earned her acceptance into the group:

I didn't really feel part of the floor until I made a really stupid mistake and I told them about it and everyone laughed. It was very kind laughter . . . and after that day, I felt really accepted. (3:3C:16)

While it is possible that some newcomers will deliberately use self-deprecating modesty as a means of increasing their approachability, it is more likely that they will sort of stumble onto this technique and discover after the fact, "Things were different after I told them about my goof. I guess it sort of made me seem more human."

Another way in which new graduate nurses are let in on the back region is by picking up on subtle cues often transmitted to them in their audience role. This frequently happens when one begins to enact some behavior that is not quite the accurate textbook performance. One new graduate recounted the following experience that occurred after she had worried for several weeks about whether it was necessary to call doctors to obtain permission to refill medication orders while on night duty:

> I went to coffee with Lil today and confided to her that I had repeated Mr. Jones' Demerol last night without an order. I told her I was worried and felt guilty about it; did she think it would be OK? She said not to worry. Then she opened up and really gave me the dope—not only about this med situation but lots of other stuff too. I felt like I'd made it. The older nurses can really make things easier for you if they want to.

> (One week later) I feel good. Mary [an RN] stopped me in the hall, smiled, and said I was really getting with it. Then she asked if the med problem had worked itself out. I said "Yes." Then she winked at me and said "Good." She also told me some of the other things you can do with different doctors' patients. I don't know what I did, or why they're finally really telling me; I guess I'll just count my blessings and let it go at that[10].

One piece of evidence that makes it very clear whether one has become a member of a team or not has to do with one's perception of "secrets." There are different types of secrets, each having its own specific purpose, but here we are talking about what Goffman labels "inside" secrets. These are secrets whose possession marks a person as being a member of a group and helps the group feel separate and different from persons who are not "in the know"[11]. In a sense, these inside secrets are proof of subjectively felt social distance. In the following two excerpts, we see clearly that the speakers were aware of secrets being kept from them, and at least to some extent of the function and purpose of secrets to membership in a group.

> They [the older nurses] really keep secrets from you, such as how to take off orders. They could make things a lot easier for you, but they keep everything a big secret and don't let you in on all the little short cuts.   (6:1A:2)

> How do you learn important things such as which doctor wants his patients in the treatment room by 8:00 A.M., and which one wants a certain kind of tray at the bedside; how do you send a patient to the OR in University; how tests are to be carried out? These are things that the older nurses could really help you with if they wanted to. But it's like a big sorority club; they keep all their secrets and knowledge among themselves.   (8:2:2)

Even after one has been more or less admitted to the back region, a lot of learning must go on. The newcomer discovers that there are rules, regulations, and norms operative within the team that must be adhered to. Everyone knows them by informal means; often they are not made explicit until they are broken. Some are not worth fighting, but others new graduates think are.

> Nothing is written but there are things. You don't do this and you don't do that, but it isn't written. Nobody tells you and nobody tells you why . . . This one nurse has a special chair—she has to go look for it if it isn't there. If you sit in her chair she throws you out. (5:3A:34)

> I'm shocked and surprised at how a nurse will just abandon—that's how I feel—her patient, and let somebody else take over . . . and they won't even say goodbye when they leave the floor or anything. I think, wow, that's really hitting rock bottom. And to me, that's not nursing care. That really upset me . . . I get involved with my patient, and somebody there, the same nurse that's been giving me problems, actually looked down her nose at me one morning because at 7:30, I was finished but I wanted to see what my patient was going to have, whether it was a boy or a girl, she really wanted a girl, so I was standing out by the delivery room waiting, you know, until she delivered. She goes, "What are you still here for?" in a very sarcastic tone. And I go, "Well, I want to see what she had." And she looked at me and said, "What do you care?" I said, what do I *care?* I *worked* with that patient for eight hours, and I REALLY CARE! And she just laughed at me and shook her head in a disgusted sort of way and said, "Pretty soon, all of the patients will expect us to wet nurse them like that." Oh, some of the thoughts that go through my head at people like that! (2:2B:26)

## Back Region Discoveries

Specific back region discoveries and new graduate nurses' reactions to them cannot always be separated, but the first series of seminar excerpts to be presented in this section will concentrate on the content of backstage reality; then we will focus on the emotional reactions to the discovery of this reality. The content will be presented under seven subthemes:

Nobody cares.

Some nurses are incompetent.

Continuity of care is a farce.

Check and double-check? Not any more!

Rules aren't for everybody.

Nursing judgments? What are they?

Can't anything be done?

Power, power: who's got the power?

*Nobody cares.* One of the dominant discoveries of what "it's really like" expressed by the nurses in the seminars was the lack of enthusiasm, caring, and liking for the work of nursing they perceived on the part of the nursing staff.

I think one reason for the poor care around here is that the nurses are just so task-oriented. They come in and they do things bam, bam, bam. Much faster than I do. But I don't think they put much thought into it . . . [Goes on to describe an incident in which she explained to the relieving nurse her rationale for placing a newborn in a certain position, and the other nurse laughed at her and said "You don't have to have a reason."] I really felt like she put me down. I see the other nurses as getting things done very quickly, but they do just exactly what they have to do, without much thought or compassion.  (9:2B:5)

It's sad to get out in the real world and find out that everybody else isn't patient-oriented. In school you're taught to be working for the patient, and here people are just working for the money.  (9:2A:38)

New graduates were also surprised to discover that not all nurses were interested in learning.

We had a nursing conference today—it was right during lunchtime. A perfect time to have a conference. All the students were there and the instructor and myself and another float nurse came to the conference too. So here we are. Me a new graduate and the float was a new graduate too and there out at the desk were the two old grads sitting on their little pedestals watching people eat. They had all been invited and there was nothing doing out on the floor, but they wouldn't come. They just didn't care to learn. (5:3B:23)

*Some nurses are incompetent.*    The discovery that not all nurses are competent was mentioned by seminar participants from virtually all regions of the country.

That's one of the things that really amazed me—the idiots that are nurses. They don't know anything. You ask them a very basic question and they can't answer you; they just don't know. They're working the floor and running way over shift. They're on but they don't know what they're doing at all. They've forgotten everything. "What is this medicine for, do you know?" You ask because she's given it twice on her shift. "No, I don't know, but I was going to look it up," and you know she's not going to look it up. They don't care.  (9:2A:30)

One night I came on and one of the nurses had emptied all the chest tube bottles. Every one of them. [shocked comments from group] Very calmly in report she said, "and the chest tube bottles have 50 cc's." And I looked up and said, "What? 50 cc's? Did you empty those bottles?" And she says, "Oh well, you know," and then she's beating around the bush telling me she didn't empty the bottles when she just told me what was in the bottles. So I flew out the door and the bottles were empty. She just gets her coat and goes home—didn't phase her a bit.  (9:2A:30)

*Continuity of care is a farce.*    Particularly upsetting to the neophyte nurses, probably because it was so much at odds with school-taught ideals, was the seeming lack of concern for continuity of care. Other considerations, such as availability, geographical proximity, and staff preference frequently took precedence over the ideal of staff assignments that would foster continuity of patient care.

> Gail was working back in the isolation unit, but now they've put me back there two times sporadically—kind of because there was nobody else to go back there. I worked a double shift on Saturday, and for one of the shifts I worked back there, and for the other I didn't. I worked the floor on Monday, off Tuesday, back there today, floor on Thursday, and back there Friday. It's real crazy and stupid. How can I give continuity of care to those patients by just being drawn back there maybe a couple of days a week or something? (1:4B:10)

> I'm beginning to understand why the nurses don't write care plans on our floor—I mean, really, what's the point? You work with a patient once, or maybe if you're lucky two days, and then bam—you're assigned to another team. I know the care plan is supposed to provide the continuity, but paper isn't a good substitute for the continuity that a person would provide. Why should I put all that effort into a care plan if I'm not going to be taking care of the patient to see the results? (5:4:1–3)

*Check and double-check? Not any more!*    There were a number of discoveries of shortcuts or modifications in procedures that the new nurses had been taught were unmodifiable. Such modifications are particularly upsetting to the newcomers. At a time when most new graduates are very unsure of themselves, they crave structure; they want to be able to hold on to some kind of certainty. In many of the following excerpts, you will observe that this certainty has been shaken.

> Passing pills, too. We were always taught to stand there and watch the patient take them. But in the morning sometimes, I notice that there will be a little cup of them sitting on the table all night, and the nurse passed them at 6:00 A.M. and didn't bother waking the patient up. And then the next time you go in, they'll be on the floor somewhere.

> I had a hard time adjusting to the medications too, cause I was always taught—we had little cards for each drug and you had your little tray and all your little cards for each pill, and you triple-checked and you checked with the identi-band and all this kind of stuff. And now, if you have one patient to give meds to, say, at odd hours, you don't push the cart all the way down there. You take the pills down to the patient, and you don't have any identification of what it is, or who you're taking it for. Really, you just go down there and give it. (4:2:14–15)

> When I was in school, I was really proud. You knew exactly what was wrong with each patient, what and why the patient was going to need something, what his meds and treatments were . . . But now when you're working staff, you're not going to know every med that you're giving, so you should look it up. But I just don't have time to do it. I was telling her I feel

really bad about it. She said, "Look. I know you've been told you have to know all the meds. Forget it. You won't, and you won't have time to look them up." "I know you're not supposed to sign them off until after you've passed them, but you'll be here all day if you do that. So stop, and just sign them off and be done with it." I was really shocked, and I still feel bad about it, but I see that I have to do it. (3:3A:19)

I can ask the doctors for renew orders daily. I put renew, renew, renew on the chart, but it's not done. The next one, I scratch out the date, and I make it real obvious—*TODAY* would you please renew . . . I once tried not giving the med and I really got jumped on, hard, by the doctor. So now I just go ahead and give it. (9:1C:28)

*Rules aren't for everybody.* Along with the backstage discoveries relating to violations of standard procedures was the new graduate's discovery that there are rules and procedures prescribed by the organization that are not always followed. Probably because of the uncertainty and ambiguity that is so pervasive for new graduates, particularly at the beginning of their employment, the newcomer tends to grasp and hold sacred any kind of structure she can see. Therefore it is not surprising that it is particularly disturbing to her when this structure or format is not followed. Many instances of this were discussed in the seminars.

I'm still very frustrated about the laxity in charting medications and IV's. I don't know what happened, but I had ordered up the IV's and labeled them, but the next day somebody got them mixed up, and didn't chart them, and the physician was mad . . . days will go by and shifts will not do their charting . . . When I brought it up—I went to the head nurse first and said, "You know the IV's aren't charted," and this happened first when I really noticed it. When I really said, "OK, no more of this," was when the blood wasn't charted right. It said, one unit of red cells, and it was supposed to be two units of packed cells because I had put the order in, so I knew. And the head nurse just said, "Well, not everyone that came here had learned that you're supposed to chart IV's; they just never did it at all. You just have to give them time." So we have a procedure, but it's not being followed and she's not enforcing it. (4:3:2-4)

What happens to the incident reports once they're filled out? They're put in the nursing office. So why bother? If I write an incident report, why give it to the nursing supervisor? If she doesn't want to turn it in—if she doesn't buy it, who knows what happens to it? . . . Oh, they (people on the floor) hear about it from me because I talk about it. This upsets them because I talk about it, but I feel they should know about it. But they don't hear about it from the supervisor. (9:3C:25-27)

*Nursing judgments? What are they?* New graduates discover that there is a discrepancy between what they were taught and what nurses actually can and cannot do, the judgments nurses are allowed to make.

There's also a difference between what you get in your orientation and what you find really on the floor. I've gone round and round again just about hair shampoos. They told us in orientation that we do not need an order for them, then I go on the floor and they say "you absolutely need an order for that."

No, you don't.

That's what they tell me.

[All talk at once.]

Nursing can't make that judgment. Like if the patient's got pneumonia or if they've had something done cervical spinewise, then of course not, but every time I bring it up they all say "You have to get a doctor's order" and I go, "Well, in team leading they told us we didn't," and they go, "yes, you do," and so what am I to do? . . . Also, what about diets? You know, they say that they write a certain diet, well you can advance the diet as you assess the patient, and that was what I was taught in school too. Well, I tried to do that and my charge nurse said "Absolutely not. That says clear liquids." I said "This guy is ravenous; he is *so* hungry and he doesn't want jello."

I heard that you could decrease the diet, but you can't take them forward . . .

Oh no, oh no, she wouldn't even let me give him orange juice. It's not a clear liquid, you know.

We give diet as tolerated . . .

[All talk at once.]

You could have called a doctor to get the order changed.

I could have gone ahead and fed him while the head nurse was on break. [general laughter]

But you're saying an awful lot there.    [murmurs of assent from others]

Yeah . . . I begged her. I kept saying "He's hungry; he's so hungry; he's not sick to his stomach, you know. There's no reason he can't have a regular dinner." (2:6A:32)

*Can't anything be done?* Another expression of this subtheme is: "There must be something you can do." This expression is in response to a backstage reality discovery that was particularly upsetting to the new nurses. It is perhaps best described as a means-goals conflict, the discovery that modern science simply does not have all the knowledge and techniques needed to accomplish its goal of optimum health care for all. We simply do not possess the means to help everyone get well. Many new graduates are aware of this in the abstract while they are students in a school of nursing. But somehow it is different when they graduate and start working with *specific* patients on longer-term basis. Then the reality hits that no matter what the doctors and nurses do, some patients are simply not going to get well—and that sometimes we even make them worse in the hospital.

> I came here really feeling blue about modern medicine, and at school I was taught all these things and I read all the stuff in the textbooks. You know, "If somebody has this, you do this for them, and then they will get well." And now I see all these people with this and this being done for them and they're getting worse and worse, and it's really depressing. (1:2B:8)

> The doctors oscillate between treating her vigorously and then dropping back and saying, "Well, she's not going to make it." And you know, it's just really hard for me to deal with that. (1:2C:7)

*Power, power: who's got the power?* A somewhat surprising discovery by new graduates is that some of the backstage reality that they had been warned about was, in fact, true.

> I've heard that the auxiliary personnel have more control on the unit than the nurses because they have been there longer and they know the ropes. I found that out when I worked at Cord last summer. I was so glad I wasn't an RN then because there was this one aide who had been there for 13 years and she would talk about all the RN's like she was good and this one wasn't. You really had to approach this aide the right way. They know their jobs and you'd better not cross them or tell them to do something different or accuse them of not doing their jobs. And you'd better not ask them to do something that they aren't supposedly qualified to do. They are pretty set and you don't want to break their routine. We had been told that in our trends course that the auxiliary personnel have more control than you would ever imagine, and they really do! (6:2A:24)

## Emotional Response to Back Region Discoveries

Many more examples of back region discoveries could have been selected for presentation. The ones chosen represent the range of discoveries made by new graduates as well as those with greatest frequency. In the remainder of this chapter, some of the other kinds of back region discovery will be presented, as in the following series of seminar excerpts, selected to illustrate the range of emotional reactions that the new graduates had to the various kinds of surprises and differences that were uncovered.

> I'm teased a bit and still told that I'm idealistic, but it doesn't bother me a bit because I think I'm right when it comes to some of the things I was taught. And I do them that way rather than the way they sloppily run through it. You know, like this one LPN. I was standing there with her and she was catheterizing this female and she got it, instead of going into the upper hole, she goes into the bottom hole and she misses but then she takes it out and puts it up there. I mean that's terrible! I couldn't stop her. That to me is just very poor technique and I think a lot of people probably do

that when they're not watched. I said something to her about it and she just kind of passed it off.  (2:6A:33-34)

This above excerpt illustrates the subtheme "Some nurses are incompetent" as well as showing one nurse's determination to maintain her professional standards.

Anger and frustration were expressed by the new nurses concerning discoveries related to the larger social system, which was beyond their control.

And that's the way it is on the psych floor. You must admit private patients and forget about county patients because you don't get money for county patients . . . private is always taken before the county patients, even though this hospital is the center for the South Community Mental Health District.  (9:2C:5)

Whether the emotional reaction to them is anger, disgust, or shock, one of the things that these discoveries of back region reality have in common was that they tend to be what Schein calls "upending experiences"[12]. An upending experience is a deliberately planned or accidentally created circumstance which dramatically and unequivocally upsets or disconfirms some of the major assumptions which the new employee holds about himself, his company, or his job. Although upending experiences can occur every time a person is socialized into a new position or a new organization, they are especially traumatic for a new graduate. In subsequent career positions, a certain amount of learning has taken place as a result of prior upending experiences and a newcomer is better able to read and respond to environmental cues and clues. But for the new graduate, upending experiences are especially trying and can well have a permanent effect. A typical example is given in the following excerpt. The nurses in the seminar had been talking about a young patient who had a total bowel obstruction. She had come into the hospital with appendicitis a year ago and something had happened. She now had only 10 feet of bowel and no pelvic organs because she had had so much radiation that everything was destroyed. One nurse exclaimed:

And she's just a 13-year-old kid! You know, I mean, what do you do with a child like that? She's had 27 operations and nothing helped her. There's nothing more they can do for her. If she were an adult she wouldn't have even survived . . . It's all so depressing. I try to talk to the staff people, and I say, "Well I can't blame Tracy for being like this because I would be *worse* if I were in her condition." And they say, "Well, you feel like that at first but then you'll see . . . " And they bring out all these arguments and what can you say? . . . Now I've *dealt* with this child for four months and she is manipulative, and screaming, and whining and carrying on. . . . And the staff is angry because it's [a special tube feeding] not working. And they're angry because they've got her there, and there's nothing they can do. And I can really sympathize with the staff now, because I'm the staff! . . . I mean, they never told us about *that* in school . . . And I'm so shocked at the change I see in me and my behavior.   (3:2A:21)

## Coping with Backstage Reality

Individual self-presentation or impression management can be changed or altered at almost a moment's notice. Were it not for the human desire to be somewhat consistent in our social interactions, we could literally manage and individualize the impression we convey to each person with whom we come into contact. The same is not true when we are or aspire to be a member of a team, such as a unit staff. Sooner or later a newcomer must come to terms with these back region discoveries because what are back region discoveries to the newcomer or outsider are reality to the "in" group. When the new graduate "discovers" what are areas of impression management to other audiences—patients, physicians, front nursing office—she is no longer in the posture of audience member but is now in that no man's land between being a member of the group and its reality and continuing to be an outsider. Her dilemma rests on the question, "Do I accept this reality and, if so, to what degree?" The reality that is accepted presents role expectations for self and others. Nonacceptance of reality ("What the group thinks is good nursing care is not what I think") is often the stimulus for engaging in some kind of activity as an agent of change. But since one's nonacceptance of the group's reality means one's nonacceptance *by* the group as a member, it is difficult if not impossible to bring about change.

In coping with backstage reality, one must deal with two levels. On the first level is the understanding or acceptance of the backstage reality as reality. In other words, the newcomer has to come to terms with the realization that what she is seeing and perceiving is true, that she is not mistaken in her interpretation of what is going on.

> I think the hardest part for me was getting it through my thick skull that this was really it . . . the things I was seeing—like the unsterile gloves and the meds without an order and all—that this was the *real* nursing care on this unit.   (6:4A:12)

In all likelihood, the movement from the shocked reaction to what one was seeing to the acceptance of one's perceptions as reality is what marks the transition from the moral outrage phase of reality shock to a comprehension of backstage reality as a phenomenon. However, accepting that what one is seeing is reality is not necessarily the same as accepting that view of reality for oneself, of accepting the procedures and standards of the back region's definition of nursing. The new graduate may still find it difficult to change her professional standards even after she has begun to understand the necessity for change.

Because of the larger patient load, your priority setting kind of changes, I guess. Because you think when you're in school that you'll get all the idealistic kinds of things done, that, "Well, gee, the patient is really important and, you know, emotional needs are just as important to me as physical"—but realistically when you get onto the floor and you have eight or nine patients and critical people who just require a lot of technical kind of work, you just can't do that. And it *is* frustrating! And, you know, it's just a real dilemma between what you've been taught and sacrificing those things—priorities that you have been taught in school—against priorities that are needed. (4:1:2)

There was considerable evidence that new graduates went through a sifting and weighing process in their attempts to cope with the reality they had discovered.

Some of the things that I find cause my frustrations are that the things that were so strongly stressed in school are not the things that are stressed or are different on the floor with their routine. On the floor that I'm on there are a lot of trachs and laryngectomies and the tubes need to be changed. We were taught that the technique had to be just perfect and here they aren't . . . the rationale for what they do is that the patients are going to go home and be changing their own tubes so they're doing it and teaching them the way they're going to be doing it at home. Well, when I think of what cultures come off of the tubes and they're just, you know, picking them up with their hands and no gloves or anything, at first, I just couldn't believe it, and then I thought, "Well, I'm not sure; I will really think on this matter" . . . But the way it's done is that you don't use any gloves—you try to be clean about it and each day the tubes are changed, but there's a lot of play with that. You don't have to lay them out, you don't have to tie them and strip them, and it's just little things like that, you know, that come up. And the other nurses say, "Well, you learned differently in school, but we do it this way here." And yet, that way conflicts very much with what I think to be right or what I think should be done and I say to myself, "Well, maybe they found this works best with this type of patient." Yet, I say, "Well, based on principles and all this, I don't think this is right," but then I say, "Well, how do you change it?" or "Can you kind of compromise so that you feel comfortable and that you're doing a good job, yet, you're not bucking the whole system, especially being someone new in the area or on the floor." (5:2B:12)

People do things that you're really not sure they should do, like in IV therapy . . . and the things people do to CVP lines when they're not running. You know, like sticking a syringe onto the stopcock to try to get the blood clot out, try to get the blood flowing out, get fluid, you know. I'm not going to do it but at the same time, I have to say to someone, "I can't get my CVP line to work." And they go in and do it anyhow. So you know . . . The doctors do it too—put a syringe at the end of the intracath. I mean I see it pushing the clot right through. You're standing there trying to look calm so the patient doesn't realize you're doing such an awful thing . . . then when you go up to them and say, "How can you do that? I always thought you couldn't do it for this reason, and that reason." And they'll give you some explanation that at the time you can say makes a lot of sense. But somehow, you know there's still something wrong with it somewhere, because you're not supposed to do it.   (3:1A:34–35)

While in some areas there is sifting and sorting, in others we hear some sounds of beginning acceptance of very common backstage realities.

With some doctors we feel comfortable enough to write the orders. Well, I don't—I don't do this but one nurse has said that she will—especially with this one particular doctor. She will just write down a laxative order as a telephone order when she didn't really call him. But he will come in and co-sign it. He will. He really gets mad when you call him up and say someone wants a suppository but he'll come in and co-sign the nurse's order. If you put LOC and put "TO Dr. (X)," he'll sign it.   (2:2A:22)

Even when new graduates began to conform to the team's performance or began to think about accepting the team's standard operating procedures, they often hesitated to admit to their new graduate seminar colleagues that they were conforming. Sometimes it seemed as though they were testing the response or reaction of the group before making a clear-cut statement as to whether or not they agreed with the back region practice that was counter to some deeply held school-bred conviction.

In the following excerpt, as in the diary entry quoted earlier, we see a clear indication that a new graduate has accepted some practice in the back region as her own.

I found it hard when I started here after school to learn how to establish the right priorities with patients. Because when you're in school, you only have one or two—you can really give them total care, and it isn't hard to establish priorities. But I found it difficult when I have eight or ten or whatever, to not try to give them the total care that I had been taught to give. And it took me a while just to relax and not try so hard.   (3:2A:24)

Not all new graduates reacted to the backstage reality discoveries by accepting the status quo. Notice how aware the nurse in the following excerpt is of the whole image impression process. Although she is attempting to do something about the reality she has discovered, she is still quite aware of the need to maintain the patient's good impression of the team. She's trying to change or influence the backstage reality of the team (physicians as well as other nurses) but, at the same time, to continue the unified performance of the team before the patient.

It's really a problem. The doctors don't wear masks when they are changing the dressing, but we have a solution as far as the doctors are concerned. In the morning, I asked a doctor if he wanted to see the dressings. And he said, "Yeah, what time are you going to do them?" So I said 2:00 P.M. and he said, "Fine" and he was there, so before we went in, I put on a mask and handed him one. It's something that's really important, wearing a mask, and I want to show that I'm a good nurse and do it. You can't tell the patient, "Don't let them change it without a mask," but so many of the other nurses do it without a mask. I don't know, I think it's important, but I feel the pressure from them that it isn't that important and I don't need to wear a mask, and I feel like the patient is getting double messages. Sometimes he looks at me kind of funny when I come in with a mask on. (4:4:30)

## Suggestions for Handling of Backstage Reality

Many newcomers are more distressed with the feeling of "I've been sold a bill of goods by my previous instructors" than they are with the discovery of the actual backstage realities. A second difficulty in handling backstage reality is the slowly dawning realization of the complexity of the phenomenon. Awareness of the multiplicity of roles and of the conditions for movement from front to back region does not come all at once. A cloud of confusion often compounds the negative feelings with which many new graduates respond to their discoveries of backstage reality. Another source of difficulty is the somewhat sudden realization of some of the positive or functional aspects of the image management phenomenon. What at first may have felt coercive, the new graduate now discovers she is using for her own ends.

*Initial discovery and feelings generated.* Strong feelings can immobilize a person, distort perceptions, and divert much-needed energy. For these reasons it would seem highly desirable to acquaint students with the whole process of image management and the backstage realities they are likely to encounter. For many faculty, who have had little work experience themselves, this will be difficult to do, because they themselves may not have been initiated or exposed sufficiently to the backstage realities that exist. Other faculty may have remained fixated on the surprise of backstage reality and may not have progressed toward handling and coping, and thus will also find it difficult to increase students' awareness of the process and phenomenon. Still others may be quite well aware of what goes on in the back region, but may be so disgusted by the seeming deviance of it all that they suppress or deny its existence. Probably large numbers of faculty of schools of nursing are aware of the existence of backstage reality practices—possibly not in the hospitals where they teach, but rather in former places of employment. Finding these backstage practices to be at odds or markedly deviant from the values and mores promulgated in faculty meetings, on answers to test items, preachings from the lectern and so on, they suppress this knowledge and teach only the "shoulds" in pure form. Because of faculty attitudes, it is very difficult for the young student either to learn of the existence of impression management and backstage reality from the faculty, or to learn how to handle and cope in a way that is constructive for her and her ideals.

We must stop pretending that backstage reality does not exist. Moralizing and evangelizing about its awfulness and incorrectness will not make it stop or go away. We must come to terms with the fact that impression management is a normal process of social interaction that is functional. Help students to live and function effectively in the real world of nursing by preparing them to meet it.

How best to prepare them? First, acknowledge the existence of back-stage practices. Give students some examples of differences between the general principles they have been taught and the practices they are likely to encounter in the work world. Do not teach a wholesale rejection of backstage reality practices, but rather help the student to look at the pros and cons, the advantages and disadvantages of the practice for the nurse, the patient, and the people with whom the nurse must work. Help her to see that all of these factors must be balanced.

There is a little doubt that getting a renewal order from the physician for a pain drug which has automatically been stopped after 48 hours is the safest practice for both the nurse and the patient. However, if the nurse discovers at 3:00 A.M. that a narcotic should have been reordered and wasn't, and the patient wants something for pain, what is the nurse to do? Many nurses will make a judgment and give the medication without calling the physician. New nurses tend to be unaware of this practice initially and even when they discover it, they do not have sufficient experience or information to make a judgment as to what to do. They wonder, "Do I call the physician, withhold the drug, or do I go ahead without an updated order?" Without experience and knowledge of the physician and of the situation to balance with her knowledge about drug and legal limitations, the new graduate is at a disadvantage, both in terms of analyzing what must be done and in evaluating the backstage reality practice. Students need to know that these practices exist and then need to know how to make decisions about their own actions when they enter the backstage.

Acknowledging backstage reality is a difficult task for a faculty member. Presenting students with backstage practices means presenting practices that are against the values that the faculty have been teaching. However, the student will inevitably meet these challenges and be faced with the task of sorting out her standards of practice. Take for example this exchange from a new graduate seminar:

> It's very difficult for me to sit back accepting some of the practices I think are wrong and that I don't agree with.
>
> Can you give us an example of what you mean?

Like starting an IV and using the same needle after it's gone through the skin and been contaminated. You see people using this technique, and I have to tell them that they should use a new needle, but they've been working for years!

What do you do?

Well, you know, you can be real tactful and offer them another needle. Or you can question them, pretending you don't quite understand. Is that okay to do? Like you were under the impression that maybe that wasn't a good idea (even though you really know it's not good technique). And they assure you, oh yes, that's alright. And you know it's not. And hopefully they know it's not . . .

But you've got to keep her from doing it?

Hey, wait a minute! If you do, you just make enemies and animosity. For the patient's benefit, I shouldn't be making enemies . . .

Is there anything else you can do?

Besides offering her another needle? No. She's been there for two years.

Maybe she doesn't realize. Maybe she's just not thinking. You could say, we've been taught you're not supposed to take the needle in and out. Can't you see that this is a way of contaminating the patient? . . . Because she couldn't deny that. It has to be basic, really.

Well, however, doctors do that often. I've seen doctors do it, so maybe she's seen that and thought it was okay.

[silence]   (6:2A:6)

If, after reading this conversation, you are left with a feeling of confusion, indecision, concern for the patient, but bewilderment as to what on earth you should do—both in terms of your own practice and in terms of the practice of other nurses—then you've experienced the essence of the difficulties encountered by the new graduates in such a situation. They have been taught one standard (breaking through the skin contaminates the IV needle); this standard has frequently been reinforced by the inservice educator during the orientation period. But in actual practice, the newcomer observes other, more experienced nurses not follow the standard; and furthermore, the physician, who really should know whether it is harmful to the patient or not, also does not uphold the standard that was taught.

In many instances, the standards taught by the faculty in school were not tempered by reality. Part of the maturational crises which all new graduates must undergo is deciding which of the values and standards taught by the School of Nursing faculty are truly integrated into self as nurse, and which were only temporarily borrowed from the faculty and do not exactly fit the newcomer's practice. Each person must decide for herself how to handle backstage practices. In this sorting out process the temporary community afforded by these new graduate seminars was of

almost unimaginable help. The leaders could see it happen over the passing weeks. From the initial week's "It's just terrible sticking the patient
twice with the same needle!" to the beginning questioning by some members of the group, "If it's so harmful to the patient, why is it everybody
does it?" or "My heavens, on some patients you would use 5 or 6
needles!" and then later on, "I think maybe you have to look at the
individual patient and figure out how much resistance to infection they
have. I'd never stick a leukemic patient twice with the same needle
. . . but, some other patients, yes, I would." In discussing a practice
such as this, the new graduate sorts out her values and standards and
gauges the effect and reaction of her peers to her statements, either maintaining old standards, or beginning to build new standards that are truly
hers.

Whether this sifting and sorting should all be done *after* one enters the
reality scene is a real question. Helping students to sift through their
standards of practice is not a way of encouraging students to practice less
than ideally but, rather, it is helping protect standards and principles.
Since the process will happen anyway, it is far better to provide guidance
for it than to leave students to figure out for themselves what is going on
after they enter the real world of practice.

*Awareness of the complexity of the phenomenon.*    Often it seems as
though the newcomer begins to get a grasp of the situation only to find
that it is far more complicated than it seemed at first. The signals and
messages are not at all consistent and clear. In some of the excerpts presented earlier which describe the new graduates' awareness of moving
into the "inner circle," of moving from an audience role to a participant
role in the back region, the messages were clear and overt: "We've
decided to let you in," "Here are the keys to the closet." More often the
messages are cloudy and inconclusive: "I don't know what I did, but all
of a sudden I realized I was in."

It would probably be helpful to new graduates if older staff were
advised to decrease the complexity and lack of clarity of the image management phenomenon. Make it clear to the new graduate what she must
do in order to be trusted and to take her place on the team. Make some of
the planning for team performances more overt and more easily understood by the newcomer. All of these things might help, but they are not
going to happen. Deliberate planning and clarity is not in the nature of
informal social processes. More often than not, people are socialized into
individual or team performer roles or into audience roles without ever
being consciously aware of its happening. Because of the nature of the
process, much of the action must come from the newcomer. This is not
to say that those in practice can ignore the backstage activities in the
work world. Nursing service organizations need to examine the practices
within their institutions and make judgments about these practices. If

backstage practices exist which are at odds with the standards of practice espoused, then the practices need to be corrected or the standards examined for their appropriateness.

It has been stated in the preceding section that it is probably impossible or undesirable to deny the process of image management. This does not, however, mean that one must accept or approve all of the backstage reality that one discovers. The new graduate can be immensely helped to deal with backstage discoveries by understanding the framework of impression management. Possessing a cognitive framework which one can use to analyze and interpret what is going on is extremely helpful in lessening the confusion caused by the simultaneity and multiplicity. Such a framework for analysis also helps one to dissect the events or problems causing confusion.

> The head nurse just stood there nodding in agreement while this patient goes on and on about what a wonderful doctor she has . . . And she [the HN] and I both know that Dr. Celebrity is absolutely incompetent. I think that's a terrible thing to do to a patient!  (4:2:12)

Here the new graduate expresses shock and confusion at the discovery of conflicting aspects of backstage reality. As a nurse, the new graduate performs as a member of the team as well as an individual, and at times the two performer roles are in conflict. By recognizing that the team performance when presenting a certain front is in conflict with her individually desired impression, the new graduate is in a position to handle the conflict. By dissecting the event, the new graduate can examine alternative actions. Do I go along with the team performance? Do I enact a patient advocate role and uncover the team performance with the patient? Should I go along with the team performance in front of the patient and confront the team afterward? What are the consequences of the alternative means of handling this backstage reality? The new graduate who can dissect the backstage events can then choose to act based on the situational ;ssessment of what will be best for all involved.

Another example of how a cognitive framework can allow for dissection and analysis which lead to more effective action and intervention is the following excerpt from the seminars:

> Almost every single one of our patients—especially the older ones—come down with decubiti all the time, and there are so many ways to prevent pressure sores. I know they are on bedrest the whole time but it just seems like the care that is given, if they were given a little bit more and a little better care like they should have, we wouldn't have so many . . . I found that there is this one aide in particular. She tells me how well she does patient care and I really believed her until one day I went in and checked how she was doing—she had been commenting about the evening shift and the night shift and how poorly they take care of all the bed sores and things—and she was just as bad as everyone else. She was talking but that was it. (2:1A:10)

Here we see that not only is the new graduate a performer in impression management, but others manage the impressions she receives. Auxiliary workers often carefully portray a backstage image to the registered nurse audience. New graduates, because of their newness to the organization, are often taken in by these performances. A new graduate who understands backstage reality is in a better position to analyze events. If a patient has a decubitus ulcer that is getting worse despite reports of appropriate care, the new graduate can use her observational skills to further examine the situation. By observing the care, she can determine if the treatment plan is at fault or if she has been an audience for impression management. Furthermore, if the event is impression management, is it an individual performance by the aide or is this a team performance? Once the new graduate analyzes the situation, she is in a position to intervene appropriately. Unless she has a cognitive framework from which to examine events, she may be confused by the complexity of backstage reality.

Part of the confusion of the new graduates' experience when encountering the backstage is caused by their inability to differentiate between poor practices and different practices. Just because a particular nursing practice is different from what you were taught, it is not necessarily wrong. One way of helping students make this distinction is to help them analyze the advantages and disadvantages of a practice, to become knowledgeable about the risks involved in a situation, and truly to look at the consequences. What is the probability of causing an infection if an IV needle is stuck through the skin twice? How does the probability of this risk compare to disadvantage of increased cost in using more needles, or of running to get more needles if you do not happen to have one in the room, or of delaying the start of the infusion? In educational settings, we tend to build a subtle priority system in which safety and prevention of infection are at the top of the list—to be guarded at all costs—and nurses' time and energy are at the bottom of the list—of limited concern. In the work setting, the newcomer often finds that in backstage practices, this priority system of risks and consequences does not hold up. Not all possibilities of infection are placed at the top of the priority list; nor is time always at the bottom.

With a framework for the whole image management process, one is in a position to pick and choose the aspects of backstage reality that one will accept, and those one will reject. With this knowledge a person is also in a position to identify, analyze, and weigh the consequences that will ensue if one chooses to reject or attempt to change some of the backstage reality.

*Useful aspects of image management.*    Managing the impression that others receive of us or deliberately trying to shape the image that someone else receives of reality is a normal, everyday occurrence that most of us engage in, either consciously or subconsciously. The reaction of anger, shock—"Oh, I'd never do that"—that many readers might have experienced is also common among new nursing graduates. This reaction is not infrequently accompanied by a staunch determination: "I won't play their silly games." With time and more exposure and experience, there is a cooling down, and then all of a sudden one day the newcomer becomes aware of the fact that she has fallen into step with the team performance, or that she is consciously trying to manage the impression that others receive of her. Along with this realization comes the discovery that there are aspects of image management that are exceedingly functional for achieving one's goals. There are also the adaptations of practices that make our world a more livable, workable, and enjoyable place.

Also functional are the performances that the nursing staff as a team put on for various audiences. They encourage the presenting of a united front, particularly at stressful times, or to persons under stress, when portrayal of discrepant or nonuniform information would particularly add to the stress. There is also benefit derived from the saving of time. Consider for example the tremendous amount of time that would be consumed if each member of the nursing staff attempted to find out what was actually holding up the x-rays of a complaining patient instead of using some of the pat responses usually given by the team: "Oh, it's Monday; X-ray is unusually busy because of the build-up over the weekend" or "The emergency room is busy and that always puts an extra load on X-ray." It doesn't take long before a newcomer comes to the realization that if the real reason X-ray is behind is because someone arrested down there or had an allergic reaction to the dye, these true reasons are never told to the patient, anyway. Most nurses feel that this type of impression management is best for the patient.

The point of all this is that at some time or other the new graduate comes to realize that what at first was very distasteful to her now has become a much more accepted part of her practice, and furthermore, she feels somewhat guilty about seeing the usefulness of this impression management. Concomitantly, there is the realization that there is a functional need to be a part of a team effort, and that there are times and instances when it is more functional and best for the team for the individual to submerge personal values to the team effort.

The real problem with the usefulness of backstage reality is the judicious choosing of what is useful and acceptable practice and what is not. Many new graduates more or less acquiesce to the practices they see. After the initial shock and surprise, there is a capitulation of one's values and standards and adoption of those prevailing in the environment. Sometimes this is done with the idea, "I'll do it their way for awhile, but then I'll go back to doing it the way I was taught." This kind of temporizing is unwise; many new graduates related that the backstage reality practices become habit and if adopted quickly, they are seldom, if ever, reevaluated.

Other new graduates adamantly refuse to accept *any* of the practices discovered that differ rrom their own way of doing things. The probability is very high that these individuals will find themselves permanently in the out-group, always swimming upstream against the current.

And yet another group of new graduates do learn to differentiate between poor practices and different practices; do learn to sort out standards of practice, assess consequences, and evaluate each practice before adopting it as their own. This last method of handling backstage reality in all probability will have the highest payoff for both the patients and the nurse. The acceptance of backstage reality practices moves the practices into the arena of role expectations, the next subject area to be presented in this chapter.

But even with the method of handling backstage reality described in the previous paragraph, what does the new graduate do when she has assessed the situation and determined that she cannot abide by the impression management performance and wants to alter it? This question sets the stage for the discussion of the subject area: change. If practices are going on that one judges are not for the benefit of the patient, and if one is disturbed enough by them so that they can neither be incorporated into one's own practice nor allowed to continue, then the most effective solution is to attempt to bring about a change in the practice. This is easier said than done.

## ROLE EXPECTATIONS:
## CONFLICTING, AMBIGUOUS, AND UNMET

> Joan really hasn't been here that long. But she used to talk to patients; now she doesn't. You try at first, but then you learn that there are things that just have to be done . . . You have to get your own goals and values straight, but unless someone else supports you in things, you are all by yourself . . . In two years, other new graduates will say the same things about us. We'll be in the same rut as everyone else.   (4:1A:12–14)

How sad are the consequences predicted by the new graduate above, the consequences of not meeting one's own role expectations. And this realization occurred after only five weeks of employment in her first job as a nurse. Surely, something can and must be done to help new graduate nurses deal with such unmet and conflicting role expectations.

Role expectation is a conception of how one should behave in a particular social situation. Not all of the role expectations verbalized by new graduates are necessarily accurate or legitimate. In fact, the process of assessing the accuracy and legitimacy of one's role expectation was one of the most beneficial processes stimulated by the peer discussions. However, because not all of the role expectations expressed were evaluated in this way and because a great deal of background and situational information is required in order to do this, role expectations will be presented in this chapter as if they were valid. Even if the conceptions and perceptions that the seminar participants relate are erroneous, they do constitute reality for these young people.

Beginning with a discussion of the place and importance of the subject area of role expectations within the various medical centers and the patterning of occurrence, the sections will proceed with some basic notions about role and role conflict to a presentation of a framework for the analysis of a role interaction or role episode. The Voices' experiences with role expectations will be presented within the context of this model so that the reciprocal and dynamic nature of role expectations can be seen and the consequences of role conflict and role adjustment analyzed. The chapter will terminate with suggestions of how problems and concerns in the area of role expectations might be handled.

Without doubt, the major concern of new graduate nurses is role expectations. This topic ranked number one in frequency of occurrence in six of the nine medical centers; number two or three in all of the others. Almost 20 percent of all themes discussed in the 93 seminar sessions revolved around the subject of role expectations. Most of these discussions (46 percent) occurred during the first two seminar sessions, but the pattern of occurrence for this subject followed the general patterns for the other subject areas, i.e., about 45 percent in the early seminars, 35 percent in the middle, and 20 percent in the last two seminars. There were no identifiable differences in patterns of occurrence for the various medical centers.

A total of 37 subthemes were identified under the subject of role expectations. Thirteen of these were positive, indicating in some way that role expectations were met or confirmed, or favored. For example,

Doctors take the time to teach nurses about patients.

Doctors respond to calls at any time.

Some patients want to take care of themselves and get well.

The frequency of occurrence for these 13 positive subthemes was 117. Two subthemes accounted for 66 percent of these:

Nurses help me out when I need it; we all work together.    $\dfrac{N}{46}$

Nurses are supportive of one another.    31

The remaining 24 themes, occurring a total of 304 times, were in a negative, disconfirmed, or unfavored direction:

Doctors are very difficult to get hold of when you need them, or they won't respond.

Nurses don't help me out when I need it.

Nurses don't follow through with nursing care plans.

Frequency was divided more evenly among such subthemes than among the positive ones, although the following subthemes accounted for the largest frequency of occurrence:

Others refuse or don't do the work I assign them.    $\dfrac{N}{28}$

Others perform their tasks incorrectly.    40

Nurses don't do all that they know should be done for a patient.    19

Others expect me to think or/and behave in a certain way.    18

Head nurse or supervisor doesn't do her job the way I think she should.    26

Role is a useful conceptual framework for the investigation of individual behavior within an organizational setting. It links the social structure of an organization with the personality of the individual. Although there are many definitions of role, the classic definition is that of Linton, who states that a role is what is created when a person puts into effect or action the collection of rights and duties which constitute a status or position. In this definition, as well as in the unitary conception of role developed by Levinson[13], there are three essential elements to the conceptual framework provided by the word "role." First, there are *structurally-given demands* (also called norms, expectations, taboos, responsibilities, and the like) that are associated with a given social position, say the position of nurse. Second, there is the person's *conception of or orientation to* the part she is to play in an organization, in her job. And third, there are the *actions performed* by the people who are in the role. These three elements give rise to the three primary components of the concept of role, namely, role expectations, role conception, and role behavior. Although in actuality these three components are inseparable, they are frequently split apart for conceptual analysis. And that is what we will do here. Our primary focus will be on role expectations (the formal and informal demands of the nurse's job), but we will also talk about role conceptions (what you think the job of a nurse is) and role behaviors (what the nurse actually does).

The role expectations one holds or verbalizes reflect the holder's conception of the role. Role expectations both guide a person's actions and provide meaning and explanation to the behavior we see her perform. If I hear a nurse saying, "I think someone should be in there with a dying patient and his family," her expressed role expectation tells me that this nurse's concept of the role of the nurse includes "support during crises." This expressed role expectation also guides the nurse's action as well as explaining to others the meaning of her behavior when she foregoes doing her charting and spends the rest of the evening in the room with the patient and his family. We can see, therefore, that role expectations are pivotal in the interaction process. When they are expressed, they reveal a great deal about the individual and her role value system. When role expectations are met, they confirm these conceptions of the role. When they are not met, they negate the role conception. On the other side of the interactional process, expressed role expectations are also pivotal. Not only do role expectations guide our own behavior, but the role expectations we feel from others (also called role pressures) shape our behavior. When I send out messages to another nurse that I expect her to perform the role of nurse in a certain way, these perceived messages act as a stimulus to her to perform her role the way I want her to. The stronger the message I send out, the greater will be the pressure to conform and the greater will be the shaping of her behavior. When the role expectation messages that I send out contradict her conceptions of the nurse role and hence the role expectations that she has for herself, then role conflict will result for her. This is the simplest and most basic form of role conflict. There is, however, a great deal of theory and research on role conflict which has led to a delineation of various different kinds of role conflict. Although the feelings evoked by these different kinds of role conflict are probably the same, it will help us in our analysis if we understand the different sources and different kinds of role conflict.

First, there is what is called "interrole" or "role-role" conflict. This means conflict that results when a person holds two or more roles simultaneously and the expectations of one role conflict with the expectations of the other—for example, the conflict experienced by a person who is both a nurse and mother. Her child is going to be in a school play at 4:00 P.M. and expects her to be there to see him. At 3:25 P.M., an emergency admission comes in and the nurse feels she must stay over and take care of him. This nurse-mother is now in "role-role" conflict.

A second type of role conflict is "intrasender" conflict. The role sender is the person who sends out expectation messages in intrasender conflict, delivering a double or contradictory message. Say, for example, a nurse's aide tells the new graduate that she wants her immediately to give some pain medication to her patient, but at the same time, tells her she wants her to help her turn one of the patients.

For any person in a role, there is more than one group of role senders. For a nurse, not only do all the nurse's aides on the unit send role expectations messages, but so do the other nurses, the head nurse, the ward secretary, and also the physicians. "Role-set" is a term given to the pattern of relationships and accompanying role expectations that all of one's colleagues have for a person in a role[14]. Many times the role expectation messages sent to a new graduate by the head nurse conflict with those sent by the nurse's aides, or with those sent by the other nurses. The conflict caused by different role expectation messages from different members of one's role-set is called "intrarole conflict."

A last type of role conflict experienced by many nurses is called "self-role" conflict. This happens when the expectations of the role are in opposition to one's need-disposition, as when a nurse who "can't stand the sight of blood" takes the role of nurse in an operating room or recovery room and encounters the common role expectations of cleaning up blood.

An understanding of role conflict is helpful since role expectations alone seldom present a problem to a person and it is only when role expectations are incongruent in some way or when they are not met— when some kind of role conflict occurs—that they become of concern. Role conflict feels the same, no matter what the source of the conflict is. So we cannot use our feelings as a guide to figuring out what is wrong. However, by understanding the various sources and types of role conflict, we are in a better position to analyze what is causing the problem, and then, of course, to work out some solution.

As we have seen, unmet role expectations (role conflict) usually occur within some kind of social context. The only type of role conflict that does not is the conflict between an individual's needs and the requirements of a job or role (self-role conflict). To understand the process by and through which a new graduate (or any person, for that matter) adjusts to the stresses of a new role, it is necessary to understand and to analyze that role within the social context in which it is embedded. In this way, we can see and study the whole process and perhaps figure out the vulnerable areas and offer some suggestions for coping with stresses in the area of role expectations. Kahn et al. provide a useful model for analyzing role conflict and the responses for coping with tensions which arise from role expectations being sent and received[15]. They make the point that an adequate understanding of the processes of an individual's adjustment to the stresses of an organization must consider many factors. They organize these factors into a model which has as its base a role episode, a role interaction which occurs at a given moment in time. This model, by providing a general understanding of a role episode, provides us with a way of thinking about a large set of factors and conditions in a very complex interaction. A role episode is a "complete cycle of role sending response by the focal person, and the effects of that response on the role senders"; Figure 5-1 illustrates the core of this model[16]. Looking at the model, we see that four events constitute a role episode: the experience and response of the other nurses (role senders) and the experience and response of the new graduate (focal person). Other nurses,

**Figure 5-1**

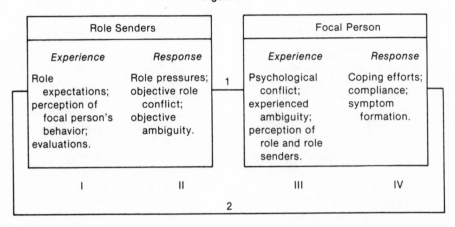

nurse's aides, et al. have certain expectations regarding the way in which a staff nurse role should be performed by the incoming new graduate. They also have perceptions of the way in which the new graduate is actually performing that role. As role senders, these colleagues consciously or unconsciously compare their expectations with their perceptions of her performance and then exert pressure on the new graduate to make her performance congruent with (or at least closer to) their expectations of the staff nurse role. These pressures perceived by the new graduate nurse induce in her an emotional experience and a rethinking of her role. The new graduate is aware that other nurses expect her to do certain things in certain ways. If these perceptions do not concur with her own conception of the nurse role, she will experience psychological conflict or emotional discomfort. This in turn leads her to make certain kinds of adjustments in her behavior—good or bad ones depending upon her past experience and upon her resources. The response of the focal person to the role expectations that others hold for her feeds back into the loop and affects the role senders' perception of the focal person's behavior, and the process begins all over again. In other words, when a new graduate reacts in some way to her perception of others' expectations of her (whether or not there is a conflict with her own expectations), this reaction or role behavior then alters in some way the other nurses' perceptions of her and how she fulfills her nurse role. These altered perceptions will affect their subsequent expectations of her in the nurse role. This loop is very important to understand in order to realize that the focal person does, in fact, have some control over what is expected of her. Many new graduates feel as though they have little or no control over what is expected of them, but that is not so. Their reaction to others' expectations of them does in a sense subsequently shape others' future expectations of them. The influence of this loop process will be discussed more later; but for now, let us use the role episode model to look at some of the role expectation experiences discussed in the new graduate seminars.

> I just couldn't believe it! Because in the middle of doing something—I had 6 or 7 patients—in the middle, she [the head nurse] came running up to me and told me, "You have to prep this lady's hip." And I said, "OK, who's going to take care of my other patients while I'm doing that?" because this lady was in traction and everything and it would take quite awhile. So I came back to her about an hour later and asked, "When is she going to surgery?" "Oh she's not going until after lunch." And this was at quarter of eight in the morning when I'm trying to get vital signs done and things like that. I got very angry because she doesn't seem to know what things are important to tell you when. And when you know what's important but then she blocks you by telling you to do stuff that isn't important at that time it's a real problem. I don't know—it's so disorganized. I just hope things straighten out because I don't know what to do about them except to get angry. (3:4A:16)

The new graduate perceived that the role function of prepping the patient's hip was expected from her by the role sender, the head nurse (box I of the Kahn model). This perception was in the form of pressures (box II). Because the expectations of the head nurse differed from her own expectations of how a nurse should perform, she experienced conflict, both affectively in the form of hostility and anger and cognitively in the realization that both role functions could not be carried out simultaneously (box III). Her response to this conflict was to cope with it on an emotional level; deliberate remedial action was not evident (box IV).

In spite of the fact that seminar participants usually related their concerns about role expectations as an entire role episode, a deeper understanding can be brought about by separation and analysis of the meaning and consequences of the four segments of a role episode.

*Role senders: experience.*   A role episode starts with a set of role expectations held by role senders as to how a particular focal person should perform. There were many discussions in the seminars in which the new graduate nurses *as role senders* identified and clarified their expectations of a whole array of focal people with whom they worked. These focal persons included patients, physicians, other nurses, nurses in charge, nurse's aides, and in a very few instances relatives, visitors, and the system in general.

One of the dominant subthemes in the area of the role expectations concerned the role expectations that new graduates held of the other nurses with whom they worked. The following list is a sampling of the kinds of role expectations held—some of which were met, most of which were not.

1. Nurses should persist in getting for patients what they need—calling another doctor when they are not getting what you want from a first physician, for example.
2. Everyone should pitch in and help, especially in very busy times.
3. Nurses should admit patients properly, welcome them, interview them, make assessments, and so on.
4. Nurses should carry out procedures properly, do treatments ordered, chart accordingly—not let IV's infiltrate, not collect specimens.
5. Nurses should follow through on patient problems and care, including nursing care plans, oral and written reports, and so on.
6. Nurses should speak up to doctors and tell them what they think, judge, and assess.
7. All nurses should read charts and know about patients.
8. Nurses should support one another.
9. Someone should back you up when you want to challenge a procedure or person.

In the new graduates' own voices, some of these expectations of fellow nurses sounded like this:

> On our shift, it doesn't go both ways. I've set up so many delivery rooms for the other people and then when I need one set up, no dice. I asked somebody who wasn't doing anything to set up the delivery room for me. She opened the packs but didn't lay out the instruments or anything. Just opened the packs—big deal—and let the pan set out. So I take the patient in thinking the room was set up. And the doctor's going, "Where's the Zylocaine?" . . . And I was so frustrated because I expected that nurses would help one another and they don't. (2:2B:20–21)

> At times everybody works together. That's what pulls us through. I don't know how we could manage it, but the RN's help each other out. Like last night when the other girl went to supper, something went wrong with one of her patients, so I was down there when she got back. And one of my patients was kind of crazy and pulling her dressings off, so she went to my patient and before we ever found out what was going on with each other's patients, we were at opposite ends, but it seems like that worked out—to cover for each other—it worked out real well. People do work together. (1:3C:5–6)

There were a lot of comments—both positive and negative—from the new graduates relative to their expectations around the theme of 'support' from others.

> The staff I work with is really nice because they don't get mad at me. They are very good at pointing out what is wrong without making me feel this

big. So that's really good . . . And the nurse I was working with on the 3-11 defended me. The 11-7 said, "You should have done it this way and bla, bla, bla. But the 3-11 just stepped in and said, "What do you expect her to do when no one tells her what to do?" And she even took some of the blame herself. She said, "I did not tell you; I assumed you knew and I didn't tell you," which was kind of nice because she supported me and backed me up, which is really helpful.   (2:2A:5-6)

Another focal group for which new graduates as role senders held rather uniform and clearly articulate role expectations was the nurses who were in some kind of charge or leadership position—head nurses, supervisors, directors of nursing. The kinds of role functions they expected of this group included:

1.  Fair play and fair treatment for everyone

2.  Support

3.  Supervision to ensure that everyone does her job properly

4.  Interest in the patients

5.  Clinical competence

6.  Keeping the unit organized, running well, with correct priorities

7.  Proper orientation of new staff or to new procedures

Some of the above expectations are illustrated in the following excerpts:

In our hospital, the director of nursing doesn't stand behind her nurses as well as she should . . . She'll tell you one thing but then when she comes up against a patient, the patient is always right. I guess because they're in there paying their money and stuff.   (9:3C:22)

The head nurse never said anything at all about the pills or hypodermic being left at the bedside . . . I asked her once about it, and she said, "Don't worry about it; we always do it." *Really* she has that attitude; she doesn't really care. Same thing like giving medication and narcotics and stuff. She goes, "Just use your own judgment. If you think they can handle it, give it to them; if not . . ."   (4:2:16)

The first time it happened, I wasn't really aware of what to do when she missed her charting for the whole side of the ward. I mean, no midnight meds charted for the whole side. So, I went to both the head nurse and the supervisor. They just didn't think it was necessary to call the night nurse and ask her, you know, if the medications had been passed or not.   (4:6:16)

It's ridiculous! It's gotten to the point where she's asleep when the supervisor comes up at night, and the supervisor wakes her up and says, "Hello Daisy," and Daisy says, "Hello," and goes back to sleep.   (1:2A:21)

You can't offend the private doctors because they'll take their business elsewhere and the supervisor will really rag you out. You'll get no support from her. When I was working at this private hospital, I had a patient who was on Lasix and her K had been 2.5 and 3 for two days. And I was waiting for him to do something and he didn't do anything. She was getting jittery, you know, really weird. So I called him up on the phone and I explained her symptoms and the lab reports and all and I said, "What do you think about giving this lady some potassium?" Well, he went and phoned the head nurse after I'd gotten off the phone (by the way, he ordered the potassium) and yelled, "Who's that nurse and what's her name; I want her reported." And then I really got it. "You don't talk to doctors like that here" and all this kind of garbage. And I thought I was real nice about it. Because I didn't say I think she needs 20 meqs of K!   (9:3C:17)

Of all of the leadership positions in the hospital organization the one that was the most unclear to the new graduate nurses was that of the supervisor. Although in some instances they did voice clear-cut expectations, there was also evidence that their previous experiences provided them with, at best, only very hazy conceptions of the supervisory role. These conceptions were then reflected in their unrealistic, inaccurate, or impoverished expectations of the supervisory role.

> I asked my head nurse just what is my supervisor's role and she goes, "Well, we've got a nice little booklet on what their role is, and you have it on your unit." She was very sarcastic; she said she really couldn't answer me what their role was . . . I know what I *don't see them doing,* and that's functioning like she cared or was concerned about what was going on with the patients on our unit. And like the head nurse said, she can't count on our supervisor to carry things out. If she wants something done immediately, she feels she has to go do it herself. The feelings I got were that she's not filling her role—whatever that is.   (7:2B:21)

> It was terrible! We had this emergency and the supervisor came and told me to tell the charge nurses that she would come back later. We really needed her and she split and never did come back. I think she should have helped us. I don't know what she's supposed to be doing if it's not that!   (7:3B:7)

One series of subthemes concerned the new graduates' role expectations of physicians. These tended to fall into two major problem areas. The first comprised specific items in which the doctor did or did not do what was expected for a patient. The other comprised incidents in which the physician did or did not treat the new graduate as she expected to be treated in the role of nurse or the role of woman. The latter problems were more general and diffuse, centering on the qualities expected in a relationship rather than the specifics.

> The OB men and us are just the same, but the anesthesiologists! They were in there and after we had worked and worked, the anesthesiologists came in and said, "Well, I'm going to take away all your pain; you're not going to feel it anymore." Just blew the whole hour we had just spent calming this person down . . . And you'd have to go and get all their supplies for them. It's their [anesthesiologists'] attitude. Like if their pen broke, they'd expect you to give them your pen.   (9:2A:24)

I had a patient this weekend who was from Germany and this girl has metastatic disease and is 26. I can really identify with her, you know, and she was three and a half days on a plane traveling down here and the oncologist knew that she was coming and all . . . I made seven phone calls before I finally got somebody to come and see her.   (1:2B:11)

The way that surgeons talk really pisses me off. "Well, we didn't find anything." They don't say "I know you must be relieved" or anything. They are very objective and noninvolved.   (7:4B:18)

Not all of the role expectations of physicians held by new graduates as role senders were negative or unmet. There was some evidence that role expectations of physicians were met. However, in contrast to the unmet expectations, note how global and nonspecific the reports were:

I really enjoy the patients, and the doctors are great. They answer all your questions; they're really nice; they'll talk to you all day because they're so involved in learning.   (9:2A:33)

A lot of the nurses on our floor really know what they're doing and the doctors rely an awful lot on them for observation of the patients. And they suggest something to the doctor in terms of what she thinks the patient might need, and he'll go do it. And stuff like that.   (4:2:21)

The only positive example of physician's role expectations that was specific was the following, and it's quite possible that this did not become an expectation of the physician's role function until after the event. This is, of course, one manner in which role expectations are altered. A role episode occurs; people behave; their behavior either fits our expectations or it doesn't. If it doesn't, we often modify our expectations so that the next time a similar role episode occurs, we now expect the new focal person in that role to behave according to our new role expectations.

It was sort of a pleasant surprise, because then after the patient died and the intern was out talking to the family, the attending man called and asked about the patient and I said, "Well, he's no longer with us," and the attending was real concerned about the intern and said to me, "Look, he's really involved in this and give him all the emotional support you can and tell him to call me if he needs any help himself or with the family." It was like everybody was really caring for everybody else. That's the way it should be.   (1:2C:15-16)

Role expectations of patients was not a major area of concern for new graduates, although it was discussed in the seminars. The kinds of expectations were mainly these:

1.  Patients should want to progress as rapidly as possible.
2.  Patients should not demand attention when other patients need it more.

3. Patients should practice health prevention and health maintenance; they should not wait to go to the doctor until it is too late or until all else has failed.

4. Patients should do all they can to take care of themselves, for example, cleaning their own dentures.

5. Patients should conform to the social expectations of the environment, for example, use the bedpan instead of the floor for defecation, not spit on the floor, not "shoot up" on the ward, not have intercourse in the open wards.

The following are some seminar excerpts which illustrate new graduates' role expectations of patients.

> I was giving report to the night nurse and I said, "Barbara's in again. She's really in bad shape." And immediately I get this, "I can't stand to take care of her." Well, it's true, she doesn't want to do anything for herself. She's an RN and she should know better. I can hardly even stand to go into that room. (9:1C:31)

> A lot of it is pretty hopeless. The trouble with my position is I don't really see how they recover . . . A lot of people wait so long I think, in the beginning because it could have been stopped and cured but as long as people wait—you read the chart and see that they've had weight loss in the past year and a half and the patient is getting progressively worse. Those are the things they shouldn't let slide by. I'm sure people were denying they were losing weight . . . but a lot of it can go on without you even knowing. I know I don't even have scales at home. A lot of these people come from lower income and they might not have scales or note changes in bowel habits and that type of thing. (6:2B:6)

The experience of the role sender—in this discussion, the new graduate—always includes an evaluative component, as well as the perceptual and cognitive components that have already been illustrated in many of the previously cited excerpts. The confirmation or disconfirmation of role expectations feeds back to help form the identity of a new nurse. When a person who is new to an occupational role such as nursing is just learning that role and is trying to establish her identity, both in her own eyes and in the eyes of others—when such a person encounters a situation in which role expectations she holds are confirmed in reality, it not only confirms the role, it confirms the self. For example, if a new graduate, after assessing a patient, makes the decision that the physician must be called, and the physician responds and initiates the kind of orders that she expects, the physician's role behavior not only confirms the new graduate's expectations of how a physician should act, but it also, and perhaps more importantly, confirms her self-image as a nurse. The external identity confirmation is of crucial importance for a newcomer to a field. It has long been established that such external confirmation must precede and form the basis for the subsequent internal identity confirmation[17]. The following seminar excerpt illustrates this process of role and identity confirmation and disconfirmation.

> The girl I worked on nights with—she's also new—had a patient die on her one night. The patient was hemorrhaging and she started a hemorrhage alarm in the middle of the night. She called the attending physician and he refused to come in, so she called the intern and went through the whole bit. And the lady kept getting worse and worse and she said that she felt like the doctor should be there so she called the attending again and he wouldn't come in. Well, by the time he got there in the morning, the patient had died. That's when she realized she'd been calling him up but it was her judgment she had to go on. And if something went wrong it was on her shoulders. She said she'd rather call and get yelled at than to have something really terrible go wrong. Which I agree with. If it's something you think could develop into a complication, it's not going to hurt to wake up the doctor. (1:2C:14)

> This kid was real sick and the parents wanted to know about their child and I didn't know. I called and called him. I felt very inadequate that I couldn't get the doctor to come in.   (5:3B:11)

> A patient started bleeding and I called almost everybody and no one seems to do anything. Finally I got the medical intern to come down. Both surgical residents were in surgery all scrubbed and they wouldn't come down, so finally the medical man came and he was really really nice and just ordered tons of things to be done right away and started the IV for us and that made me feel really good—that I had made the right decision. All the activity and things we were doing told me that I had been right in persisting.   (2:4A:12)

In the preceding section, we have seen that new graduate nurses as role senders possess and express quite clearly a wide range of role expectations for a variety of members in their role set. The expectations they hold for other nurses were most frequently expressed and centered around competence and support. Nurses in authority positions were expected to be fair, supportive, and organized in the running of the unit or service. Expectations of physicians focused on correctness of patient care and respect for the nurse as a nurse and as a person. Expectations of patients, although minor in frequency, centered around doing everything to get well or stay well. The last part of this section dealt with the very important function of confirmation or disconfirmation of role expectation in the establishment of nurse role identity for the new graduate.

**Role Senders: Response**

Role senders will behave towards others in their role-set—focal persons—in accordance with the expectations they hold of those persons' roles and with regard to some anticipation of how the focal persons are going to respond. The response behavior that is determined by those role expectations is usually manifested in the form of role pressures. As role senders, sometimes the new graduates expressed their role expectations as overt role pressures. (See for example the excerpt on page 000, when the nurse suggested that the Doctor order potassium.) On other occasions, the role expectation messages were more covert. The important point is that role expectations, no matter who held them, led to role pressures. Although it is not uncommon for a role sender to be relatively unaware that her behavior is in fact an attempt to influence another, both direct and indirect role pressures are perceived or felt by the focal person at whom they are directed.

The new graduates' seminar discussions reflected a range of awareness of difficulties in the sending of role pressures. In the following two excerpts we see that new graduates are aware of their role expectations, but there is little or no evidence of exerted role pressure.

> It's really hard to talk to an RN on the staff when she's five years older than you—to tell her that you think what she did was wrong. I ran into one—she had gotten the patient all the way up in bed. It was a hip patient and they are only supposed to be up 30 degrees. That was the first thing that I learned—that they are not supposed to be up more than 30 or not at all if they have a certain kind of surgery because the bed is too soft. I expect that she would know that. (2:1A:19)

> I had the urge last week. This doctor came in and he was doing a cut down, and he just took his tray and made a complete mess of the room; then when he got through, he took his gloves off and threw them on the bed and walked out of the room and he just went out and started drinking a cup of coffee, afterwards. I felt like going out and saying, "Look, aren't you going to clean up your mess? You really made a wreck of that room." (1:3C:3)

In the next two excerpts we see how the newcomer becomes aware both of the need to exert pressure if she wishes to have others perform their role the way she expects, and of the desirability of a united front in the application of such role pressure by members of the team.

> When I was on patient care the aides would come in and would say "I'm going on break," and they would just leave and if they still had work to do, I'd go do it . . . So I went in and did their work—not all their work—which didn't bother me to do. And then they realized that if they wanted to go on break or leave early that they could just do that and I'd cover. So, that wasn't the way to get them to do their work. (1:3B:10)

> Sometimes you'll see the aides in the tub room for two hours. They're gone at 3:00 P.M. when everybody else is there 'till 3:30, but they were the ones who had the heaviest assignment. I find it really frustrating because you don't get support from the other RN's. Nobody else will put her foot down. They all pussyfoot around or do the work themselves. I feel like I can't be

the only one to put my foot down. I feel like we make our own beds to lie
in.   (9:2A:35)

Once one is aware of the need to exert role pressure if one wishes some
focal person to enact role behavior that is consistent with the expectations one holds for that person, the next step is to exert such pressures
and to do so consistently. Here is where the newcomers expressed a great
deal of concern. The following rather lengthy excerpt is an excellent
example of multiple role pressures which a new graduate exerted on
another nurse. We see not only role pressure, but a great deal of role conflict and ambiguity on the part of the new graduate as role sender. She
was willing to exert some role pressure, but not extensively or consistently. The result is the sending of an ambiguous role message.

> She's just so incompetent. The two nights I was with her, she went home on
> time every morning, and I was there, I think one morning, a half hour over-
> time, and the next morning, 45 minutes overtime—cleaning up her mess!
> And I told the day girls, both days, I said, "I caught her on so many things
> she did wrong, and I'm just scared to death of the things I didn't catch her
> on." And what it amounted to was, I had a whole team of patients—post-
> op you know—responsible to do all the aide work for them, and take their
> vitals and all that, and also watching her every step of the way. And she's
> coming to me with some of the most obvious questions! Like, you know, in
> orthopedics, if a person's going to have a hip replacement, you don't give
> the injection where they're going to do the surgery. And you give the anti-
> biotics in two dosages because 4 cc's is too much to give in just one injec-
> tion. And you use ice. So she's, of course, giving the medication as the
> charge nurse, and there was this one patient on my team going to surgery. I
> just happened to go in to take his vitals, and there she was with her 4 cc's,
> no ice, ready to go right into the operative hip. I go, "No! Stop!" And I
> took her out and explained it and asked her if she didn't know. And she
> says, "I haven't given meds before." And I went, "Oh, no!" And so I
> asked her if she had done any team leading, and she said no, that she didn't
> like to do that, that she liked to do patient care . . . So then when it came
> time to tape, I said, "Well, I can tape for my side, but why don't you tape
> for the whole floor and get the experience?" And she goes, "No, I really
> don't need the practice." And I just wanted to *choke,* you know. And so I
> didn't say anything, because I thought that everyone was pretty well aware
> of what kind of nurse she was. I mean, I think she did great as an aide
> except for bedpans upside down, but everyone was aware of how she was
> doing. So I got a call last week, asking if I would fill out a performance
> note on her. And I wasn't really sure of what that was, so I said, "Well, I
> don't know; I have to think about it." And I looked it up in the procedure
> book, and it said, that when you fill one out, that one copy goes to the
> employee, and so I said, "No, I don't think I want to do that." Because
> she's really likeable; I think she tries hard, but it is like she's just kind of
> surrounded by a *haze,* like she doesn't really listen or realize what's going
> on . . . So, then the next night when I came on, they said, "You're being

pulled to go to West Ward." And that was going to leave her as the only RN on the floor. And I said to myself, "Oh, no; this just can't be." So I didn't want to call staffing right in front of her and say, "Hey, she's not capable," so I went over there and told them. And I talked to a coordinator on the phone, and she was really rude. She said it was that *I* didn't want to be pulled, and that wasn't the point I was trying to get across to her at all. What I was trying to get across to her was that this girl wasn't capable of having the unit all by herself. And she said, "Well you realize that you have to go where we tell you to go and you have nothing to say about it." So I just said, "OK, if that's the decision you want to make, that's fine." But then later, someone came out and told me to go back to my own floor.   (2:5B:20–22)

Besides direct, overt verbal role pressure messages such as, "No, you don't do it that way," a variety of other pressures were utilized to get other people to respond to role expectations. These varied from the use of people and tools in the system, to the calling of special meetings, to the use of "dirty looks."

I was having this problem, but I resolved it last week. Everybody seemed to go on break at the same time . . . Each time all the people would go on breaks—some of them would tell me and some of them wouldn't, and they would all be in there. And I'd look through the window and the whole staff was sitting in there, the RN's and everybody. I'm the only one out there on the floor answering lights. I went in to answer a light and the patient who needed to be fed and the tray had been there for like a half hour. There was cold bacon, and cold cereal, and everything was cold. So I started feeding her what she wanted off the tray, and I was the team leader. I had other things to do besides feed her, so I said, "I'll be back in a minute," so I went in there and I looked in the utility room and I just gave them the dirtiest look and everybody came flying out of there. It really helped! So I went back and fed the patient, and an LPN comes in and says, "Did you want me?" And I said, "Well, she needed to be fed," and she says "Do you want me to do it?" and I said "No, I've got it under control now." But it really helped. They haven't done it since. Just because I gave them the dirtiest look.   (2:4A:24)

We have the same trouble on our floor. I mean, they [the aides] hide—or take what they call "breaks" 10 minutes before they're supposed to be doing something they don't like to do . . . What we did was we had a conference on the floor . . . They had a conference with the assistants and they all came in, and the supervisor held the conference and she told them that the nurses want to know what they're doing wrong that the assistants were not cooperating with the nurses. That helped for about two days, maybe, they straightened up a little bit, but now it's the same thing . . .   (1:2C:22)

And no one on the old staff charts IV's. I go to hang a bottle and you couldn't even tell that the patient had an IV! One patient was supposed to have gotten two units of plasma and they wrote, "One unit, red cells." That was something I talked to our head nurse about in private, and she said to bring it up at the next staff meeting. It looked as though I had started the IV on that patient, because I charted that I hung a bottle. But I hadn't started the IV; it had been up for three days. And I don't like that! But the head nurse did nothing about it—just said to bring it up at the meeting . . . So I came in the next morning and looked at the chart to see if the same person had been on. So anyway, I find that all the meds were charted at 6:00 A.M. for the day before, but not to the date that's today. So I think to myself, did she give them today and chart them under yesterday? Or did she not give them today, but she gave them yesterday and post charted them? That leaves you not knowing what to do.   (4:2:11–12)

Just because role pressures were applied doesn't mean that they were necessarily effective in bringing about the desired role performance. In the following excerpt the role pressures applied were quite successful in getting the physician to comply to the nurse's role expectation.

I had a patient who was diabetic and we got his 4:00 P.M. blood sugars and it came back fairly high. He was still having sugar in his urine and so I called the doctor who was on call and he didn't do anything. He just wrote orders for tomorrow. I wasn't satisfied with that. I thought this man had to get some insulin now. He had 300 blood sugar and he had 3-plus sugar in his urine. I thought, this doesn't satisfy me, so I called the directory again and said, "I don't want to talk to the other doctor; I want to talk with the doctor I called because the first one didn't help us." She said, "No, you have to talk to the other doctor." So I said, "Well OK, I'll talk to him again." So I said, "Doctor, this patient has 300 blood sugar; his 4:00 P.M. urine was 2-plus and now at 10:00 P.M., it's 3-plus. I really think he should be getting some insulin." And he goes, "Well, OK, start the previous order I gave you tonight." And just as I hung up, the other doctor called, so we got plenty of things done. But I just wasn't satisfied with what that first doctor did. He did not do what I expected a doctor to do; he didn't seem to care. That isn't right. This guy's a diabetic who's always on insulin. He should be getting some more; he's going to surgery tomorrow.   (2:2A:20)

There was considerably more evidence of the effects of role pressure as it was applied to the new graduate, than when she applied the pressure. Shifting our conception from the new graduate as role sender to the new graduate as the focal person to whom others are sending role messages, we can examine the following examples of role pressure and its effectiveness:

As far as job satisfaction—there's no satisfaction coming from nursing. Because people make fun and say, "Oh, you got your beds made yet? They're so slow, you should be a minister, or you should be in guidance counseling. You sit and hold everybody's hand." And they make fun of you, and then you get the patients that are real belligerent or something, and nobody ever goes into the room. I don't really want to either, you know . . . But I'll make the effort to go in and get along with him. And other people say, "Oh, Trudy's our diplomat. Send her in." It's said more or less sarcastically, but sometimes, it's even said with resentment. (6:4B:22–23)

You don't want to have to be the one to say "Do we have to stay?" "Oh, no; go home." But then; you *feel* like a real you know what. When I worked here as an assistant, I never ever got out on time. But one time, we designed it so that every day somebody else would stay and cover while the others were giving report . . . Well, you know, I mentioned that the other night, and it didn't go over at all. It was like, "If you want to leave—go ahead. You don't have to stay." They say you don't have to stay, but you *do* have to stay. You just feel it. (3:1A:7)

You can be really busy and really working and really carrying it off well. And the supervisor will come up to you and say, "Did you distribute the water pitchers?" or something that's really insignificant compared to your other priorities. And you'll have to say "No" and she'll give you kind of a look and walk away. You know, you feel, I don't want to make excuses; I don't want to say "Well, I have a patient who came back from an aorta-gram, and I've got vital signs every half hour, and I've got another patient that's vomiting, somebody else's IV is running dry." That seems like excuses. (4:3:12)

I feel very guilty sitting at the nurses' station flipping through charts when people are running around going nuts trying to get all their work done. You're just sitting there and just look so cool, calm, and collected, and everybody else is working their tails off. And if you're sitting there cool, calm, and collected, they're probably thinking, "All she does is sit at the nurses' station and read the charts." Resentment builds up; so pretty soon you stop reading the charts. (9:2B:20)

If you do a care plan, they'll laugh at you; all the orderlies will laugh. You're sitting there writing and they'll go, "Ha, ha, wow, she's doing a care plan." They don't read them; it's just a joke to them. (9:2C:17)

I thought that she [the head nurse] did know that I was a new graduate, that she would be patient with me through my trial and error. And all this time she was expecting me to perform like a nurse who had been working several years. She didn't say that, but that's the feeling I received from her. (9:1B:7)

The newcomers differentiated between the way in which they wanted role pressure messages to be delivered to them and how they did not want them to come.

I think it's the way she comes across, you know. Like, if she had said it like, "Well, if I help you maybe we can get him up a little sooner," or "You just do what you have to do, but get him up as soon as possible," or something like that. But the way she said it, she made me feel that I was really slow. Well, I just headed off right there, you know. I was ruined for the rest of the day. It's the way she comes across. She makes you feel like that's not the way it's supposed to be done. And then she'll walk away and not give you any alternative. (6:5B:5)

Sometimes they "got the message" from the patient as well as the other staff.

> I didn't know how to empty the tubing and one of the other staff persons was there, and I was saying, "Well I'm just learning this," and the patient says, "Well, you're not a student, are you?" And I said, "No—well, I am in a way. I'm a new graduate; I just started." And the other nurse looked at me and said, "You're not a student any more." I said, "Well, I am in a way." And the patient just said, "You really aren't, period." I got the message that I was expected to perform as a nurse, not a student, but I really felt like a student because I was learning something I hadn't learned before. (3:1A:28)

But not all role pressure messages are unpleasant:

> The nursing assistants that I have been working with on evenings have been helping me to remember that I'm not an assistant up here. They'll say, "You go ahead. I know you have to go and do some more pre-op teaching. I'll take care of this. You sit down and eat dinner, now." Cause I worked for two years while I was in school as an aide and I'm just accustomed to being busy and when something needs doing, doing it, and not always remembering to delegate. And then I get caught behind. And you know, they'll say "Gee, we don't want you running late giving report or something. We like you to get out on time. Go do your job. We'll handle it." It's nice. (1:2B:24)

To understand the prevalence and nature of role pressures, the expectations behind the messages sent by each role sender in a role-set must be investigated separately. It cannot be assumed that role-set members such as nurse's aides, other staff nurses, head nurse, patients, and physicians are all sending the same messages or exerting the same kind or degree of role pressure on the new graduate. The degree of role conflict a newcomer will experience is dependent upon the total configuration of role pressures applied by all of these role senders. Likewise the clarity or ambiguity of a role is dependent not only upon the communicator, but also upon the availability of relevant information. If the new graduate is unfamiliar with the role of supervisor or does not know what it is a nurse aide can or cannot do, she is at a marked disadvantage in terms of exerting role pressure on these members of her role-set to get them to meet her expectations for their performance.

**Focal Person: Experience**

Continuing with the analysis of a role episode with the new graduate as the focal person (rather than a role sender), let us now consider how the total set of role pressures will affect the immediate experience of such a new graduate. This experience is perceived both cognitively and emotionally. The new graduate will come to know or understand what various role senders expect of her, and will also feel psychological conflict if these pressures are not in line with her own role conceptions. If other nurses, aides, and physicians are generally supportive of the new graduate's performance, she will probably perceive that support and her response will be primarily one of satisfaction and confidence. If, on the other hand, the pressures from her associates are strong and directed toward changing her behavior, or if some pressures are contradictory to others or to conceptions she holds, then the experience is likely to be heavy with conflict and ambiguity, and tension, anger, or indecision will be felt.

For many of the new graduates it is quite likely that role senders were communicating supportive messages. These experiences would be quite satisfying and positive, and hence, quite understandably, were not the instances that the newcomers chose to talk about in seminars. Therefore, no examples are available. There were, however, numerous discussions of conflicts engendered by unmet expectations, differing role expectations, or unclear and ambiguous role expectations. See, for example, the following excerpt:

> It makes me really mad! It really does, because I find the aides do it more than anybody. When the patient needs to be turned on the orthopedic floor you have to maintain their position. But they'll just take them and push them over, stuff some pillows under them and leave. They won't even ask them if they are comfortable. I've been in the room at times when the patients get these expressions on their faces and they don't want to say anything because they don't want to get anybody in trouble. But then, after I leave the room I say to the aide, "Didn't you notice . . . " and they say, "Oh yeah, but you can't be so compassionate that you spend all your time in that room." That's their excuse! . . . It's not that they don't know what to do; it's that you can't be compassionate! (2:1A:5)

The discussions of the conflicts experienced as a result of differential role expectations were almost equally divided between 1) those that emanated from differences between what the new graduate expected of herself and what she found she could realistically do in the work setting and 2) those from differences between expectations of self and what others expected of her. An example of the first kind of conflict is as follows:

> I expected that I would know things after I graduated. I thought when I was in school that when I got out of school I'd know the answers to the questions that I didn't know then . . . Today, one young girl of 19 died of leukemia, and another man who's 50 is dying and his wife asked me today whether or not she should bring the children in to say goodbye. And you know, I didn't know what to answer her. I don't know, which is what I told her, but, I just really feel bad that I don't know the answers to the questions that people are expecting me to know. (3:2A:2)

In the next example the conflict that results from differences between one's own conceptions of one's role and that perceived to be important by others and transmitted in the form of role pressures is evident.

> Like tonight was my all-time low. This is the first time I ever left work in tears. And I've been thinking about it all day today instead of sleeping, cause I couldn't sleep, and I have this big conflict with the attitude of the people that are in charge down here. I have this thing about everything being on the chart in case that chart goes to court, everything is there. I feel that if an order says "Vital Signs q 30," there should be vital signs on that chart every thirty minutes. And I'm always told, "Don't worry about it," or "Well, what do you want *me* to do about it?" "Well *I* can't do anything about it." When I ventilate how I feel . . . And I guess it's the attitude more than anything else that I just can't stand. I was ready to say, "I've had it!" So I had a talk with my coordinator this morning about transfer-ring shifts and I went up there in tears, so it was a little obvious that some-thing was wrong. So she asked me what happened. I say, "It's just the way I feel and when I get back the attitude—Don't worry about it; what do you want me to do about it?; there's nothing I can do, forget it." It's just such an inner conflict that I can't come to grips with it . . . Cause I had three patients I was watching, and I went in to start an IV for Susan and after I started the IV, I went to help Dr. Adams do an epidural on one of Marcia's patients. The whole time nobody's done anything for my patients. Two of them and no vital signs, no anything.    (2:6B:8)

In addition to rather clear-cut differences in role expectations which engendered outright conflict, there was also the problem of ambiguity. There were four major sources of the ambiguity associated with role expectations: 1) different expectations of different statuses or people, 2) different messages from different role senders, 3) unclear messages from the same role sender, and 4) shift in emphasis on whose role mes-sages to follow. The following two excerpts illustrate different expecta-tions because of different statuses or people:

> I'm being treated as a peer by all the RN's, which is a bit overwhelming since some of them have worked on the floor for three, four, five years, and I get treated just like I was equal though I know myself I don't have any of the skills that they have.    (4:1:5)

> I worked there as a nursing assistant; I'd worked as a temporary one day a week. But, you know, I need something just to get back into the feel of things. And it was like, "Oh, you know it." And it was funny, you know, because before that they really questioned that I knew different things . . . but the minute you come in as an RN, they really expect you to know everything."    (4:1:7)

In the next excerpt different staff nurses have different expectations of the new graduate.

It's very confusing. On evenings, when I work with (X) you know, I'm supposed to pass my own meds and all and really do everything for my wing,
make my own decisions, call out the docs myself, everything. But then
when (X) is on, oh, boy, watch it. If you do one single thing that she doesn't
know about, she'll be on your back.    (5:4:9)

Differing and unclear messages may come from the same role sender.

He told me to call the medical man, so I called him and he gave all the
orders. Then the next night, there was another patient having problems, so
since I knew he didn't want to be called, I called the medical man. But I
couldn't get a hold of him so I called this doctor and he says "I want all my
calls. She is my patient: I want every call." I mean you don't know what to
do. It just depends on what mood they're in . . .    (2:4A:35-37)

Sometimes there is a shift in emphasis as to whose message to follow.

I'm sick of doing, or trying to do my best all the time, but still feeling frustrated. According to the expectations of other staff, I'm doing a good job,
but . . . nobody has really spelled out any expectations to me. No one has
said anything to me about what they expect . . . In any new situation you
find yourself in, it's a matter of meeting others' expectations but primarily
meeting your own at first. But then the others', or rather my perception or
what I perceive others want me to do, gets in the way of me meeting my
own.    (3:5C:12)

The specific reactions of a focal person to a situation will be determined by what that situation means for her. Some new graduates found
ambiguous situations to be more troublesome than outright conflicts; for
others it was the reverse. In some situations, the nurse could respond to
conflict or ambiguity by attempting rational problem solving; in others,
particularly those in which the confict and tension were very severe, they
reacted with defensiveness, tears, or other coping techniques. The choice
of reaction was to a large extent affected by situational and personality
factors.

### Focal Person: Response

A person who is confronted with role conflict or ambiguity must respond
to it in some way. One or more role senders is applying pressure to get
her to change her behavior in some way, and she must cope with this
pressure. Whatever response the focal person adopts may be viewed as
an attempt to find or recapture some degree of job satisfaction. Coping
responses which people frequently use in situations such as this have been
identified. Kahn et al. discuss five[18]. A person can cope by 1) complying to the strongest force, 2) persuading the different role senders to
modify demands that are incompatible, 3) avoiding the sources of stress,

4) distorting reality so that the anxiety caused by the conflicting demands is relieved, and 5) forming emotional or physiological symptoms which help to relieve the stress. These five responses are somewhat general. Merton's ideas of how conflicting role expectations from different members of one's role-set are brought together build upon these five techniques but are more specific, and hence more helpful[19]. These will be used to look at the coping responses of new graduates experiencing conflict in a focal position.

First of all, the conflict situation is helped by different degrees of involvement in the relationship among the people who constitute the role-set. This means that because certain role relationships are more important to some people in the role-set than to others, the role pressures applied will differ, and hence it will be easier to ignore some of the weaker pressures. For example, when faced with a situation of two-hour vital signs ordered by the physician but deemed unnecessary by the nurse, and another patient's need for preoperative teaching, the nurse must make a choice as to which role pressures from the members of her role-set will take precedence. Depending upon which role relationship is more important to her—the physician or the patients—and consequently which role pressure is more effective—the physician or the patient—she makes a choice. The tension generated by the conflict is reduced with the choice and by concentrating future involvement with those members of the role-set whom the nurse has decided are more important to her. This differential attention to role-set members can also be seen *within* a role-set, as in the following example.

> It all depends on who's applying the pressure! If Dr. [X] wants something done . . . even though I think what I was doing is more important, I'm more likely to do it than if some other attending asks. What Dr. [X] thinks is more important than what the others think—to me it is.   (4:4:21)

A second way of decreasing the tension of conflict generated by differing role expectations and pressures is by considering the distribution of power of the people making the demands. Members of a person's role-set are not likely to be equally powerful in shaping that person's behavior. However, this does not mean that the persons or group most powerful separately are necessarily more successful in imposing their expectations upon the focal person. Coalitions of power may be formed which will make a difference in the use of power balance to relieve conflict. The counterbalance to any one powerful member of the role-set is at times provided by a coalition of lesser powers in combination. When conflicting powers in the role-set neutralize one another, the focal person may then have relative freedom to proceed as she intended to do in the first place.

There were no examples of the use of this social mechanism to allay or deal with role expectation conflict, although it is possible that power may have been a factor in the preceding excerpt if Dr. X was in a more powerful position than other attending physicians. Although the seminar participants discussed power quite freely—others' power over them and feelings of powerlessness being very common topics—there were no instances in which conflict reduction through differentials in power was specifically illustrated.

The third mechanism—insulating role activities from observability by members of one's role-set—was much more in evidence. Put in the vernacular of today, this means that when you feel conflict from differing role expectations, you do your own thing out of sight of other people.

> What do I do? When I'm in a bind, I just quietly go ahead and do it—even though I know others won't approve, I just go do it. Do you chart it? No. It's no big deal. (3:5A:13)

Calling attention to conflicting demands is a fourth mechanism that can be used to decrease the tension from this kind of conflict. As long as others in the role-set are happily ignorant that they are making incompatible demands on a focal person, each of them can press to get her own expectations met. The problem and the conflict therefore rest with the focal person. However, if the focal person makes known to all members of the role-set that these role expectations are conflicting and contradictory, the problem and hence the conflict are shifted, and tension on the focal person is eased.

> The staff that's up on 9 is really good, because at least I feel like, if I really want to just sit down with a patient, you know, and someone walks by the room . . . in other places I have felt like if I was sitting down and talking and another nurse or aide would walk by, she would say or think, "OK, she's really not doing anything" or something like that. But it's not that way up there. I was giving a guy his breakfast and he started to open up and talk, and the aide came and wanted me to help her turn someone, and the other RN wanted me for something else. *You just have to let them know all the things that the other people want you to do, as well as what you yourself want to do.* It was really important to listen to that guy. It's a matter of priorities and explaining, in a nice way, of course, all the different things that people expect of you. (3:1A:18)

A fifth mechanism used to reduce conflict caused by the different role expectations held by different people in one's role-set is social support by others in similar positions who are experiencing similar difficulties in coping with an unintegrated role-set. This mechanism presupposes the idea that others who are in the same position will have much the same kinds of problems in dealing with their role-sets. Another way of putting that is that hospital staff nurses all over the country will have similar problems in dealing with contradictory role expectations of respective role-sets—physicians, patients, other nurses, aides, and so on. Sharing of these difficulties, and the social support engendered by this sharing, permit a person to better withstand the pressures which depart from her own concept of her role. By so doing, this mechanism serves to counteract the instability of role performance which could otherwise develop.

It will be recalled from Chapter 1 that such peer support was the whole purpose of the new graduate seminars. There was considerable evidence that this social mechanism was used by the new graduates as an aide for coping with the conflict of differing role expectations.

> That one time; that did it. Someone said to me, "You can always say 'No'. " And I've learned to say "No" now. Now I know just where I can take off, just where I should be, and what my priorities are . . . You think first of the patient. That's why I was there till nine o'clock in the morning. I'm the one who changed the IV bottle; I was the one who added the med; I was the one that held her hand when she was crying; when she wanted something to drink, I was the one who gave it to her. And I should have been out there signing off my books and things like that. Because once you give report, the other nurses *know* what is happening and that they should take over. But they just disappeared. They were off in Room 1 and I was down in Room 20. That's where all the bad patients were . . . so I socked them for overtime. [laughter] That's the only compensation you can get, you know. No one is going to say thank you to you. But I felt that I was there when the patient needed me. That was my role. [general murmurs and comments of agreement]    (2:2B:25)

A last mechanism for coping with role expectation conflict is to disrupt the role relationship. This method of coping is possible only under special and limited conditions. It must be possible for the focal person to break off relationships with that member of his role-set who is placing the incompatible demands, and it must be possible to do this without damaging one's relationships with the other members of the role-set. This is not usually a mechanism available to a new graduate in a staff nurse position. It would be very difficult for her to break off role relationships with a nurse's aide with whom she was in conflict without damaging the relationships that she has with the other aides, her head nurse, and others. Its being difficult does not mean that it was not tried, however.

> I just couldn't stand it anymore. This aide I had to work with on nights thought she was the boss; she was the one in charge, and she expected me to do all the aides' work. I had to get away from her, so I told the head nurse that I would not work permanent nights anymore. Now all the other nurses are mad at me because they will have to rotate nights.    (7:5:12)

Although a few examples of coping mechanisms have been given to illustrate some of Merton's options, for the most part, the new graduates in the seminar discussions seemed unaware of the existence and range of such options. Their efforts to deal with the conflict and ambiguity of conflicting or contradictory role expectations were almost solely limited to 1) identification of a problem but with nothing they could do, 2) compliance to the force perceived to be the strongest, or 3) symptom formation. The following excerpts show the variety of situations describing identification but no coping.

Well, I thought about it because it made me really angry. I was running to the kitchen five or six times every mealtime and the people in the kitchen are always at coffee. Every time I walk by the coffee room, they're sitting there. Then I began to realize that I can't expect them to work as hard as I do. Because they don't get paid as much as I do. And you know, the conditions that they work in aren't really as good as the ones that I do . . . But, I don't know, I do expect them to do their job. And they don't and there's nothing that I can do about it. There's nothing. I called down to the diet kitchen one day because every day for a week, I'd been trying to get this special diet for the anorexic patient and couldn't get it . . . You can't get angry with the people in the kitchen either. You have to sort of send down good vibes, because otherwise, they won't do anything for you, or give you any special trays.   (3:3A:36)

There were patients that people don't really get along with. And it would get to the point that the attendants would say, "I won't work with that patient; I just will not work with that patient. I worked with that patient and I just can't work with him again." And they wouldn't even say it kindly. They'd say, "If you assign me to that patient, I won't do anything with him." And you just don't know what to do. If you reported everybody that did that, everybody would be fired. Not all, but a lot of them. (6:2A:26)

That is the hardest thing I've found coping with. The doctors you can't get to do anything. We had this one patient and her heels were breaking down; the doctor put her in a cast and now this heel cannot even be checked. She complained about her heel hurting and the other one was breaking down and you know, that the one in the cast is going to break down. And the nurses won't do anything about it. Being on shift, I don't get to talk about it to the doctors and I pass it on and ask the other nurses, "Did you ask the doctor about the cast?" And the nurse will go, "That is not my responsibility; the doctor will take care of that." And I am just dying because I know her foot is just decaying and the doctors don't do anything about it. That really upsets me . . . You're reporting and doing your nursing part but you can only do it so far. And the doctor doesn't even care, even though he did the surgery.   (2:1A:22)

This "what's the use, nothing can be done; I have to learn to live with it" coping mechanism seems to be entertained as a long-range style of coping.

I'd be really interested in hearing what you all think—there's this one person on the tape I listened to, where she said that the other nurses on her unit were more concerned with the technical aspects. The ones that had been there for a longer period of time weren't as concerned with the patients as they were with getting their work done. And I would be really interested to know, whether nurses that have been working two or three years have the same concerns that we are talking about, or are they just into a routine way of doing things. What are their feelings? Because we feel so frustrated, and maybe they still feel the same way but have just learned to live with it, or carry it around inside of themselves.   (3:3C:4)

Sadly, most of the other seminar participants agreed with the preceding conclusion that "Yes, you have to learn to live with it, to carry the tension and conflict around inside of yourself."

The second dominant pattern seen for coping with role expectation conflict and ambiguity was that of compliance. When one encounters conflicting demands, particularly those between the self and others in the role-set, the tension is relieved by complying to the role pressure of others.

I don't really know what you could do, because like I said, they tried assigning the attendants more patients, but they refused to do anything. They just go on the way they have been. They get the baths and stuff done in the morning and they help with some of the beds, but then as soon as they get their patients done (and that's well before noon with all of the nurses helping), the attendants sit back in the utility room and talk while we answer all the lights and try to get our charting and the treatments done . . . You can report it but if you push too hard, you're going to get nothing. When they work, they really are a big help.   (7:2B:11)

The tone of voice in which situations such as the preceding one were related would seem to indicate that the seminar participants were not particularly happy with this way of coping. Neither were they happy when their coping efforts resulted in symptom formation—their becoming physically or emotionally ill because of the conflict.

I asked the other nurse to help me and she said she didn't have time. It's "Well, I can't come now because I've got to do this and this." And then she said, "Do you know the procedure?" And I said, "Yes, I've seen it done." And she said, "Well, why don't you go ahead and do it?" And I said, "No, I'd like to be checked out on it first." So, it wasn't done; the procedure didn't get done! And the patient lost out, and I got so sick over it. I had a terrible headache when I went home that day.   (3:4A:21)

A last and very prevalent coping effort described in the seminars, one not usually described in the literature, might well be entitled "Do it yourself. If others aren't meeting your expectations, then do what you want done yourself." There were many examples of this kind of coping effort; the following is quite typical:

I work night, and the nurses in postpartum at night, I really don't think are safe. So many times there's been such obvious neglect—really patient neglect. It's really horrible. Sometimes I had to take a patient over who's delivered. If we're not busy and there's any suspicion that she might bleed or something, I'll keep her for a couple of hours because I just don't trust them. This one woman was very severely pre-eclamptic and her BP was going up and up. One of the night nurses was giving report in the morning . . . and one of the signs that they're going to convulse is substernal pain, and the night nurse says, "Well, she has a stomach ache, so I gave her some hot tea." And we went [opens and drops her mouth]. An hour later, the patient convulsed. The night nurse hadn't done anything about it because she thought the patient had a stomach ache . . . One time I'd taken a patient over and she'd started bleeding. I went back to check on her on purpose because I didn't trust them. It was about an hour later. The nurse was scrubbing the floor in the kitchen. I said, "What's so and so's vital signs?" And she goes, "Oh, it's not time to take them yet." I said, "When was the last time you took them?" She said, "Well, you took them before you brought her over." So I went into the room and took them and she was really bleeding and they had to do a D & C. *But it wasn't time to take them!* I really don't know what to do in a situation like that. Everyone knows about it, but no one seems to care. (9:2A:31)

In summary, therefore, we see that although a variety of coping possibilities are available to persons in a focal position in a role episode, in response to contradictory role demands, for the most part, new graduate nurses appeared to be stymied or fixated in the posture, "I don't know what to do" or "That's what you have to do." There was some maladaptive coping by way of symptom formation, as well as the "Do it yourself" coping effort, which may or may not be maladaptive.

The analysis of a role episode according to the model presented at the outset in this chapter is not as yet complete. Remember the all-important *loop,* wherein the response or the coping effort of the focal person feeds back into and forms the basis for confirming or altering the role sender's subsequent perceptions of the focal person's behavior. The loop ensures that if a new graduate complies when role pressure is applied, the probability is increased that her role senders will increase that pressure to gain further compliance. For example, if she copes with role pressures by doing other's work for them, then those role senders will incorporate that behavior into their future role expectations of her. In short, a role episode is a part of a process which is cyclic and ongoing. The response of a focal person to role pressures feeds back to the senders of those pressures in ways that alter or reinforce their expectations. The next role sendings of each member of the set depend upon the senders' evaluations of the response to their last sendings, and thus a new episode begins. Understanding this loop process is crucial to knowing how to go about changing the role expectations that others have for us. Let us now look at the extent of awareness of the loop process shown by the new graduates.

In this first excerpt, we see an instance of how role expectations are shaped or molded by others. Envision the speaker as the role sender who is sending out messages to the other seminar participants (the focal persons) on what Jane's behavior should be and how it should be interpreted. The behavior of the focal people (the other seminar participants), in not agreeing with the role sender, seems to bring about some alteration of the role sender's conceptions and future expectations.

> Twice today I was told by different people that I was seeing too much good in people—which I didn't understand at all. You know, that hit me funny: in a matter of two hours! I guess I was making excuses for people . . . I'm supposed to practice being charge nurse today and one of our GN's, I guess, just took off for about an hour and a half. And we couldn't find her. I didn't think much of it; it did mean, you know, more work for us— you have to fill in her gaps, but we weren't that busy. But the ward secretary, almost the entire time, was going up and down the hall looking for Jane, calling out, you know, in the bathroom and everything. It was like the most important thing this morning was to find Jane; this was the big project. And finally—I had looked around for her and I didn't see her— the head nurse says to me, "Find her." It was like, you know, this was the big project for the morning. And we had so much else to do, it was really silly. Well, I said, "I think she's down at her break still." "Still? It's 11:00 A.M.!" And I said, "Yeah, I know. But maybe she's having a bad day." And they said, "Well, she's not having any more breaks." I don't know what kind of comment that was, but it really kind of scared me. You know, what does that mean, that she's not having any more breaks . . . And I just explained it, "Well this is one of her off days, you know." If she feels the need to take that long a break—it was way too long, I have to admit—it's better if she's not on the floor than for her to hang around the floor and not do anything."
>
> Well, I don't know. I don't know that I agree with you. I know about having off days—don't we all—but I think you have to expect people to be there when they're supposed to be.
>
> Yeah, I think if she was having that really bad a day, she should have gone home.
>
> But then you wouldn't have her help at all.
>
> Well, she wasn't any help sitting downstairs for a long break, was she?
>
> Um, no, but if she could pull herself together in a little while . . . (6:5A:18)

In this next excerpt we see that the past behavior of the RN in question has led the speaker, as role sender, to modify her expectations at least of this RN.

> On my floor I found that the new people will not answer lights. The old staff is beautiful, the aides and the LPN's. I'll try to answer lights but there are a few of the newer ones who will not answer a light . . . She will not

answer lights unless it is her patient. She refuses. She says it's out of her jurisdiction. She just refused to answer a light unless it is her patient. What are you going to say? She's an RN.   (2:1A:19)

In the next excerpt a new graduate describes in more specific detail how and to what extent her expectations of the performance of others have been modified by their past role behavior.

Now that I've seen how people do their jobs, I realize that you can't expect when you work with a staff that everything is going to be perfect. You've got to get the most important things perfected first; then you think about the minor ones. Because every day, someone forgets to do this, or doesn't do that, that is expected. But they're small things. As long as they don't seriously affect the care of the patient—that's the only thing that bothers me—then you really don't have to hold people to that expectation . . . You'll always find one that's not enthusiastic about patient care, one who's slow, one who'll try to push it off on you, one who gives you the attitude, "Well, what are you telling me that for?" But most of them do their job, and do it properly.   (2:4B:30)

## Other Factors Involved

Analysis of the experiences and responses of the role sender and the focal person in a role episode helps a great deal to understand a person's adjustment to role conflict and ambiguity. However, the context within which the role episode occurs must also be considered to obtain a complete understanding. Obviously this context will differ with each role episode, but there are three factors which are always present. These, and their points of influence on a role episode, are shown in Figure 5-2[20].

Unlike the momentary nature of the components of the role episode, the three factors of organization, personality, and interpersonal relations represent enduring states of the organization, the person, and the relationship between the focal person and her role senders. The properties and traits which make up these three factors are generalizations derived from past and recurrent events and behaviors. For example, saying that a head nurse has a friendly relationship with her staff means that past interactions between these two parties were pleasant, supportive, and so forth. It is the repetition and patterning of behaviors and events which provide the history so necessary for understanding each new role episode.

Organizational factors are all of those structural qualities, functional specialization and division of labor, formal reward systems, and so on which dictate the content of a position in an organization. They dictate, at least in a formal sense, what a person in a position is supposed to do. There is a causal relation (line 3 in Figure 5-2) between these organizational factors and the role expectations which are held about and exerted toward a particular position. In a decentralized organization, for exam-

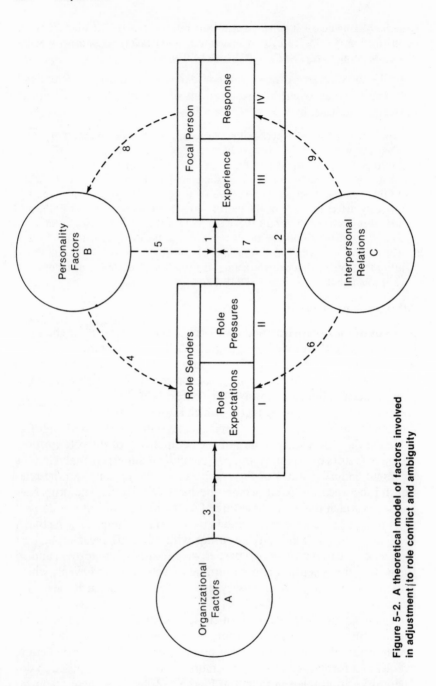

Figure 5–2. A theoretical model of factors involved
in adjustment to role conflict and ambiguity

ple, the role expectations held for the head nurse will be different from those held for a head nurse in a highly centralized organization. In the following excerpt, a new graduate speaks of the effect of the organizational factor of reward systems on the role expectations and performance of the nurse:

> Somehow the system—I don't like to use this word but—*hardens* them or they become task-oriented and they feel that if they're doing that, then they're good nurses and the system's rewarding them and they're moving up and becoming senior staff nurses. And that's what makes them happy. But does that mean that the patients' needs are still being met—all the patients' needs? Their own needs are certainly being met, you know, because they're going up the totem pole as far as seniority; they're getting more pay. But somehow I wonder if that's even a good system, as a reward system for nurses . . . And maybe that system has to be reevaluated as to how nurses become secure in their positions and usually it's through monetary value that they do—because they're rewarded monetarily for their amount of time there, for the type of job that they've done, which is usually evaluated on things one can see rather than the time I spent with a patient who was very anxious and I really met that patient's needs. That's very often overlooked and that's part of being a good nurse too. But things like that usually never get noticed or considered as part of an evaluation when a nurse is up for moving up in a position.   (9:3C:11)

Personality is used broadly to refer to all those factors that describe a person's tendencies to behave in certain ways, his motives and values, his sensitivities and fears, habits and so on. All of these factors can affect role episodes. Some traits of a person tend to elicit certain responses from role senders—an aggressive personality is likely to elicit strong role pressures from others because they have to be strong to have any effect on him. Also, because of these personality traits, some people will experience role pressures differently that others—a highly sensitive person will probably feel a great deal more tension under mild pressure than will a more "thick-skinned" person under intense pressure. It is likely that certain personality types lead toward certain kind of coping responses (line 8 in Figure 5-2). The "thick-skinned" person, for example, may be more prone to use defiance as a coping strategy than the sensitive person. In the following dialogue from a new graduate seminar, the personalities of the different speakers emerge somewhat. So also, the effects of these personalities on resistance to role pressure and on types of coping efforts employed can be seen.

> I don't have time to sit and talk with the patient any more, so I don't worry about it.
>
> Did you lose help or something?
>
> No, but I'm working evenings now and I'm the only nurse on the floor; I have only two other people to help me. I don't have to worry about that anymore; I just have to get my work done.

Then you're a good nurse, right?

Uh huh.

In whose eyes?

The eyes of the rest of the staff.

Is that what you think too?

Uh huh.

Why?

Because I get my work done and don't cause any problems for the head nurse and the rest of the staff. I don't cause any problems for the supervisor. She doesn't have to worry about if I'll get things done. It's not worth the trouble to fight to do it your way. You're a good nurse if you do it their way.   (6:5B:23)

The first speaker seems to be of a conforming, nonassertive personality, which explains in large measure the minimal resistance to role pressure and the compliant coping response.

## Interpersonal Relationships and Role Conflict

The "interpersonal relationships" factor refers to the more or less stable patterns of interaction between a person and his role senders and to their orientations toward each other. These patterns of relationships include such dimensions as: 1) power or the ability of one party to influence the other, 2) affective bonds, or the degree of liking and respect of one for the other, 3) dependence of one on the other, and 4) the style of communication between the focal person and his role senders. Interpersonal relationships function somewhat like personality factors with respect to role conflict and ambiguity—namely, in the areas of the kinds of role expectations held and corresponding pressures exerted (line 6 of Figure 5–2), the interpretation of the pressures (line 7), and the person's behavioral reactions (line 8). The head nurse, because she is in a superior position in the organization, will hold different role expectations and will present her demands differently to the new graduate than she will to a veteran nurse on the unit. Likewise the newcomer and the veteran will interpret the role pressures from the head nurse differently depending on whether they have established affective bonds with her. In other words, "I'll do what you want me to do because I like you," may be an experienced nurse's response to role pressure from the head nurse, but not the response of a new graduate who hasn't established such an affective bond yet. And lastly, some kinds of coping response, such as overt aggression, may be virtually ruled out when the protagonist is our superior in the organization. The effects of a host of interpersonal relationship factors on role conflict and ambiguity are heard in the plaintive voice of the new graduate in the following excerpt:

The doctors [the interns and residents] think all the nurses are just mother hens and worry warts—you know, what's our problem? They don't believe us; if we say something about the patient's condition, they'll say, "You're crazy, where'd you get that idea?" Or they'll laugh all the time, and that really irritates me. Like right now, we have a patient and he's got no urine output, no nothing. And so they'll come in and instead of being concerned—all the nurses are just being torn apart—they'll come in and laugh and think that's so funny. And it's so irritating to me I could just run over and wring their necks.    (7:2C:6)

Here we can see that past interpersonal relationships between the doctors and nurses are governing and conditioning current behavior and conflict. The nurses are unable to exert sufficient pressure on the physicians to get them to meet their role expectations (to do something about the lack of urinary output) because of the preestablished "mother hen" view of the nurse. This leads to the ineffectual coping response of further "worry wart" behavior.

The explication of a role episode is now complete. We began with an analysis of the four primary events occurring at a given moment in time. Role senders, holding expectations, send out pressure messages to a focal person which lead to conflict and ambiguity, which demands some kind of a coping response. These responses or role behaviors are perceived and evaluated in relation to expectations (the loop) and the cycle resumes. The enduring states of the organization, the person, and the interpersonal relations between the role sender and the focal person will impact upon and help to determine how conflict engendered by differential role expectations will be resolved.

### Suggestions for Handling Problems in the Area of Role Expectations

Despite the fact that role expectations were such a dominant concern for new graduates and that the area is very broad and diffuse, all suggestions for handling these concerns can be consolidated into four. 1) Teach people to understand the process of how role expectations are formed, verified, and modified. 2) Provide needed information relative to kinds of role conflict, coping mechanisms available, and techniques for exerting role pressure. 3) Make role expectations clear and overt. 4) Appreciate and plan for the interrelation between crises and structure.

*Role expectation process.* Role expectations are formed from a variety of sources. Organizational factors such as job descriptions, procedure books, and policy manuals are a predominant formal source in the work world. Expectations derived from this source are joined by two other sources: one's conceptualized ideal, that is, the role conception that is developed during the nurse socialization process, and ongoing observations of what we see others do in the role.

A primary consideration regarding role expectations is the delicate balance between legitimacy and realism. In establishing these characteristics, the source of the role expectations must be considered. Role expectations derived from job descriptions, while high on accuracy and legitimacy, will tend to be quite general and nonspecific, and lower on realism than will expectations derived from the observation of others' performances. Role conceptions derived from school are likely to be legitimate in the school world, but lower on legitimacy and realism in the work world. In formulating workable role expectations, new graduates must learn to assess them on the dimensions of legitimacy and realism. By striking a delicate balance between these two, they are in a much better position of having their role expectations fulfilled. It also gives them a guide as to what role functions they can reasonably expect from others, which expectations are likely not to be met, and so on. For example, in deciding to give digoxin to a patient with an apical pulse of 56, the nurse will probably consider the formal job description as a legitimate but unrealistic source of role expectation because of its nonspecificity. It probably only says something to the effect that "The nurse will engage in safe patient care." The school-bred role conception will probably be considered legitimate but perhaps unrealistic, and the observations of other nurses' practice, a realistic source, but perhaps not quite legitimate. New nurses need to be assisted in analyzing the sources of role expectations for legitimacy and realism. By so doing, they will be in a much better position to make decisions relative to retaining, modifying, or dropping their role expectations.

Verification of role expectations is of paramount importance because of the all-important function that such verification has in the formation and confirmation of one's role identity. Awareness of this process, which was described earlier, is of paramount importance for those who are involved in and responsible for the early postgraduation socialization of the new graduate nurse. Physicians, head nurses, and more experienced staff nurses need to appreciate the fact that every time they disconfirm a newcomer's expectations of how they should enact their roles, they are not only causing conflict for the newcomer, they are also affecting her identity of herself as a nurse. This is not to say that all of the newcomer's role expectations are worthy of confirmation. But we need to be aware of what we are doing when we disconfirm, and to try to practice selective and judicious disconfirmation.

By helping students, staff nurses, and others to understand the role episode model and to utilize it in the analysis of role conflicts and role expectations, we can help to bring about planned and deliberate, rather than happenstance, modification in role expectations. The forming, verifying, and modifying role expectations can also be expedited by clarifying roles. Ambiguity of a role is brought about not only through obscure communication, but also because of the lack of availability of relevant information. The two roles that appear to be the most ambiguous for new graduates are those of the nurse's aide and the supervisor. There is a real fuzziness in the minds of new graduates as to what differentiates an aide from an RN. "An experienced aide is just like an RN; they can do just as much if not more than an RN," new graduates might say; but then on the other hand, they criticize the aides for not functioning or charting like an RN. One way to solve this problem is by making available relevant information about this and other roles—both in the preservice and in the inservice settings. By so doing, the newcomer will be put in a much better position to formulate legitimate and realistic role expectations and to exert the necessary role pressures to bring about the desired role behavior.

And last, but not least, considerable help would be forthcoming if the functions and duties expected of the newcomer were spelled out clearly. As one new graduate so aptly expressed it: "One of the major problems is that no one really spells out their expectations, so I have to operate on my perception of others' expectations of me"(3:5C:12). Although job descriptions are common and certainly are a legitimate source of role expectations, they are nonetheless unrealistic because of their necessary generality. Specific role expectations are far more useful and operational.

In conjunction with this spelling-out of specific role expectations, both the new graduate and the veteran staff must realize and make clear the temporal quality of role expectations. Role expectations are *situational demands*. Just as a situation does not remain static, neither do role expectations. What is a legitimate and realistic expectation of a nurse during a normal, moderately busy workday may not be so during a heavy crisis-filled day. So also, the behavior expected of a newcomer during the first three months of employment is not necessarily the same as the role expectations at six months.

*Role episode information needed.*  There are three specific kinds of information regarding role that would be particularly useful and beneficial to the newcomer, as well as to more experienced nurses. Knowledge and understanding of the major kinds of role conflict would be helpful in assisting an individual to understand the source of actual or potential conflict. In this way, strategies for avoiding or resolving the conflict can be developed. For example, if one recognizes that one has need dispositions that are contrary to the requirements of a certain kind of job, then one is begging for "self-role" conflict by accepting that position. A nurse who abhors a fast-paced, technique-oriented work environment would be foolish to choose to work in an intensive care unit.

The second major kind of role episode information needed is concerned with coping responses. By raising the nurse's awareness of the usual kinds of mechanisms by and through which an individual copes with conflict, a whole new vista is opened for her. In some instances the person may want to incorporate a particular mechanism into her own repetoire; in others, the value simply may be to help her become conscious of what is already being used. By so doing, the person is in much better control of the situations and can make a deliberate choice with respect to the consequences of each mechanism.

Particularly difficult for new graduates, an area that would benefit markedly if newcomers were presented with needed information is the area of role pressures. The new graduates had a great deal of trouble in exerting role pressure. A lot of it seemed to stem from the feeling of not having the right to do so. Others could exert pressure on them, but they felt "too new" to do so even when they were in charge and had the responsibility of seeing to it that the work got done. The truth of the matter is that, in all likelihood, it is not a question of whether "to exert or not to exert" pressure, but rather whether to exert it overtly or covertly. As long as we hold role expectations (which are inevitable if we have any kind of role conception at all) we are probably transmitting some kind of role pressure; it is far more desirable and effective to make these expectations clear and plain instead of setting up a guessing game. If a new graduate expects support from her head nurse for a new project that she has undertaken, then it is far better for the newcomer to spell out what this support means so that the head nurse will present the project at staff meeting and will verbally and behaviorally encourage the other staff nurses to participate and so on, than to leave this expectation of support covert and veiled. There is no dearth of role expectations among new graduates, as we say earlier in this chapter. The problem is in making these expectations known. Role pressure can and should be exerted to do so.

A good deal of the frustration in self-other role conflict is the vagueness of the expectations. In working with physicians, for example, the usual sequence is as follows: a patient's condition worsens and the nurse calls the physician to notify him. She expects that the doctor will not only answer his page but will also do something to stabilize or improve the patient's condition. The physician answers his call; the nurse tells him about the patient; the physician says OK and hangs up. From that point on, the nurse is frustrated, angry, and upset. Not only were her expectations not met; they were so poorly communicated that in all likelihood they were not even picked up by the physician. It would be far better for the nurse to make these expectations overt by saying something like: "Shall I expect that you will be coming to see her?" or "Will you be needing anything when you get here?" If the physician says outright that he is not coming, the nurse might respond by saying, "What is the next development in the patient that I should expect to see?" Then if it is necessary to call the physician again, the nurse can start out by saying:

"You indicated that I should expect X, but that is not what happened. Her condition changed to Y, so that is why I'm calling you." By making expectations clear and overt in this way, there is much less chance that the role pressure will not be felt and responded to.

A third suggestion that may be of help either to new graduates themselves or to people working with them is to analyze unmet role expectations in terms of the effects deviation from expectations will have on one's own performance of a role. How will others not performing their role according to my expectations impinge on my role performance? By asking and answering this question, we are in a position to approach others, to apply role pressure. Role pressures will be more effectively and satisfactorily received if expectations are made known by emphasizing the effects that deviation from these expectations will have on the role sender's performance rather than by advocating compliance to role pressure simply as something that is positive or negative or should be done. For example, it is generally expected that at change-of-shift reports, the status of IV's will be clearly and accurately communicated. If this is not done, a nurse will be more successful in applying role pressure to get it done by communicating the effects that such unmet expectations will have for her practice and for the patients ("When you tell me that the IV is on time and I find it's two hours slow, that's hard on the patient because I have to speed it up to get it on schedule"), than by a positive or negative remark about the individual or about the role ("That's your responsibility. Good nurses keep IV's accurate and on time").

The last suggestion that will be likely to help the newcomer in dealing with the area of role expectations is concerned with the interactive effect of stress and structure. There can be little doubt that the first job experience is a stressful experience for many new nurses. When confronted with such stress, the human organism must utilize energy and coping resources to restore equilibrium. Too much stress over a long period of time will lead to exhaustion.

When anyone is under stress, some measure of relief can be obtained through a structuring of the environment. Such structuring enables an individual to deal with stressors with a minimal use of precious and limited resources. By this husbanding of one's resources, one will have more resources available to deal with other stressors and situations that cannot be structured. Therefore, it is often very helpful to the newcomer in managing the conflict of unmet role expectations if initially as much of her environment can be structured as possible. We often see new graduates doing this for themselves when they construct "crib sheets" to get themselves organized, to give a clearer, more logical report and so on. This intense desire for certainty, for structure, for uniformity is also one of the dynamics behind the newcomer's intolerance of rules and policies that are not applied consistently and fairly. It is strongly suggested that this need for structure during initial stress and crisis be recognized and structure provided to help the newcomer cope. It must also be recognized, however, that after the stress of newness has been overcome, such structure is no longer of such importance and may in fact be counterproductive to creativity and individuality.

The preceding discussion of role expectations could logically lead to either of two subjects discussed by the new graduates in the seminars. One of these is friction; the other is change activity and concerns. The former occurs when there are persistent, continuous, and vaguely defined unmet role expectations with a high emotional charge; the latter occurs when a person attempts to influence another's role conceptions or role behavior. Friction, a minor theme, will be discussed before the major theme, change activity and concern.

## FRICTION

Friction, or the interpersonal rubs between different parts or subsystems within the larger organization, was a minor area of concern discussed in the new graduate seminars. Although the subject came up at least once in all of the medical centers studied, there was a definite concentration of concern over this subject in four places—the two West Coast medical centers and the two private hospitals—where 80 percent of the 106 discussions involving friction occurred. Ascertaining a reason for this is relatively simple when one looks at the content of the frictions described. What was different about the four medical centers was increased discussion of racial and union tensions. This does not necessarily mean that the remaining five medical centers did not have racial or union problems, but that either they did not produce friction or they were not discussed.

Friction ranked tenth in terms of frequency of discussion in the seminars. Most of the discussion occurred in the first four seminars—equally divided among them—with only 15 percent occurring during the last two seminars.

### Causes of Friction

Whenever a job or task is broken up into components, with each component the responsibility of a different group of workers, friction is inevitable. In each department or group of workers there is some degree of the "mine-yours" phenomenon, some degree of claiming for self various components of the job. These components must be coordinated if there is to be satisfactory completion of the task. Coordination thus requires that there be specification of the portion of the task to be performed by each group of workers. For example, in the care of the hospitalized patient, the nursing, dietary, housekeeping, X-ray, lab, and other subgroups must know what portion of the job is theirs and must coordinate the achievement of this task with the other departments. This requires that some agreement be reached as to what functions belong to each subgroup. Thus, a certain degree of the "mine-yours" phenomenon is necessary and required by the division of labor of a task into component parts.

However, while there is a division of responsibilities among the subgroups, there is also some overlap of function. Although the dietary staff is responsible for the patient's dietary needs, are they responsible for the actual delivery of the food to the patient? Housekeeping maintains the physical environment for the patient, but who is responsible for cleaning up an emesis if it should land on the floor? Functions which could potentially belong to one or another department create gray or fuzzy areas of responsibility. These gray areas of overlap are the source of much friction.

In addition to the subgrouping of tasks into different departments within the hospital, there is also a further division of tasks within the subgroups. Within the nursing department, there are the nurses, the LVN's, the aides and orderlies, as well as the unit clerks. There also exists the groups of people who work days, evenings, and nights. Each set of workers must perform portions of the nursing function for the nursing staff to accomplish its total job. Both allocation of specific functions for each worker and gray areas of function exist within the nursing division as within the overall hospital structure. Thus the potential for friction within the nursing group is the same as in the overall organization.

There are at least three possible points of friction. The first is in the area of "mineness." If a subgroup defines a specific function as its domain, then the other subgroups must agree and relinquish the function. If there is no agreement as to the appropriate domain of a function, then rivalry and friction can result if more than one subgroup is performing the function.

The second point of friction is in the "yourness" of a function. If there is mutual agreement as to the location of the function then there is no problem. If a subgroup constantly disclaims a function which they do not want but which others say belongs to that subgroup, then friction ensues.

The third potential area of friction exists in the gray or fuzzy functional areas. When more than one group is capable of performing a task or function, then the lines of demarcation are not as clear as for the "mine-yours" tasks. If there is overlap of function, then just where one subgroup begins and the other leaves off is troublesome. The potential for friction is high.

There is much speculation as to why friction exists in nursing. Some say the friction results because there is a high proportion of women in nursing and women do not get along as well as men. Others say that the stress resulting from dealing in "life and death" situations creates the friction. These factors may contribute to the amount of friction in nursing; however, it is more likely that the universality of skills among the nursing staff as well as the possession of some of these same skills by the ancillary personnel who work with nurses is the predominant cause of the friction. When more generalized skills of patient care are possessed by the nurses on each shift as well as by the nurses on the same shift, then disagreement and friction as to who will perform the function is highly likely.

Some examples of friction discussed by in the new graduate seminars will now be presented. First we will look at the progression of involvement of new graduate nurses in friction or organizational discomfort, and then at the range of subunits affected by and involved in friction with the nurse.

Friction differs from conflict, from unmet role expectations, in its nonspecificity and highly emotional overtones. Although we might become upset when our views conflict with those of another nurse on how to handle the family of a dying patient, or when the head nurse fails to meet our expectations that she should post the time schedule two weeks in advance, these feelings are different from those experienced from friction caused by poor articulation between the different parts of an organization. The friction we are talking about here can be defined as organizational discomfort[21]. Discomfort is the negative feelings experienced by any one or group of individuals in the organization that are beyond their desire or control. Such discomfort may be labeled tension, anxiety, rivalry, frustration. This kind of discomfort does not refer to the tension that may occur, for example, when one is striving to achieve goals; it refers only to a state of negative feelings. One very important characteristic of this discomfort is that the precise causes of it usually are not known, although it is not unusual for the individual or group to attempt to assign causes to it.

The characteristics of discomfort—nonspecificity, high negative feeling tone, and fault-finding or blaming—can be seen in the following two excerpts in which the new graduates describe the friction they perceive:

> It's tension from the time you walk in on that ward 'till you walk off. There's never not any tension. Occasionally you might get a laugh from an intern and get a couple of yucks from the doctor or something, but other than that it's constant tension with the aides . . . It's kind of like a game too. They're trying to see which of the nurses they can get rid of. They [the ancillary staff] have been there for years and they kind of get a big kick out of it: "Let's see who we can stick the knives into and let's see who we can upset the most, and who we can get out of here." (9:2C:18)

There's almost constant bickering. Each shift finds things that the shift before didn't chart. Like the evening shift did it or the night shift. They keep putting blame. Nobody's happy until the fault is fixed, and that doesn't really make them happy either.    (2:1A:3)

It is interesting how the new nurses became aware of the presence of friction. Organizational discomfort is not usually the kind of thing that is announced during orientation. Furthermore, the stance taken by virtually all of the nurses in seminars was that eventually they knew about it but did not want to get involved themselves. As we can see from the following series of excerpts, however, involvement was only a matter of time. In the first excerpt, a new graduate seems to be getting a general awareness of the discomfort present on the unit through the experiences of a coworker.

There's a lot of things going on among the people on the staff on our floor . . . We had a guy who started a month before we did and he's transferring out. All the little things started getting to him more than he wanted to handle them, more than he wanted to deal with them. And I can really see what he means. It's so petty. Little things like forgetting to put your initials over the medication, or something like that. They're so many little bitty things that you have to, you know, they're important little things but they're just that, little things. And they bug you to death on them . . . It's like, everybody is watching, to catch everything that isn't done. Everybody's out for everybody else.    (1:3C:7)

Later, it seems like she is personally encountering and experiencing some friction.

I'm getting kind of frustrated because, you know, you're working really hard and you're doing a nice job, but then in report they pick on these petty little things that didn't even matter, you know, and you feel like you're a terrible nurse because you give good care, good patient care, but because you didn't clean the little bags on the bedside tables, or something like that. It might be a lot more important that someone got a back rub, because those are the priorities you set up, but they'll hassle you because if you don't replace the little bags, they have to. They won't see that they should give the back rub if you don't.    (3:4C:10–11)

She eventually seems to have arrived at the conclusion that involvement is inevitable.

You almost have to get involved in the hassles on the floor. The first night I felt like an observer, but now everybody's getting tangled in because you've got to choose sides, and you just can't sit in the middle of the road. So you either go left or right. Or if you don't say anything they're going to put you where they want you to go anyway.    (1:6C:20)

And in this following excerpt, there is full-blown involvement in the nonspecific, emotional-laden problem of "watching yourself" so that you don't get written up on an incident report:

You ask how could something like that be detrimental to a person? Well, I'll tell you. It makes me feel very tense. You should learn to be comfortable in what you're doing and every day you should learn something new, but when you think someone is always writing up an incident report, it makes you tense. It shows up in your work. There's this one particular person who is always looking over your shoulder and watching. So you know she is going to be looking for every mistake that is made—not just mine— she does this to every nurse. So because of this, you are going to try to rack your brain with every single thing you are doing . . . On each shift we all know who they are. We all watch out for them. We're all careful for what they do every day. No one has ever corrected them because they are really, actually within the law of the hospital . . . The supervisor and the coordinator know who they are too. They are always writing things and people up, but no one has ever said anything to them, like, "Why don't you sit down and talk to the person instead of writing up a report all the time?"    (2:1B:4)

Every member of an organization, in each subunit, is probably capable of perceiving and reporting various degrees of discomfort. The following series of examples necessarily reflects the new graduate nurses' perspective. The first is an example of personal friction, or discomfort between two individuals. The lack of specificity of the issues and the relating to the nurse as an occupant of a position are what makes this friction rather than a specific conflict.

Do you know what happens? If I say, "I'm not going to do that right now, I'll stay an extra half hour and do it later. This person needs me to sit down and talk to him for a few minutes." You can't do that; you'd get laughed out of the place. You'd have a head nurse on your back all the time. She's the kind of person I listen to and then I go and do whatever I'm going to do anyway. But you never say, "I won't do it." You just do what you think is right. You don't ever come into direct conflict with this person because she has to win. That's part of her problem. I just do what I have to do. I think that's how a lot of people deal with her.    (9:2A:25)

In the next excerpt, the subunit or part of the organization involved in the discomfort is broadened from a single nurse to the new graduate as a member of that part of the organization called new nurses, or younger nurses.

Bicker, bicker, bicker. All the time. I was thrown into it last Friday night. I was the one longest on the floor so I had to take charge. I'm hit with it and I have to do it; I have to do my best. I thought I did OK. I know I made a couple of mistakes but nothing that would have killed a patient or anything . . . I sent the wrong slip down to the lab, and my supervisory report was late, stuff like that. But then yesterday when I came to work, somebody said, "Oh, I heard from the night shift that you made a couple of mistakes the other night." I felt really terrible . . . This one certain nurse was so mad. She's always crabbing about the young nurses. It made me feel really bad because I figured, "Can't they have any room to give you some leeway to make a mistake?'' If you're thrown into it, what could you do? See, that's your problem too because you have some guilt feelings and that's something you have to deal with too. Because I did make the mistakes . . . I went home and thought I had done a good job . . . I mean I did, but afterwards I thought about it as I was working last night. And I thought, that nurse, she always finds something wrong with everybody. (9:3B:34)

One of the largest areas of discomfort experienced by the new graduates in the seminars was friction between shifts. Each of the usual three nursing shifts can be viewed as a separate subunit or part of the organization. The evidence would seem to indicate that there is a lot of difficulty in articulating these subunits.

I don't like it but there seems to be a lot of animosity between the day and 3-11 shift . . . They are always trying to find something on one another. I always get caught in the middle because I'm new and I don't feel like I can say anything . . . Little errors. One shift would say that they ordered a special food for a patient and then you'd find out that they didn't.   (2:1A:18)

There was some mention of friction between physicians and nurses, but not much. Most of the rubs between these two subunits were specific, with an identifiable focus, and hence were more in the area of unmet role expectations than friction.

We just started behavior rounds, which is kind of exciting. We had behavior rounds on this kid, and I think the medical staff was having more difficulty with him than the parents were. The orthopedic guy would come in and write things down or take the kid out of traction and put a brace on him, and the medical staff wouldn't even know that that was going on. The nurses would decide that he was best handled with a firm hand, but then the doctors would come in and be very permissive . . . The nurses were kind of caught in between because these people would always be walking in to see the kid and asking questions and we wouldn't even know who they were. You'd have to ask and they'd say, "Well Dr. (X) called me and said . . . ," or "Dr. (Y) is over here," And we wouldn't even know that Dr. (Y) was on the case much less Dr. (X).   (7:2B:18)

Another rather extensive area of organizational discomfort was tension and friction between floors or nursing units within the organization.

One thing I found was the terrible friction between floors. They do it one way on one floor and then I go up to the recovery room and someone will say, "Well, I don't know why they don't start doing this downstairs so it's done for us by the time the patient gets up here," and you feel like saying, "Well, sometimes ladies come in complete and you take them to the delivery room and everything happens so fast you don't have time for things before you take them to the recovery room." . . . From now on, we have to do them and everybody is screaming at us because now we've got one more thing we gotta fill out while somebody's delivering! (2:3B:18)

Interdepartmental hassles produced their share of discomfort also.

> The kitchen people hassle us and the patients all the time. I mean, I used to be nice, but they treat you like every request is an enormous imposition . . . We had a patient and his menu came up and he said he marked it; he does not want rice; it constipates him. So his food came up today and he had rice on his tray. He asked for beef; he had chicken. I just couldn't believe it. I just started here, but I was astonished at how poorly everyone gets along. And now, I'm in it too. I feel the same way.    (3:3A:35)

> We have bad relations with CSR. The girl from CSR comes up and insists that you search from room to room if anything is lost.    (7:3C:31)

> First Housekeeping gives us a bad time for not calling sooner and then they send up this derelict to clean the room. He was so dumb, he had to ask us how to do everything.    (7:3C:32)

Discomfort which the new graduates perceived as being caused by racial differences or union membership was prevalent throughout the organizations.

> You really get hassled by the patients and by the families. You'll hear about it. If the patient doesn't say something, the family will. You know, like sometimes I wouldn't get to do a patient until after lunch. And I'd ask them if they'd mind waiting, and oh, boy. They'd say, "You're making me wait because I'm Black."    (4:4:16)

> The head nurse was on vacation at the time that I came. So the nurse that I met initially was not the head nurse. The morning that I came to the floor and the head nurse was back from her vacation . . . I came into the office and I took my seat and everything. I didn't know who this strange person was and nobody was telling me who she was. It was about time for report so I took a chair and sat down. The relief charge nurse had already informed the head nurse that a new nurse was on the floor . . . After report was over, the head nurse turned to me and asked, "Oh, are you the new LVN?" Because the expectation was that my being Black, I was going to be an LVN. And I said: "No, I'm not an LVN, I'm an RN" . . . So from that point on, I didn't get very much help from the head nurse—just a lot of grief. There were a lot of little things like that that happened, and I knew they were going on because I am Black, and I knew there was a lot of resentment, my being Black, and educated.    (9:1B:28)

The new graduates reported a variety of ways in which some attempt was made to deal with friction and organizational discomfort. The most prevalent solution was to hold a meeting to discuss the problem.

> A lot of feelings got hurt, the way it was handled. So it came out that if something's not done why don't you do it yourself and, you know, not worry about the nit-picking, or the shift before not having done it because they may have gotten into a bind and couldn't do it. Which is true. We should all work together, but right after the meeting, you could tell it wasn't going to work. Everyone went right back to where they were before.

A lot of people are on the defensive right now and that makes it even worse. They're striking out for their own selves, and that's about it. It's really a mess, and more so now after the meeting than before. (1:4C:7)

Sometimes these were group sensitivity meetings led by a psychiatrist or psychiatric nurse.

It was tried at a meeting, but I really think it should have been said to her privately, not at a meeting. The girl really lashed out and defended herself. And now everyone talks about it behind her back. I don't think those group kinds of thing work at all. (6:5B:8)

Organizational tools such as incident reports or anecdotal notes were also fairly commonly-used devices to attempt to isolate the problem if not to solve it.

Some people are just very, very picky people. I don't know, I haven't really believed that those performance notes are all that hot. I think they're just a way for a person to get back at you. First the person writes it and then you get it and read it and then you write something back and then in the meantime all this resentment starts building up between you. You know, I practically had to force myself to say hello to her. It's just the feeling between us now. We even talked about the first one after it was over, but it's still there, the feeling, it's still there. Somehow, I'd rather just sit down and talk with the person—I think the notes do more harm than good. (1:3B:6)

I'm all for incident reports as a documentation of an incident, but I just think it is sick the way people go, "We're going to write one out on Nursery." And then Nursery retaliates: "Well, we're going to write one out on Labor and Delivery. Nah, Naah!" Obviously, incident reports are being misused, but they don't really get at the problem. They're sort of used like a vendetta. It's not like, "We're going to document this incident for future problems"; it's more like, "We're going to get them, now, and let them sweat for a couple of days." (2:4B:32–35)

A common bit of advice that new graduates offered to one another as a solution to the tension and friction felt was "not to get involved" in it. The following conversation is typical:

They're so many grapevines around here.

Just like everyplace else.

Yes, but the hassles here are unreal!

Like anyplace else you work.

I've found hospitals to be more so—maybe because the tension is higher.

Oh, I don't know. I worked in a department store and the friction was real bad there. I never got caught up in it though, because I just laughed when I'd hear some.

Yeah, I think that's the best way to handle it here, too, just don't get caught up in it. (6:6B:33)

Unfortunately this strategy, like the others, was seldom, if ever, seen as effective. What then is the answer? How can individuals or groups who constitute a subunit or part of an organization deal with organizational discomfort, with friction?

There are no magic answers to the foregoing question, but a few suggestions can be proffered. First, organizational discomfort or friction is an emotional reaction; it is a state of negative *feelings*. Dealing with feelings through strictly cognitive means such as group meetings or incident reports will almost certainly be ineffectual. As explained in the opening paragraphs of this section, the real cause of organizational discomfort is some kind of lack of coordination between the parts of the organization. When this lack of coordination is felt or perceived by the workers, all kinds of compensating mechanisms are brought to bear to fill in the vacuum, to take up the slack—mechanisms such as shoving off on the other person that aspect of the task that we don't want to do, building up our own importance and status by finding fault with others, and so on. For the most part, it is ineffectual to deal with the symptoms of the problem (the back-biting, fault-finding, hypercritical behavior, and so on). It is far more useful to identify and define those areas between subunits which are lacking in coordination, and to correct the problem at that level. It is certainly to the organization's as well as to the individual's advantage to do something about organizational discomfort, as such discomfort leads not only to psychological distress, but also to organizational ineffectiveness.

It must also be recognized that some degree of tension and friction between subunits of an organization will probably always exist. Even in the best run organizations there will always be some area in which overlap and ambiguity of function will exist. Providing people with an opportunity first to vent hostility and feelings, and then to go on to objective cognitive handling of the problem, will be a great boon. Many of the techniques and strategies outlined in relation to the principles for constructive conflict resolution[22] will also be applicable here. Development and use of empathic behavior will help in dealing with the emotional feelings that often get in the way of being able to deal cognitively with the problem. But above all, what is to be avoided is the use of preexisting tools, such as incident reports, to hunt down and document the aberrations. Incident reports are fine and useful for the purpose for which they were designed. When used to solve the problem of organizational discomfort, they often lead to the development of the witchhunt syndrome so aptly described by Henry[23].

Let us turn now to change activity and concern. In contrast to friction, change is much more of a deliberate, cognitive, and focused process. Although emotion is encountered, particularly when resistance is met, change is not primarily an emotional response as is friction.

## CHANGE ACTIVITY AND CONCERNS

"Happy are those who dream dreams and are ready to pay the price to make them come true."

In 1974 during a nursing school graduation address, Peplau stated very clearly the contribution expected by the nursing profession of its newest entrants:

Each new graduate who enters the profession of nursing contributes to its renewal. The vigor of the profession is replenished, in part, by fresh viewpoints of new graduates. The recency of your education promises the inclusion of new theories and practices—some of which were not known a decade ago. And there is, of course, your youth, enthusiasm, and energy . . . Renewal comes from discussion, listening, compromise, and blending of refreshing new viewpoints . . . with those of all other nurses . . . The profession anticipates the help you will provide in fixing the shortcomings of the health care system[24].

That same year, a young new graduate and six of her colleagues went to work on a pediatric medical unit in a thousand-bed municipal hospital. They had been given written and verbal assurances that they would be free to innovate and to initiate nursing care policies that differed from the norm within that institution, policies such as those promoting open visiting hours for parents, 24-hour coverage by registered nurses, team nursing, parent's classes, appropriate play materials, interdisciplinary health teams, continuity of care. Their goals were simple: to better the care of children, to put our classroom ideals into practice, to prove that apathy doesn't have to be, to be agents of change[25]. Eighteen months later, all of them had left, tired, defeated, discouraged—casualties of a battle with authoritarian and stifling nursing administrators. The support for change that had been promised them was not forthcoming.

What a dilemma! Nursing needs the ideas and enthusiasm of new graduates, but the young nurses just mentioned, like many in the new graduate seminars, stated that they could not or were not allowed to give their suggestions, ideas, inputs. If we couple this problem with the fact that many schools of nursing across the country deliberately attempt to socialize student nurses into being change agents—that goal, in fact, being the NLN criteria for accreditation of programs leading to the first professional degree in nursing—we can see one of the major causes of the guilt feelings often expressed by new graduate nurses.

I know I'm supposed to be a change agent. We had all that stuff in school. But I can't! I'm barely holding on as it is and everyone is so set in their ways. I can't possibly be a change agent. And this makes me feel so guilty, so disloyal to my school and the faculty. I don't want to go back and face my former teachers. I feel like I'm letting them down, not being a change agent.  (4:2A:12)

So, we in nursing are left with a multiple dilemma. We have new graduate nurses who feel they have something to offer to improve the health care system, a system (hospitals, nursing service) that says it wants the input, another system (schools of nursing) that says it is preparing nursing students to provide the input, but prospective change agents (new graduates) who say that the hospital system will not permit the input they want to give, and who feel guilty because they are not effecting the changes they are expected to make. What can be done about such a dilemma?

To help in better understanding the dilemma and associated problems, this section will depart somewhat from the approach used so far throughout this book. Because of the homogeneity and paucity of subthemes on change the subject area does not lend itself to the treatment accorded to the other themes discussed in this book. Content analysis of the 110 instances of discussion of change showed that virtually all excerpts could be channeled into two major subthemes, the first having four subparts:

1. I can't make any changes or suggestions because
   a. the system is too rigid.
   b. people have been here too long.
   c. I'm too new.
   d. I have no power.
2. I tried to make changes or suggestions but failed because . . .

The only other subthemes ("I haven't tried"; "I was successful in making a change"; or "There is change going on") combined accounted for only 15 percent of the total of 110 change discussions. The relative infrequency of this topic is a very disheartening reality, particularly since there is so much to say and do regarding change activity, and second, because a lot of people are counting on the new graduate to introduce change into the system. For these reasons, this section will go beyond the experiences voiced in the new graduate seminars and will present a total framework from which the dilemma of change can be viewed. The sentiments and experiences of the new graduates will still be used where applicable, but the reader will find that the scope of theoretical material presented here will be much broader than that substantiated by the discussions excerpted. As usual, the section will terminate with some suggestions on what might be done to work toward resolution of the dilemma.

In looking at change, we will first inspect the occurrence and patterning of this subject area in the new graduate seminar discussions. Then we will look at the various types of changes. Then utilizing a systems framework, we will examine two of the essential components of a system that are of particular relevance for the change process— boundary permeability and mutuality of relationships—and some of the conclusions that can be drawn when human needs are used as a basis for analysis of change activity. We will hear the new graduates tell us of some of the change agent strategies they used in effecting change, and then we'll examine in some detail the kinds of resistance to change that they encountered.

Change ranked ninth with respect to frequency of discussion in the seminars. This might seem surprisingly low compared with the heavy emphasis placed upon change agent functioning and difficulties, both by nursing service and by nursing education. It must be remembered, however, that the new graduates in the seminars were only five or six weeks into their first jobs at the beginning of the seminar series. It is quite possible that they were not yet sufficiently established to get as involved in change activities as they might later on. There is some support for this contention when we look at the patterning of occurrence of the change theme. Contrary to the usual pattern of most subject areas more of the change discussions occurred in the late seminars than in the middle ones. The distribution was as follows: early seminars, 41 percent; middle seminars, 25 percent; and later seminars, 34 percent.

Although it had a relatively low frequency of occurrence in the seminar discussions, change was considered to be a major theme throughout the nation. Discussions on this theme occurred with highly similar frequencies in all medical centers. Its rank in the individual medical centers ranged from sixth to tenth. The discussions of change tended to be longer discourses than, for example, those of unmet role expectations. It takes a longer time to present and clarify information about a change agent activity than it does, for example, to vent one's feelings of incompetency. This is probably the major reason why the frequency count of change themes was considerably lower than those of the other major national themes.

### Types of Change

There has been so much written about change that it would be very easy to forget that not all change is planned change. Actually, various types of change can be identified, based upon the extent of mutual goal setting, the deliberateness of the change, and the power ratio between the change-agent and the person-system to be changed[26]. The essence of these different types of change is presented in the following chart:

Identifying the type of change one is attempting is crucially important for one to proceed in any kind of logical fashion. Such distinctions were not particularly noted in the change discussions in the seminars, however. For the most part, the speakers made no particular reference to the kind of change they were talking about. There was some indication however, that power was the most troublesome variable for them in mak-

| Type of Change | Mutual Goal Setting? | Deliberateness | Power Ratio? |
|---|---|---|---|
| Planned | Yes | Both sides | Equal |
| Indoctrination | Yes | Both sides | Unbalanced and forced* |
| Coercive | No, or only one side | One side | Unbalanced |
| Interactional | Yes | No, but may be subconscious | Equal |
| Socialization | Yes | Yes, at least on part of socializer | Somewhat unbalanced |
| Emulative | Yes | Both sides | Unbalanced but desired* |
| Natural | No | No | Unknown |

* The major difference between indoctrination and emulative change is that the latter is associated with formal organizations in which change is brought about through a form of identification with and emulation of power figures by the subordinate.

ing changes. There were frequent references to the subtheme, "I can't make changes because I don't have enough power."

> Seems like, you know, it's taking us awhile. We don't really have any authority within the group, in our staff. Until somebody comes up and says, "Sue, you're the team leader," or whatever, it's hard to throw out ideas or to make any changes . . . When you try to, you wonder if you're treading on somebody's toes or if it's going to come across as competition or what . . . I've only been around a couple of months, but there were a lot of things that needed airing—problems and such. So I asked to have a staff conference. So we finally had one on Monday; the supervisor called it, and I had to get up there in front of everybody, but no one would listen to me. I told the supervisor that ahead of time. They would listen to her because she's got the power, but no one's going to listen to dumb little me. (1:4B:6)

> I've been thinking about this a lot, and I was thinking well, you know, the head nurses, they want the team leaders to be the ones to show leadership. They really want them to do things, but I think that possibly the aides realize that we [the team leaders] really don't have any clout to back up our words. We're not responsible for their hiring or firing and all that, and they know it. So what can you do? We really can't introduce any new things, or really get them to do anything they're not already doing. You can only suggest something so many times, and then if you have no power, that's it—no change. (1:2C:23)

Whether what was desired was *more power* than the other person or group, or simply *enough* power to be equal to others, was not clear. From the foregoing excerpts, it would seem that what the new graduate desired and valued was more power than others, so that coercive changes could be made.

On the other hand, the very, very frequent reference to the subtheme, "I can't make any suggestions or changes because I haven't been here long enough," provokes speculation about power. Notice the pervasiveness of this theme in the following series of excerpts:

> All these things that you can't let yourself get upset about, things you'd really love to change in the system, but you know as a new grad, coming into a new job, you just can't, because of how the whole system is set up, the pecking order and what not . . .   (9:3B:15)

> Oh yeah, I notice those things, but I wouldn't say anything. I'll just go in there and start washing backs because after awhile I just can't stand them letting the patient sit in it, or cleaning them up but not washing them clean. It happens all the time, it really does. They just go off and take their break. I've never expressed it; I've never given anyone the details because I haven't been there long enough to start screaming yet.   (2:1A:5)

> I feel new; I've only been here for a few months. As soon as my 90 days are up and I'm permanent, then I'm going to say something. But not until then.   (2:3B:25)

> I haven't really tried to implement any changes because I feel more the intruder on the floor. I'm just beginning to feel a little bit accepted, for myself rather than as an intruder, a new young graduate coming in and trying to change the world. So I really haven't tried to implement anything yet because I'm still feeling my way.   (9:6A:7)

> It's very hard to approach people and say: "Why are you doing it that way?" or "Don't you think? Have you ever tried it this way?" Especially when you're new. It's really hard. Sometimes I'll say, "Well, how about doing it this way?" and see how it's taken and go on from there. But it's hard, and to really be honest, it's not going anywhere.   (5:2B:28)

What is it about being "new" that inhibited the new graduate from making suggestions? We can't tell for sure from the seminar excerpts, but it seems quite likely that what the newcomers were expressing was a perceived power imbalance. What they seemed to be saying was that they had to be in the job long enough so that they would feel that they had sufficient power and be on an equal footing with others, and that then they would be in a position to make changes within the system.

In any event, it is quite clear that the new graduates were aware of the elements of power of position, and power through numbers that is frequently involved in coercive change.

> We have a new head nurse on our floor and she's young—about 27 or 28 and she's just gung-ho to change everything. Like she has really great ideas. She's started a lot of patient teaching, like giving insulin. She's bringing in charts that they can read and films that they could look at all about their illnesses and stuff like that. Ward conferences and stuff like

that, whereas our old head nurse was really passive and really didn't get
into that much. A lot of people are really upset by everything being turned
over all of a sudden; things really beginning to change and jump a little
more . . . I personally think maybe she's pushing a little too hard. I think
she should go a little slower.

Yes, but see she is in the head nurse position. She has to be in that kind of
position in order to start changes.

I guess that's why as a new grad I really feel frustrated. I think if there were
two of her kind as regular staff nurses, you could really get in there and
make changes. By yourself, it's almost impossible. But if there were at least
two, it may be a little slow, but I think you can get some changes made.
Numbers and position are power to make changes.   (9:3B:16)

In the preceding dialogue, it is clear that the first speaker applauded the
changes that the head nurse was making by virtue of the power of her
position, but that she was also aware of the negative drawbacks of coercive change—namely, resentment of the use of the power differential.

The interactive change that is usually seen among friends and married
couples seems also to a large extent to be the type of change that new
graduates were attempting to use with their coworkers.

Some things have changed already. After they've already labeled a patient,
then I go in and talk to the patient. And they'll see me talking to this
patient. And then all of a sudden I'll see people being nice to these patients.
Some people, you know. I can see it happening after I do it.   (6:4B:28-29)

There're certain things you learned in school that you do. I can't sit here
and preach to everyone and say, "Look, when you put an antibiotic in an
IV you have to label the bottle." Most people don't seem to do that. It's
one example. So I thought, "OK, I'll just go ahead and do it." And then by
my example—if I run across someone directly who's not doing it, I'll say
something . . . I think you have to maintain what you think is really important and go ahead and do that, and hope it gets across to other people that
you think that's an important thing.   (9:2A:17)

Here, although we see no evidence of mutual goal setting, congruence of
goals can be inferred from the terminal behavior. Power appears to be
equal and there is little evidence of the predeliberativeness of effecting a
change. What deliberation there was on the part of the new graduate
seems to have been unconscious during the episode and recognized only
afterward.

Although Bennis, Benne, and Chin[27] talk about technocratic change
as a type of change, it really is more understandable as a *means* to bring
about change. After a client or system identifies a particular problem as
caused by lack of knowledge, the technocrat change agent brings about
change by the collecting, interpreting, and providing of such data and
knowledge to the client or systems, who then bring about the desired
change. The following is an instance in which a technocratic means of
change was evident:

They weren't about to change anything. So I slowly and methodically began to collect the facts. I noted every time that there were med or IV errors made because the charting wasn't done, not to mention the amount of the nurses' time trying to hound around and find out what had and what hadn't been done. But I collected the error data and presented it at a staff meeting, and it really seemed to impress them. I think they were surprised to find out what a big problem it was. Everyone vowed that they'd do their charting from now on, but it's too soon yet to tell. Have to wait and see if they really do change. (8:3A:4)

Other than coercive, interactive, and technocratic changes, there were no other clearly identifiable types of change evident from the new graduate seminar discussions. Generally, in most schools of nursing, the type of change that is most strongly emphasized and advocated is planned change. Bennis, Benne, and Chin identify planned change as "a deliberate and collaborative process involving change-agent and client-systems. These systems are brought together to solve a problem or, more generally, to plan and attain an improved state of functioning in the client-system by utilizing and applying valid knowledge"[28]. This type of change is frequently advocated mainly because it is not incompatible with the values and norms of a democratic system and therefore allows for adequate, mutually satisfying, and socially wise solutions to conflict and problems. It is also the type of change that has been found scientifically to be most effective and long-lasting[29].

Although different models and systems for developing and analyzing of planned change have been explicated[30], they all essentially involve three stages with several steps under each phase. Most of these models are some kind of extension of the dynamic-change model developed by Lewin in the 1940s[31] and they include the following stages[32]:

*Stage 1*

| | |
|---|---|
| Unfreezing | Create the motivation to change. |
| Steps or mechanisms | (1) Create a felt need for change. |
| | (2) Induce "guilt-anxiety" by comparison of actual with ideal states. |
| | (3) Create psychological safety by reducing threats or removing barriers to change. |

*Stage 2*

| | |
|---|---|
| Changing or moving to a new level | Develop new beliefs, values, and behavior patterns on the basis of information obtained or cognitive redefinition. |
| Steps or mechanisms | (1) Identify with a particular source of information or person. |
| | (2) Scan multiple sources of information and redefine through new integration of information. |

*Stage 3*

| | |
|---|---|
| Refreezing | Stabilize and integrate new beliefs, values, and behavioral patterns into the rest of the system. |
| Steps or mechanisms | (1) Integrate new responses into the total personality. |
| | (2) Integrate new responses into ongoing relationships through reconfirmation by significant others. |

To be successful, change programs must be particularly attentive to stages 1 and 3. It is not enough just to develop new ideas and to expect that others will take them up. Many such ideas are doomed to failure because no motivation for change was created first, and there was no attention to ensure their integration within the system or the person trying out the innovation. Above all, a cardinal principle is that no change will ever occur unless the members of the system feel that it is safe to give up the old way of doing things[33]. Although information such as the preceding is frequently taught to student nurses in schools of nursing, there was no evidence in the new graduate seminar discussions that such phases or steps were being consciously or deliberately used by new graduates to effect change.

## Process of Change

*To effect change* is a powerful phrase. What exactly does it mean? The word "change" produces emotional reactions. It is not a neutral word. Cartwright, in fact, writes that for many people, change is threatening. It conjures up visions of a revolutionary, a dissatisfied idealist, a troublemaker. There are more polite words, or euphemisms, that people use to refer to the process of changing other people—words such as education, training, orientation, guidance, therapy. Most people are more ready to have others educate or train them than to change them. Why is that? Cartwright believes that a large part of the emotional reaction to change lies in the fact that the safer words, such as education or therapy, carry the implicit assurance that the only change that will be produced will be a good one, acceptable to the person within a currently held value system. Change, on the other hand, implies no such respect for values. It might, in fact, tamper with one's values. For these very reasons, Cartwright believes that it will foster straighter thinking if we use the word change and force ourselves to struggle directly and self-consciously with the problems of value that are involved[34].

Heeding Cartwright's advice, we will proceed to look at the process of change, keeping in mind that all change activities in some way are an attempt to impose new values on other people or to get them to change their values in some way.

For some time, systems theory[35] has been used to analyze and understand both individual and organizational change. Initially, however, social organizations were regarded as closed rather than open systems[36]. Now, their conception as open systems is firmly established [37]. A system is a set of parts or units with relations among them. Each unit is, at least partially, dependent upon the state of other units. However, the whole is greater than or less than the sum of its parts. The parts of a system may combine in ways that enable them to be more; or, conversely, the parts may undermine each other, so that collectively they are less than their sum. The latter case can be seen, for example, in a staff unit team that is rife with dissension. It would not be surprising in such a case to find that the unit group as a whole puts out less work than the sum of the work each individual in the group could produce.

By definition, an open system is one that is open to the environment; it is not totally separate from its environment. An open system engages its external environment through the exchange of matter, energy, and information. All living systems are open systems and depend for their survival on the exchange with the environment. Not only does such a system take in material, energy, and information (inputs), it also discharges material, energy, and information (outputs) in the forms of waste and product achievement. The throughput is what an open system does to the input in order to produce the output. It is the transformation of the energy, the reorganization of the input to achieve the desired output.

One of the major characteristics of systems is their disorder and disorganization. Although systems strive for equilibrium, their differentiated structures or parts tend to move toward dissolution as the elements composing them become rearranged in random order. This disorganization is irrevocable over time and inevitably, in a closed system, will lead to decay. Open systems, however, can counteract this decay or entropy by absorbing inputs or energy which have greater complexity than the system outputs. This process is called increasing the negentropy of a system. Through its exchange with the external environment, an open system can thus forestall its death and even increase its vigor and vitality over time. Which of these tendencies will actually predominate will depend upon the balance of entropy and negentropy within the system.

The following dialogue from one of the new graduate seminars documents a shift of balance toward entropy or decay. The newcomer who is the primary speaker, finding that the system was essentially closed, decides to decrease her input of new, fresh ideas markedly. The system, deprived of this kind of input, will eventually move toward dissolution.

> I'm going to try not to react to it. I figure that the people who've been there are not going to change their attitudes about their thing, so I guess I'm going to have to change my attitudes about my thing.

So, we have to give in to them?

Yeah, and say, "Well it happens," and shrug my shoulders . . .

Are you going to feel good about that, then?

No, probably not.

Are you going to be able to live with it then, if you do it?

Well, right now I'm getting upset and not being able to sleep all day and that doesn't help. I can't live with that either.   (2:6B:29–30)

Although we have been speaking of systems in general, it is important to understand that individuals, groups, and organizations may each be conceptualized as open systems. Individuals regularly exchange matter, energy, and information with their environment through such processes as ingestion, expulsion, and communication. Groups and organizations can surpass individuals in their potential for indefinite life, because they can continually take in new members as senior members leave or retire. The exchange through expulsion and communication is the same for groups and organizations as for individuals.

*Boundary permeability.*   Two key facts of systems, boundary permeability and mutuality of relationships, have been identified as having particular importance in the understanding of change[38]. Survival and growth of a human system depends not only on whether the system is open to the internal environment, but also on how the system regulates its exchanges with the outside world. The external boundaries of a system regulate the flow of input (matter, energy, and information) between the system and its environment; the internal boundaries regulate the input and output of subsystems of a system. Because of the importance that external and internal boundaries play in regulating the flow of what goes in and what comes out of a human system, they are crucial in determining what is and is not a system, what is inside and what is outside of the system. The boundaries are also crucial in understanding any possibility of change within a system.

Boundaries can either be objective (concrete) or subjective. Examples of objective boundaries of a person would be clothes or skin; of a group, the members composing the group; of an organization, physical structures such as gates, walls, and fences. For an individual, ego boundary is an example of subjective boundary. Concepts such as cohesion, involvement, identification are examples of group and organizational subjective boundaries. It has now been fairly well confirmed that the establishment of objective boundaries promotes the formation of subjective boundaries, and the establishment of the subjective promotes the development of the objective.

The characteristic of boundaries that has particular importance in understanding the processes of system vitality and change potential is permeability, the extent to which information, matter, and energy can flow into and out of the system. If the permeability of a human system is near zero, the system is essentially closed and will tend toward deterioration and death. On the other hand, if the boundaries are fully permeable, there is no vitality either. The system will be indistinguishable from its environment and hence not a system at all. The greatest system vitality and potential for change will occur in systems where boundaries are definitely present but not fully permeable. The following excerpts from the new graduate seminars exemplify good boundary permeability in a social system:

> I have a pretty good feeling about my job. I feel like the only restrictions that are there are the ones I put on myself. At first I was sort of afraid to try things. I thought well, if I try something new, is this person going to think, "What's she trying to do? Look better than the rest of us?" But I didn't get that at all from anybody. It was like "Yeah, that's a neat idea," and then maybe they'd go on and do something too. (9:1A:23)

> It worked out quite well, the change. I suggested that we keep the flow-sheets at the bedside. There used to be three or four places to write down the same information. Now we keep the sheets at the bedside. Everyone is pretty open to ideas on my floor. There are no great hassles in terms of change. (5:4A:38)

Unfortunately, there were almost six times as many examples of low boundary permeability. To a large extent, the decreased boundary permeability was usually attributed to high staff stability, which produces an almost closed system.

> You can't, above all, change the bathing policy. People have to have a bath every day and their bed made—not because the patient needs it, but because the staff has been here 15 years and have always done it that way. (5:5A:32)

> The main problems are new ideas with old staff. Like we had a 65-year-old head nurse and a charge nurse in her late 50's. And it's been done this way for the last 12 years, since the hospital was built! I think they came in in the truck with the rest of the equipment. (9:1C:26)

> I made out the scheduling and I put down lunchtimes just like you learn in school—not everybody can be off the floor—kind of even staffing when you make lunchtimes so I worked real hard for a half hour to make out the assignment for lunchtime. I come the next day and Alice, who is an excellent LVN, says to me—she's been there over 12 years—she says, "Who put these lunchtimes down?" I said, "Well, I did." She goes, "Well, I always go to lunch at 1:00 o'clock and so does Linda and I don't care what you put down." Meanwhile this is at 12:30 that she told me this, "And I don't care what you say, I'm going at 1 o'clock." So at 1:00 o'clock I'm the only person down there for 24 patients and what could I do? I went to the head nurse afterwards to discuss it because it was a very traumatic experience for me. (9:3A:11)

New graduates also presented an example of the ineffectiveness of an attempt to produce change when the boundaries are almost fully permeable:

> It's too bad in an institution like that that there are head nurses like that. Because theoretically there shouldn't be. This is a university hospital; it's supposed to be innovative and all. It shouldn't be restricted to medical things, but should be, you know, open to changes and improvements in nursing. For being a research hospital and all, there's very little, if any, nursing innovation going on here.
>
> Uh huh, that's true.
>
> Staff turnover is one reason why.
>
> Yeah, that's right. Why should you make changes when you're going to leave in six months? They said during orientation while we were sitting there in groups, "Fifty percent of you won't be here in six months." Now that is a phenomenal turnover. You can't make change effectively if you're just trying to stay afloat—if the people you try to work with in changes aren't going to be here in six months.  (8:6:12)

There can be no vitality in a group such as this because the group is barely distinguishable from its environment.

*Mutuality of relationships.*   The second key facet of systems that is of importance in change is relationships—the process through which and by which matter, energy, and information are exchanged across boundaries. Relationships established across internal boundaries of a system provide integration, coherence, and coordination between subunits or subsystems. Relationships established across external boundaries provide the opportunity for the system to export waste and products and import nourishment and stimulation.

Relationships differ in their degree of mutuality, that is, the extent to which energy and information is freely exchanged across boundaries. For example, if the product of exchange were suggestions for improvement of patient care, high mutuality would be the expression and acceptance of both agreements, disagreements, positive and negative feelings both within the system (say between the nursing staff of the unit who comprise a group system) and between the system and its environment (the unit staff with other nursing units, with nursing administration, the physician group, and so on). Low mutuality occurs when there is a holding back of relevant cognitions and/or feelings across either internal or external boundaries.

In the following excerpt, we see an example of low mutuality of relationships. The new graduate was unable to express either fact or feeling directly to the nurse's aide. Because of this low mutuality, the group's boundary was impermeable to her input concerning a way of improving patient care.

The aides are doing it and I don't know how much a new grad can say to an aide. That's my biggest problem. How much can you say to someone who has that many years over you? She's 40 years old and what are you going to say? I don't know whether it's age or experience or what it is but I really can't go up to her and say, "I know you're giving poor nursing care." She's one of the ones that sets up the bath and then leaves the patient for an hour without helping them while the water gets cold. I have mentioned this fact, you know, to the people on the floor in general, and it still has not helped. I've said it as a general statement. This is what is being done and we ought to improve it. It was kind of a matter-of-fact saying it like that. It didn't help at all. (2:1A:16)

The following is another example of low mutuality of relationships. Although there was some attempt to increase mutuality, the negative reception made the speaker even more reluctant to express her thoughts and feelings.

I don't know about you guys, but I really don't have that much time, when I get home at night after working 10-hour days, to go in and do a research-type project. My idea of inservice is someone coming to the unit to give us information on certain drugs, certain products that we use a lot. That's what we all asked for. So the head nurse brought it up at the meeting that in order for us to have more inservices, we were going to have to do them ourselves. We asked her why don't we ask Dr. So-and-so to talk on the drugs that he works with. You know, and anesthesiologists, because that's the type of inservices that we were used to. Like the inservices that you guys get. And that's what we wanted. And she goes around and hits us with this; so consequently one of the nurses who has a couple of children and works part-time—she says, "I do not have time when I go home to do a project like this"; she says, "I have a family and two children." And the head nurse says, "Well, there are plenty of evenings here when there are no patients." OK, if you look at the books, we have not had a free evening— it's been a long time, when we haven't had anybody in there. OK. But she kept telling her, "Well, it's been a long time since we've had a free evening." And the head nurse kept saying, "Well, I know there's time when you can do the research here." And she just left it at that. And she said that three times, and by this time, the girl was red in the face, and she just shut up completely. And she said to me later, you know, she says, "I'm going to keep my mouth shut from now on." Those were her exact words. (6:5B:9–10)

It would not be at all surprising to find that the new graduate, in the excerpt related above, would quickly adopt the closed-mouth posture which appears to characterize the ward staff group where she works.

Not only is each of these concepts of importance in its own right, but their interaction is also of crucial importance to understanding the process of change. For example, notice in the following excerpt how the new graduate's perception of low mutuality in relationships inhibits her from causing changes:

It's a medication; it was ordered and it was supposed to be given. It was a mistake and the system very much needs to be changed so it doesn't happen again. But other people don't want to see, to hear, and I really have some feeling that I'm too new to start causing changes and trouble.   (4:3:6)

The degree of permeability of the internal and external boundaries tends to match the degree of mutuality of the relationships between and within systems. Optimal boundary permeability, that is, neither excessively open or closed, is associated with a high degree of mutuality in system and subsystem relationships.

Understanding these relationships is crucial to understanding system change. There are three possible conditions that could exist[39]:

|  | Condition 1 | Condition 2 | Condition 3 |
|---|---|---|---|
| Boundaries | Excessively open | Optimally open | Excessively closed |
| Mutuality of relationships | Low | High | Low |

System change is a complex affair involving internal and external boundaries, internal and external relationships. Some theorists[40] propose that the primary source of change is external to a system, while others[41] are of the opinion that there is a very high interdependency between them. In either event, these conditions illustrate the three primary system conditions involving change.

Condition 2 is obviously the condition of choice, the one it would be desired for the others to move to. In condition 3, the system boundaries are intact although the system may be functioning very inefficiently. Communication within the system and between the system and its environment are probably characterized by distrust, mutual suspicion, withholding of information, and so on. Although a group has formed and it exists, it probably is unable to communicate effectively either internally or externally. To get such a group to change, to move toward the desired condition 2, the emphasis must be in the area of increasing the mutuality of relationships.

In the following excerpt from one of the new graduate seminars we can begin to see some movement such as that described above. Commencing from what sounds like very closed boundaries (and presumably low mutuality of relationships), we detect in the second part of the excerpt some increase in the openness of communication and therefore at least in the mutuality of relationships between these two people who form a sub-unit of the system. Along with the increased mutuality, there is also some indication that there will be an increase in boundary permeability.

It's true, but the nurses on the night shift are so old that it's hard to get them off these habits. Every time I suggested other things, they'd say,

"Well, we never do it that way," or "Mrs. So-and-so always did it this way." And I say, "Well, I'm not Mrs. So-and-so," you know. That's my answer to them. But that is what I always get as feedback if they don't like what I'm saying and insist upon doing it the old way.

I think that they know that you're new though, and that they can get away with it.

Yeah, that's true, but one girl said to me last night: "How old is new?" and I said, "It depends on whether you trust me or not. It's convenient for you to say I'm new just as it's convenient for me to say I'm new. It works both ways." She looked at me and grinned and said, "Well, I guess I can trust you enough to listen to you." (2:3B:28)

Condition 1 exists when a group which should have formed has not, or when a group is breaking apart because of internal conflict or external stress. In trying to change a condition 1 group to condition 2, the first priority must be to aid in strengthening or establishing the system boundaries, to make the group a group. Since system boundaries that are formed under high degrees of stress are likely to be excessively closed, it is likely that when such boundaries are formed in a condition 1 group, the group will first move into condition 3, before it can be changed to move in the direction of condition 2.

In summary then, although it is possible to change or to move groups in the desired direction, because of the interdependency of boundary and relationship conditions, it is difficult. Each condition tends to be self-reinforcing. If movement is to be attempted, however, analysis of the kind of condition the group (or individual) is in is a starting place in deciding where, in the system, intervention will have the highest pay-off.

*Steady states.* Although systems change, they also establish and maintain steady states. The same theoretical concepts which help us to understand change are also relevant to steady states. Through an analysis of a wide range of research on individuals, organizations, and groups, Alderfer[42] indicates that there is support for the following conclusions.

1. For individuals, groups, and for organizations, there is evidence that optimally permeable boundaries are associated with mutual relationships, while excessively closed boundaries are associated with nonmutual relationships.

2. Internal and external conditions parallel each other.

3. Systems with strong permeable boundaries and mutual relationships show a greater tendency toward survival and health and productivity of novel and worthwhile products than systems with rigid boundaries and nonmutual relationships.

4. Individuals provide the primary internal unit in groups; groups are the major unit in organizations.

Because of the latter condition, and because of the parallelism noted in conclusion 2, there can be disequilibrium between internal and external conditions. For example, when a relatively open person meets a relatively closed group, much disequilibrium will occur. This disequilibrium is the key to effecting change. We will turn now from Alderfer's conclusions regarding steady states to an examination of changing states.

*Changing states.* For a system—be it a person, group, or organization—to change, it must move from one steady state to another. It either can move toward optimally permeable boundaries sustained by high mutuality of relationships, or it can move toward relatively closed boundaries with nonmutual relationships. All attempts at planned change activities either directly or indirectly aim human systems toward the first alternative.

The various approaches which have been used to change human systems can be classified according to the primary human needs aroused or worked with in the change process. Alderfer conceptualizes human needs in terms of existence, that is, what one needs for survival; relatedness, that is, what are mutually satisfying interactions with significant other people; and growth needs, that is, a person's or group's desire for challenge and stimulation, for opportunities to use capacities to the fullest, and to enlarge and enrich the person's or group's potential[43].

Utilizing this human need approach, Alderfer examined and analyzed available research on individuals, groups, and organizations to see how relevant boundaries and relationships change when a system undergoes change. From the analysis of studies of needs for existence, he concluded that although persons outside the system played an important role in most of the change programs, lasting change could not be brought about unless internal conditions were adequately prepared for change[44]. In terms of needs for relatedness, it was found that whether the unit of analysis was the individual, group, or organization, change programs aimed for more mutual human relationships tended to be most effective when the unit was favorably predisposed toward change before the program began. In other words, nothing quite makes up for readiness and motivation to make a change. It was also found that satisfaction of the need for relatedness was a necessary, but not always sufficient, condition for sustained and constructive planned change. Whether the change was in task performance, attitudes, or interpersonal behavior seems to make the difference as to which level should be approached for the change. Attitudes and interpersonal behavior changes were more effective at the individual and group level; task performance changes at the organizational level. Analysis of research on the needs for growth demonstrated that appealing to people's growth needs can be a highly successful approach to change. One way in which this is done is the development of job enrichment programs. Such programs, however, that focus almost exclusively on the job itself without giving adequate attention to the relevant human relationships fall into the trap of violating the key and necessary ingredient for effective change: mutuality of relationships. When such programs failed, interpersonal and intergroup relationships played an important part in diminishing the benefits of the intervention. Furthermore, it must be borne in mind that job enrichment programs on any level in an organization will always have an impact on the level immediately above and immediately below the "enriched" level. Care must be taken to take into account this interdependency of roles before making changes designed to appeal to the growth needs of an individual or group. Alderfer's conclusions provide us with some direction for how best to effect the change process to bring about maximum rewards. Before presenting this direction in the form of suggestions, let us look at some of the new graduates' attempts to be agents of change. Although there was little evidence of knowledge or use of change-agent process and theory in their discussions, it was apparent that they saw the need for and wanted to make changes.

### Experiences with Steady States and Change States

How did the new graduates go about moving the systems in which they were working from a steady state to a changed state? For those who did attempt to implement some kind of change, probably the most frequently-used method was through example, or perhaps it could be called role-modeling.

> There are lots of different ways to effect change. You could get very upset and say you're going to walk out and hope that that might change something. But when you know that's not going to work, then there are other ways. Like I just took it upon myself when I had a few extra minutes to start—I didn't have to tell anybody—I just started to do a few patient care plans and improve them and add to them and change them and things like that. Not that I told anybody, but slowly they were noticed. That's a way I found of effecting change. You can still be a new person and still do things that can really be effective, rather than be boisterous about it or be very loud. (9:3B:24)

Sometimes this method brought about change, but not exactly for the reasons desired.

> How do you do care plans? I must've done about six care plans and another RN comes up and flips through them and says: "Oh, my God, did you do all those?" Then she says, "I've gotta take some and do some so I look good too." So then they all started doing them. (4:2:14)

The new nurses were also quite cognizant of some of the problems that arose from this method of effecting change.

> I had a patient who went bad, had a cardiac problem. You get people back and they have to have special vital signs and special scanners that you need to watch closely. Well, others just sort of take the sheet and turn it over and scratch everything on there. But that was confusing to me, so I made out this special sheet and somebody says to me, "Well, don't do that." And I said, "Well, it's easier for me and if anybody wants to see how the patient is doing, they can see at a glance." And she said, "Well, *don't do* that." They didn't want me to start something that maybe they'd have to do after that. They said, "Well, we'll probably have to do that from now on." You know, somebody sees it and likes it . . . But I just did it. I'm gonna do it the way I want to do it.   (4:2:13)

As we can see, the newcomer might have effected a change, but it was done at the expense of possibly alienating the staff. This will make it much more difficult for any future attempts at bringing about change.

The role-modeling or "Just do it" type of change probably falls somewhere between what Bennis, Benne, and Chin call "emulative" change and what they call "interactional" change. It seems as though the newcomers thought that by their "just doing it," others would emulate them and change would result. Unfortunately, this is not how it works. Emulative change does not occur unless there is a superior-subordinate relationship and unless the subordinate identifies with and desires to emulate the power figure. It is possible for a new graduate to bring about emulative change with a nurse's aide or LPN, but with another RN, interactional change is probably more feasible. Interactional change is the nondeliberate change brought about by friendship and close interaction. The "just doing it" method could bring about this kind of change if the change agent were a respected and integral part of a friendly work group. There was no indication that the new graduates were aware of any of these requirements in their efforts to bring about change by the method of example.

In the following excerpts, newcomers attempted to bring about change through different kinds of interpersonal style. In the first excerpt, it appears that teasing was used; while in the second, the method appeared to be calling someone's bluff.

> If you start getting sarcastic around them, they think it's real cute. Like the day I mentioned, "You read my neat nursing care plans?" And she says, "No, I haven't had time." I said, "Oh" and looked real sad and she says, "Well, I'll go read them when I have a minute." It's a joke though; it's not as if I'm getting to them because of that.   (2:6A:3)

> It's been going pretty well with me. Maybe it's because I refuse to view the reactions as negative. I take things as a matter of fact. If people hit me with "Why are you going to do it that way?" I tend to look them straight in the

eye and say, "That's my way of doing it. How else shall we do it?" Then if they haven't got an answer that is better than my rationale, we are on the road to change. If they have got an answer, we talk about which sounds like a better idea . . . I just face up to them and don't buy that routine: "We've always done it that way." (9:2B:21 and 9:1A:23)

The new nurses seemed to be quite well aware of the advantages of effecting change through and with groups of people, rather than individually. In the first two of the next three excerpts we see a lack of success because of a lack of group support, while in the last we see success because of group support.

If you're the only one, even if you have good ideas, it's impossible to make changes. I see a lot of changes that need to be made for the night shift, but I'm the only one speaking up about them. Since I don't have my supervisor to really support me, I'm just one speaking and no one goes for the ideas. (9:3B:17)

I remember when I first started, my head nurse wanted me to do team conference and patient nursing care plans. But when no one else does it, you don't have any role model to follow and it's just "do." It's really kind of hard. It's hard for you to do it, unless someone else does it . . . Things will be started but nobody carries them out. And that's what's really hard. (9:1A:25)

It's a nice change and really good. I was kind of surprised. When they first introduced this new way of taking care of patients [modular nursing], just when I was getting used to the old method, I really didn't think I'd like it. But they presented it to the whole group of us and then the girl who was really in favor of it cornered the oldest nurse's aide on the unit—the one who's the real powerhouse—and really got her to understand it. Soon, just about everybody on the floor went along with it. And when they saw how it was working, they all really pushed it—even people who have been up there for 19 or 20 years think it's great. I guess I just got pushed along with everyone's buying it and the enthusiasm. (6:2A:3)

In some instances, the graduates specifically shared with one another how they went about effecting change.

What time did you do it?

About 10:30 to 11:00.

What did you do? Exactly.

Well, first I figured out that they weren't doing the care plans because they really didn't have too good an idea of how to do them or what they should look like afterward. So, first I chose a patient, you know, that I felt really needed a good care plan, cause it was not on the cardex and he needed a lot of care. And after, you know, organizing a care plan that I thought was good and telling a few of the others about it so that they would make some suggestions in the meeting, I invited them all to a conference and suggested that everyone come with some ideas in mind of what they could add or change about the care plan that I had written. Giving them a chance to think about it ahead of time. And then I posted the meeting and people showed up.

More than just two of you?

Yeah, they were all there but one. It was real good and lots of participation but I had to cut it off after about 30 minutes, because I didn't want to be taking up more time. I think everyone would have liked to have continued, and the next day, we got three more care plans started.   (6:4A:35)

There weren't too many examples of successful change agent activity described by the new graduates during their seminar discussions. In fact, out of the 110 discussions, there were only 11 instances of positive experiences with change activities. The following excerpt demonstrates one of these. Here we can see that the high mutuality of relationships fostered boundary permeability and the input of new ideas into the system.

The thing is that when you have an idea, you don't have to be afraid to express it. Like I brought up, OK, there's some Black children on the floor, and a lot of times their hair is not combed, and like you can go shampoo white children's hair, but you can't do that to many of the little Black girls. Because they have their hair pressed. So I taught a class on it, on the type of things to use and what is needed. So they went out and bought the hair dressing and a dryer and a thick comb and things like that. And they're on our floor now, so that when these kids come in, they can get the total care they need.   (9:1C:24)

One of the major impediments to bringing about changes within the system, in addition to the newness theme discussed earlier, was a lack of knowledge on the part of the new graduate as to how to go about effecting change.

Everyone shuts up, gets real closed mouthed on the unit when a lot of sad things—people dying and all—are happening in the unit. I don't know what to do to change that. I know it's not good. We need to talk about our feelings more. I'd be willing to do something about it, maybe to try and get some group meetings started, but I just don't know how to go about doing it, making changes like that.   (7:3B:23)

Sometimes the new graduates would directly ask for help in how to go about effecting change.

I'm having problems not so much with performance as with attitudes. How do you change something like that? You have people who have been there for years and they see the same patients come back in on a medical floor, time after time, and I have problems with, you know, I get a call from admissions, you're getting thus and so patient. I turn around and I say, "We're getting thus and so patient." "Oh, my god, Mabel's back!" they say. And so the attitude starts from there. You know Mabel's going to get crummy care. And how do you work with that? I need help on how to get the staff away from that. I find that the attitude starts affecting me. I've tried to change their attitudes by saying, "You know, look at her life, what a crummy life she's had," or "Poor lady, or poor man, can you imagine what it must be like to do this kind of thing!" And it's not just Mabel, you know, we've got a whole string of them. I don't know what to do with that kind of attitude.    (9:1C:26-28)

In other instances, it was apparent from their discussions that they wanted to see some changes made, but they were very unclear as to exactly what they wanted to see happen.

There's so many people I hate to see go home. I just hate to see them go home, but you don't want to keep them in, you know how expensive it is for them to be there, their doctor is satisfied with the progress they've made and they're sent home to either a hopeless situation—like lots of adolescents come in and they're mainly in there for psych reasons, but their admission diagnosis, for instance, like this one girl who's 16 with bronchitis, right? Well she never had respiratory involvement the whole time she was there. I mean she was a psych patient. She came from a split home; she was a very nervous girl; she had dermatitis; so finally I asked her why she was admitted and she said "for a diabetic work-up," and there was never one test done for diabetes. Not a blood-sugar level, nothing. She was in with horrible sores that would not heal all over her hands. Her hands were swollen; they gave her cortisone and her hands stopped swelling, right? The inflammation went away. She never was seen by a dermatologist. She had a psych consult for two days. She didn't like her psychiatrist—wouldn't talk to him. Well, who would, in a room with a patient right on the other side of the curtain? I mean a 16-year-old girl isn't going to open up to some strange man, and that girl was sent home to the same situation, you know. There are so many things like that. I want to do something to make things right, make them better but I just don't know where or how to start.  (2:6A:29-30)

A second major impediment to effecting change was resistance— resistance from a variety of people. This was the dominant subtheme, encompassing fully 70 percent of all seminar discussions in the subject area of change.

### Reactions to Change

When a person who has not been formally delegated authority to institute change attempts to effect change, reform, or innovation within a unit group or organization, the probability is very high that she will encounter resistance. This resistance can take many forms. O'Day[45] provides us with a useful way of looking at systematized resistance, particularly those reactions on the part of middle management to change attempts made from the lower level of the organization. This particular analysis fits the situations of the new graduate quite well, since it is usually either her own peers or the middle management level of the nursing administration that evinces the most resistance to changes and innovations that new graduates suggest.

In understanding resistance, it is helpful to view the attempted change from the perspective of the middle hierarchy in an organization, or from that group of people who are not effecting change but experiencing it. What does change look like and mean to them? First of all, most attempts are perceived as threats. It can be a threat to one's competence—after all, if newcomers want to change something, then the way I'm doing it now isn't ok, and therefore I'm incompetent. It might be a moral or ego threat: "If this is something that needs to be changed, then I should have been aware of it and initiated the change proceedings myself." Or it may be a threat to one's relationships with those above one in the organization, who might say "Can't you keep order and keep everything under control in your own bailiwick?"

In reaction to these threats, middle management or older staff may exert some rituals of control—efforts to control the person advocating change so that she does not succeed in recruiting support for her idea and plan, to discourage the person from continuing to seek reform, and to exercise control in such a way that middle management or others who are being "changed" will not look "bad" or be accused of wrongdoing. O'Day describes two major phases of these control or intimidation rituals[46]. The first phase, indirect intimidation, includes the rituals of nullification and isolation; the second, direct intimidation, the rituals of defamation and expulsion.

*Nullification.*    This ritual of control is the first one used. When the change agent approaches supervisory or older staff members with a suggestion or idea, they will assure the new graduate that, because she doesn't understand the situation, her suggestion is invalid. A frequently heard response is: "We've always done it that way," with a tone suggesting that there is authority and perfection in traditional ways of doing things. Often, it is hoped that the newcomer will be so awed by the authority and wisdom of age that no further attempts at change will be made. If, however, the change agent persists, her superiors will agree to "look into it." The results of this investigation will usually be such that the newcomer suggesting the change will see that her suggestions or perceptions of the situation are groundless or unworkable, but that her suggestions have been duly noted by the people who really care about the effectiveness and efficiency of the organization. The message is: "You don't know what you are talking about, but thank you for telling us anyway. We'll certainly look into this matter, and we appreciate you being interested in the organization." There is always a carefully managed image of reasonableness that leaves the change agent feeling somewhat good about the whole situation.

There is even a strong possibility that the whole ritual of nullification will get not only the organizational representative but also the newcomer change agent "off the hook." By making the suggestion for change to the authorities the newcomer is able to shed some of the personal responsibility for the problem that is being addressed. The change agent can quite justly have the feeling, "Well, at least I tried."

The new graduates encountered nullification, as can be seen from the following excerpts:

> This is what they tell you: "This is the way it's always been and . . ." Either you're going to fight the system or you're going to accept it. And the system is bigger than you. So you're going to have to learn to accept it and be flexible.　(2:3B:23)

> I think she's really good but I think she's into so many things that she can't finish or really do one thing and if you talk to her about something she says, "Yeah, I'll check into that," but you never see her again, or hear about it.　(2:1B:11)

> I told her about it several times. The last time, I even gave her the names of all the patients who didn't get their meds. She said she'd look into it, but I don't know if she really will. Permanent night nurses are hard to find and I guess they'd rather keep her than have to look for one who would do the job right. But I feel better in a way that at least I really brought it to their attention—all the facts and everything.　(7:3B:4)

> I just like mention it to whoever's on the unit, every time it happens. And they just all go, "There she goes again," and sort of shrug their shoulders and walk away. I think everyone recognizes the need for change, and they're always going to look into it, but nothing ever really gets done.　(6:4A:28–29)

Repeated exposure to the nullification ritual can be translated into the "banging your head against the wall." Eventually this will wear down most would-be reformers, and convince them that their voices, their suggestions are not truly welcomed. The change agent is expected to take the hint and cease and desist from further suggestions of changes, but if she doesn't, the next ritual might be applied.

*Isolation.*　If the nullification ritual was not effective and the newcomer persists in her efforts to cause changes, the next step is to separate her from peers, subordinates, and thereby minimize the effect that the person and her suggestion will have on the organization, and also make it extremely difficult for her to mobilize any support for her position. This same kind of isolation can also be accomplished by swamping the individual with work of a kind that requires so much time, energy, and concentration that she literally has no reserve left for change activities.

Other attempts at isolating the reformer might include the closing of communication links, restricting freedom of movement, or limiting her use of available resources.

Systematic unresponsiveness to a change agent's criticism and suggestions is a particularly effective form of isolation. This form of resistance to change and suggestions was noted by Turner in a study of a large number of undergraduate students in a major university. In response to the question, "During the past month, has there been anything you wanted to say, any viewpoint or opinion you wanted to express—that you haven't felt free to express?" a surprisingly large number of students responded that their freedom of expression was impaired because "No one listens; no one cares; no one understands; people have all made up their minds; the system won't change; the system can't be changed; people in my position don't carry enough weight to make any difference; I couldn't get enough support to back me up; I don't know how to go about it"[47]. Unresponsiveness would seem to be quite an effective social sanction and a form of isolation, meant to convince the potential change agent of the invalidity of her position. In the new graduate seminars, it sounded like this:

> There's no point in trying to make changes. You talk to some people that came just before you came—you know, like last year this time, and it's the same thing with them. Your feelings aren't all that unique. They wanted the same things I want now, to make the same changes. They fought their little battles and the same things are still going on. They haven't gotten anywhere. What's the use; why even try?   (1:4C:19)

> If you start yelling about these things, they think that you're idealistic, that you can't see the reality of things and that things take time. You can only say so much as a new grad. I have found this out. I mean really, and they play so many games, you get the runaround all the time. My head nurse is the biggest talker in the world. She says nothing. When it comes to things that are suggested to her that need to be changed, she keeps saying that we'll get to it, but nothing ever happens.   (2:6A:36–37)

If a person presses her right to be heard, unresponsiveness will usually generate in her a tremendous feeling of impotence and powerlessness. Not infrequently this serves as a stimulus to cause the potential change agent to overreact in order to get some sort of response from the people she is trying to change. Then the overreaction is used against her to demonstrate how unstable she is, how wild her ideas are, and hence that she shouldn't be listened to or followed.

In general, the ritual of isolation is designed to convince the change agent that it is futile to try and initiate change until she is specifically instructed to do so by her superiors. When subjected to such isolation, most people usually cease their advocacy and join the many other silent participants in the organization. If the newcomer further resists doing so, and instead mobilizes support for her position, she may be subjected to direct intimidation in the form of defamation.

*Defamation.* This ritual attempts to control the change agent by cutting her off from potential supporters. It does this by attributing the attempts at reform, or the suggestions offered to questionable motives, underlying psychopathology, or gross incompetence. This method of control is effective because it transforms a sympathetic following into a mistrustful group who may feel as though they have been "sold a bill of goods" and have been deceived. Often both the implicit and explicit messages are: "You can't even do what we can do and yet you want to change things all around," or "You're new around here; wait till you've been here awhile and then you'll understand why it's done that way." It is also quite possible that the comment frequently heard by new graduates, "Didn't they teach you anything in school?" might also be part of the defamation ritual.

The new graduates presented several examples of this type of intimidation ritual as a response to attempted change on their part.

> A couple of older nurses are about ready to retire. You just can't suggest anything to them. And if you say something with some type of authority, like you do know what you're talking about, they look at you and say, "Well, what do you mean talking to me like that!" (3:1A:22)

> Some people won't listen to you and they'll say, "What do you know? I've been doing this for a long time. You're new!" (1:2C:9)

In the ritual of defamation, the goal is to bring about retreat and passivity of the change agent by threatening the destruction of the person's reputation, reliability, and competence as a nurse. If, however, this goal is not met, then the final step of intimidation must be taken.

*Expulsion.* When all else fails, the final measure of control is to attempt to force the change agent's "voluntary" withdrawal from the organization. This is obviously an effective measure of control and resistance because not only does it remove the person and her offensive ideas, it also serves as a warning to others and as a confirmation of the unfitness of the potential change agent in the first place. If at all possible, voluntary withdrawal—that is, resignation—is preferable to forced expulsion. The latter is undesirable because it permits, even fosters, public inspection of records, and potentially embarrassing cross-examination.

Although there were times in the seminars when the discussions relative to effective change ended on a very sad note, and a few times when new graduates verbalize the feeling, "What's the use! I might just as well leave this place," there were no actual examples of individuals being expelled or forced out of the system because of change agent activities or suggestions. For the most part, it appeared as though these newcomers were being held in check either through 1) the first three intimidation rituals, 2) their lack of knowledge of how to proceed with change, 3) perceptions that the system was closed because of its low boundary permeability or low mutuality of relationships, or 4) their lack of power due to being new in the system. Therefore, we are still confronted with the dilemma described in the opening paragraphs of this section. What can be done so that the system can receive the input from new graduates, thereby energizing itself and enabling its vital growth?

## Suggestions for Effecting Change in Open Systems

One of the most consistent and conclusive research findings has been that effective change requires simultaneous internal and external stimulation. The establishment of insider-outsider teams has been demonstrated as one of the most effective means of helping an organization or group to become more open, and more effective in making desired changes. Outsiders, such as new graduate nurses during the first five or six months of employment, who have not been fully socialized into a system provide fresh perspectives and stimulation. A person is a new graduate nurse on her first job only once in her whole life. At no other time will a new graduate have as unique, fresh, and sensitive a perspective as she does at that time. By formally pairing such an outsider with an established nurse insider—someone who has the knowledge and empathy of the system which can be gained only through extensive experience with it—and by designating this outsider-insider team as the official "change agent" team of the unit, much could be done to bring about ongoing, unit-level change. If, within a very short period of time after the new graduate's arrival on the unit, such a change agent team were designated, and if such a team were held accountable to initiate planned change activity, the system could reap untold benefits, both in terms of increasing the permeability of the group's boundaries and the subsequent input of the new ideas into the system, and in increasing the mutuality of relationships.

As a preliminary step in any kind of change agent analysis, we need to begin by identifying and understanding the type of change desired. There may be times when one wants to make other than a planned change. For example, during crises, it is not uncommon for group members to respond very positively to coercive change. It may, in fact, be the almost constant crisis footing of the modern-day hospital which makes it unusually ripe for coercive changes. But there are other types of change that can be quite beneficial as well; for example, interactive and emulative changes definitely have their place in the success of human endeavors. The important thing is that people need to be aware of the different kinds of change and be able to recognize when they or others are employing or need to employ various change strategies.

One of the most important things that needs to be done to solve the dilemma noted in the opening paragraphs of this section is to be complete and realistic in what we teach students in schools of nursing about change. They need to be taught how to distinguish the various kinds of change and to differentiate the positive and negative aspects of each. By recognizing the type of change that is being used, they are in a much better position to evaluate and select courses of behavior, to conform or not to conform. Although there is no question that planned change is the most democratic form of change, the most long-lasting and effective, ours is an imperfect world. Different people will use other forms of change. To recognize these is to take the tyranny and frustration out of them.

There are other aspects of change that it would be well to teach to students and practicing nurses alike. Before commencing a change activity, it is extremely helpful to identify the extent of permeability of the boundaries of the group with which one wishes to work, and to estimate the degree of mutuality in the relationships of the group. By so doing, one can conjecture what condition the group is in, and where movement is desired. And then perhaps most important is deciding upon which basic human need the change agent wishes to appeal to. By following some of these very basic steps, the change agent will be in a much better position to be effective.

A primary goal must be to establish relevant boundaries, to open closed boundaries, and to move relationships from less to more mutuality. To establish a boundary where one previously did not exist means that the relationships between those parts must be developed and opened up. To make a boundary more permeable means that the amount and kinds of material flowing in and out of the system or subsystem must be increased. When one tries to move a relationship toward greater mutuality, then one must work on balancing the flow of relevant information, energy, and matter between parts of the system, or between the system and its external environment. For many hospital work groups, this means that effort must be made to open up the communications between shifts, between units, and between the ward staff group and the hospital at large. Encouraging total unit staff meetings, instead of meetings with day staff, evening staff, and night staff separately, is one attempt at opening boundary permeability. As we have seen, the new graduates were particularly aware of a great deal of friction between the nursing staff on different shifts. At the same time, it can be noted that there is an increasing tendency to conceptualize a nursing unit as a single group under a head nurse. There is some fallacy in this practice with respect to both system boundaries and relationships. Particularly if the evening and/or night staff is permanent, it is quite possible that these staff members will feel more a part of the permanent evening and night staff on other units than a part of the day shift on the unit assigned. In other words, the actual group boundaries may not be the same as the formal boundaries. What must be recognized is that more change and more effective change will be brought about by working with the staff through their existent informal groups, irrespective of the formalized group boundaries which in many instances are boundaries on paper only.

Perhaps it will have been noticed that all of the preceding suggestions very clearly address the process of effecting change with a group, not with an individual. It has been well documented that group change is far more effective than individual change[48]. Virtually all individuals in a work environment are members of one or several groups. The new graduate or others as change agents would do well to remember this, and always to plan on affecting change with and through a group rather than individually.

Students and practicing nurses alike need to understand that it is almost predictable that change attempts will engender resistance and conflict. Knowledge of the intimidation rituals of nullification, isolation, defamation, and expulsion will help the change agent a great deal in understanding what is happening when it is happening. Through this understanding, the change agent is in a much better position to forestall the intimidation ritual than if she did not know or understand what was going on. For example, during isolation, the newcomer making suggestions practically guarantees her defeat if she reacts to systematic organization unresponsiveness with anger and confrontation or by increasing the pressure to bring about the desired change. Such intensification of efforts and confrontation are self-defeating because of the intense frustration brought about because of the change agent's belief that the unresponsiveness violates her basic rights of freedom and expression and carries with it the implication that she is personally an ineffectual person [49]. If the change agent can forestall the impulse to lash out against this unresponsiveness and can redouble her efforts with her constituency to continue with the change practice rather than to get new adherents, the intimidation attempts to get the change agent to behave irrationally and emotionally can be foiled. So also with the defamation ritual. If the change agent can understand and appreciate the fact that it is precisely the validity of the things she is suggesting that motivates and drives those who are opposed to her ideas to attempt to destroy the credibility of the originator of those ideas, she will then be able to see that the most effective counteraction to defamation is a temporary withdrawl and refocusing. By temporarily withdrawing from efforts to push through the desired change, coupled with a redoubling of effort to establish her competency and credibility in those areas valued by the group of people whom she is trying to convince, she can ensure that the change desired will be carried in on the shirttails of competency and credibility.

A few other aspects of resistance and intimidation will also help the prospective change agent. First, it is helpful to understand that people may resist suggestions, new ideas, and changes because:

1. They perceive themselves as being cast into an unfavorable light when contrasted with the enthusiasm, energy, and heightened activity of the change agent.

2. They may fear that the change agent's activities will be successful, and they are afraid of some of the implications of the change for their own job or practice.

3. Others may fear that if they cannot match the newcomer change agent in zeal and enthusiasm, that they will look bad, and that eventually the newcomer will replace them in their jobs[50].

Generally speaking, people actively or passively resist changes because the pain of the status quo is less intense than is the fear of the unknown. Prospective change agents must understand and work with the realization that if more of their coworkers would be willing to turn their various dissatisfactions with the practice of nursing as it is today into concentrated effort and activities to change those practices, then intimidation rituals would lose much of their power. Nurses must stand up and must stand together to bring about much needed change in nursing practice.

Nursing must also come to grips with its own version of the well-ingrained reflex of flight in the face of crises and change which has been noted to characterize North American society since colonial days[51]. It is time that we stop running to change jobs every time the going gets rough. For years there has been such a marked discrepancy between the supply and demand markets of nursing that it was relatively easy for a nurse to change jobs and get another one, always looking for greener pastures. Large formal hospital organizations and all of their desirable and undesirable by-products are going to be with us for a long time to come[52]. We are going to have to learn to devise ways of making them more functional, patient-centered, and responsive to the needs of client and nurse alike. There simply is no place to run to anymore.

Encouraging new graduates to be change agents, to try to change and improve the health care system for the betterment of patient care, is a risky and foolhardy thing to do unless these aspirant change agents are taught not only the change process as described in this chapter and elsewhere, but also the basic interpersonal skills of constructive conflict resolution. They need these skills to be prepared to handle constructively the conflict that will in all probability result when they attempt to bring about change. As was mentioned early in this section, all change attempts in some way or other are concerned with value changes. Values are something very near and dear to most people. They are not given up or changed without a fight or a struggle. To expect the newcomer to make these kinds of changes, to bring and to implement new ideas into the work setting without a firm grounding and skill development in conflict resolution, is setting her up for failure. (For a discussion of values and the part values play in change activity, and for a presentation and discussion of conflict resolution principles, see *Path to Biculturalism* [53].)

In addition to teaching students the principles and techniques, the planned change, and the theory and practice in empathy and constructive conflict resolution, another very important preliminary step that nurses must be taught is to make assessments of the values of those with whom they work—patients, physicians, and coworkers alike. This is a preliminary step to developing empathy. Persons unable to recognize values as they are reflected in behavior and verbalizations will be unable to interpret behavior, hence unable to exert effective influence by getting into the shoes (values) of the other person. The process of and strategies useful in value assessment are discussed in *Path to Biculturalism* [54].

Many schools of nursing include aspects of change agency in their curricula. Not infrequently, this includes an assignment wherein each student must execute and write up a change agent project. The purpose of such an assignment is to provide students with some real practice in effecting a planned change. These change agent activities often run into difficulties because the school term is too short for students to complete the project. Very often they identify a need for change, they plan the change, meet with unit staff to present the change idea, the staff agrees to the change, the student initiates the new practice once or twice, and then the school term is over. The student may well complete the term believing that she has effected a successful planned change. The real proof of the pudding is the extent to which a real and more or less permanent change in behavior has been brought about—whether the change has been refrozen, to use Lewin's term.

To overcome this truncated and distorted view of the change process and simultaneously to bring about effective changes in nursing practice, what is suggested is that the student's change agent process begin at the end, rather than at the beginning. Since it is common practice for student group to follow upon student group, the change agent activity initiated by one student can become the starting point of the change activity for a student in the group to follow. For example, if a student in the first rotation initiated as her change activity the use of a teaching plan for diabetics, then the initial activity of the student in the next rotation who comes onto that ward would be an assessment of how successful the previous student's change activity has been. Are the staff still using the teaching plans? If not, why not? How long did they use them before they stopped? What were the barriers to their use? Following this assessment, and if the decision is made that the teaching plans are still a good idea, the student in the second rotation picks up where the first student left off and follows through as the agent of this change activity. In this way, there is a much greater probability not only that students will have practice and experience in all aspects of the change process, but also that some real changes in nursing service might be brought about.

Although new graduates are generally not involved in total organizational changes, there are a few suggestions that need to be made about them. Again, the insider-outsider approach has been found to be most effective. For the most part, sending people out of the organization in order to be changed is not as effective in bringing about a total organizational change as is bringing in a change agent team to work with the staff. If staff members are going to be sent out to be changed, previous work has demonstrated the wisdom of sending at least two people at a time.

With respect to total organizational change, it must be remembered that changes, particularly job enrichment programs, cannot be introduced on one level only. If job enrichment will encroach upon or realign already existing functions from workers at one level to workers at another level, caution must be exercised. Failure to take into account the effect of changes on one level on the efforts of people at other levels in the organization can undermine otherwise successful enlargement efforts. A classic study by Rubenstein and Lasswell[55] demonstrates this phenomenon quite well. An experimental effort to change the nature of patient roles at the Yale Psychiatric Institute was highly successful except for the fact that as the patients became more involved in their care, were more engaged in full-time and part-time jobs, it became increasingly evident that the nurses were the most displaced group. Some of the activities which previously the nurses alone had done, like gathering information about the patients, were now being done during the patient-staff meeting. What happened to the nurses is similar to what happens to those persons who have the most immediate and direct contact with the employees whose jobs are enriched. When the lowest level jobs are widened, the next level position is threatened unless efforts are made to take account of the interdependency among roles.

This is not to be understood as an indictment against job enrichment programs. When properly undertaken and executed, such programs must be considered a highly successful change strategy benefiting both the individual and the organization. We certainly need many more of these in nursing. And it is highly probable that through such programs, more and more nurses would find their jobs to contribute much more to their personal growth than they do at present. In this way, we hope, nursing as a whole will be in a much better position to cope with the dilemma of making full use of the talents and new ideas of new graduate nurses. It is sincerely hoped that some of the suggestions offered in this chapter will be implemented so that in the future we will see new graduates who dream dreams and yet are ready and willing to pay the price of making them come true.

## REFERENCES

1. Goffman, E. *The Presentation of Self in Everyday Life.* Garden City, New York: Doubleday Anchor, 1959.
2. Schneider, D. and Turkat, D. Self-presentation following success or failure: Defensive self-esteem models. *J. Personality,* 43(1): 127–135, 1975.
3. Goffman, E. 1959, pp. 10–11.
4. Gergen, K. and Wishnov, B. Others' self-evaluations and interaction anticipated as determinants of self-presentation. *J. Personality Social Psychology,* 2(3): 348–358, 1965.
5. Goffman, E. 1959, pp. 17–21.
6. Glaser, B. G. and Strauss, A. *Awareness of Dying.* Chicago: Aldine, 1965, pp. 32–34.
7. Becker, H. S. and Geer, B. The fate of idealism in medical school. *Am. Sociological Rev.,* 23: 50–56, 1958.
8. Goffman, E. 1959, p. 20.
9. Blau, P. A theory of social integration. *Am. J. Sociology,* 65(6): 545–556, 1960.
10. Kramer, M. *Reality Shock.* St. Louis, Mo.: C. V. Mosby, 1974, p. 141.
11. Goffman, E. 1959, p. 142.
12. Schein, E. "Organizational Socialization and the Profession of Management" in Kolb, D., Rubin, I. and McIntyre, J. (Eds.), *Organizational Psychology.* Englewood Cliffs, N.J.: Prentice-Hall, 1974, p. 4.
13. Levinson, D. Role, personality and social structure in the organizational setting. *J. Abnormal Social Psychology,* 58: 170–180, 1959.
14. Merton, R. K. *Social Theory and Social Structure.* New York: Free Press, 1957.
15. Kahn, R. et al. *Organizational Stress: Studies in Role Conflict and Ambiguity.* New York: Wiley, 1964, pp. 26–34.
16. Kahn, R. et al., 1964, p. 182. Reprinted with permission.
17. Kelman, H. Process of opinion changes. *Public Opinion Quart.,* 25(1): 57–78, 1961.
18. Kahn, R. et al. 1964.
19. Merton, R. K. 1957.
20. Kahn, R. et al., 1964, p. 187. Reprinted with permission.
21. Argyris, C. *Integrating the Individual and the Organization.* New York: Wiley, 1964, p. 131.
22. Kramer, M. and Schmalenberg, C. *Path to Biculturalism.* Wakefield, Mass.: Contemporary Publishing, 1977, pp. 248–304.
23. Henry, J. "Attitude Organization in Elementary School Classroom" in Charters, W. W. and Gage, N. L. (Eds.), *Readings in the Social Psychology of Education.* Boston: Allyn and Bacon, 1963, pp. 254–263.
24. Peplau, H. An open letter to a new graduate. *Nursing Digest,* 3(2): 6, 1975. Reprinted with permission.
25. Genn, N. Where can nurses practice as they're taught? *Am. J. Nursing,* 74(12): 2212, 1974.
26. Bennis, W., Benne K., and Chin, R. *The Planning of Change.* New York: Holt, Rinehart and Winston, 1961, p. 155.
27. Bennis, W., Benne, and Chin, R. 1961, p. 11.
28. Bennis, W., Benne, and Chin, R. 1961, p. 11.
29. Alderfer, C. "Change Processes in Organizations" in Dunnette M. (Ed.), *Handbook of Industrial and Organizational Psychology.* Chicago: Rand McNally College Publishing, 1976, pp. 1591–1638.
30. Schein, E. H. and Kommers, D. W. *Professional Education.* New York: McGraw-Hill, 1972; Arndt, C. and Huckabay, L. "Change" in *Nursing Administration: Theory for Practice with a Systems Approach.* St. Louis, Mo.: C. V. Mosby, 1975, Chap. 7, pp. 152–167; Bennis, W. et al. *The Planning of Change.* New York: Holt, Rinehart and Winston, 1961; Havelock, R. G. *A Change Agent's Guide to Innovation*

*in Education.* Englewood Cliffs, New Jersey: Educational Technology Publications, 1973.
31. Lewin, K. Frontiers in group dynamics. *Human Relations,* 1(1): 5–41, 1947.
32. Schein, E. H. and Kommers, D. K., 1972, p. 76.
33. Schein, E. H. and Kommers, D. K., 1972, p. 78.
34. Cartwright, D. Achieving change in people: Some applications of group dynamics theory. *Human Relations,* 4(4): 381–392, 1951.
35. von Bertalanffy, L. "General Systems Theory" in *Yearbook of the Society for the Advancement of General Systems Theory,* vol. 1. 1956, pp. 1–10.
36. Katz, D. and Kahn, R. *Social Psychology of Organizations.* New York: Wiley, 1966.
37. Alderfer, C. 1976.
38. Alderfer, C. 1976, p. 1593.
39. Alderfer, C. 1976, p. 1597.
40. Katz, D. and Kahn, R., 1966.
41. Alderfer, C. 1976.
42. Alderfer, C. 1976.
43. Alderfer, C. 1976, pp. 1614–1632.
44. Alderfer, C. 1976, p. 1617.
45. O'Day, R. Intimidation rituals: Reactions to reform. *J. Appl. Behavioral Sci.,* 10(3): 373–386, 1974.
46. O'Day, R. 1974.
47. Turner, R. Unresponsiveness as a social sanction. *Sociometry,* 36(1): 1–19, 1973.
48. Cartwright, D. 1951, p. 387.
49. Turner, D. 1951, p. 387.
50. O'Day, R. 1974, p. 383.
51. O'Day, R. 1974, p. 384.
52. O'Day, R. 1974, p. 384.
53. Kramer, M. and Schmalenberg, C. 1977.
54. Kramer, M. and Schmalenberg, C. 1977.
55. Rubenstein, R. and Lasswell, H. D. *The Sharing of Power in a Psychiatric Hospital.* New Haven, Conn.: Yale University Press, 1966.

## BIBLIOGRAPHY

Arndt, C. and Huckabay, L. *Nursing Administration: Theory for Practice with a Systems Approach.* St. Louis, Mo.: C. V. Mosby, 1975.
Deutsch, M. Reflections on some studies of interpersonal conflict. *Am. Psychologist,* 24(12): 1969.
Festinger, L. A. *A Theory of Cognitive Dissonance.* Stanford, Calif.: Stanford University Press, 1957.
Johnson, D. W. *Contemporary Social Psychology.* Philadelphia: Lippincott, 1973.
Katz, S. and Burnstein, E. Is an out-of-role act credible to biased observers and does it affect the credibility of neutral acts? *J. Personality,* 43(2): 1975.
Morris, B. Reflections on role analysis. *Brit. J. Sociology,* 22(4): 1971.
Munson, P. and Kiesler, C. The role of attributions by others in the acceptance of persuasive communications. *J. Personality,* 42(3): 1974.
Rizzo, J., House, R., and Lirtzman, S. Role conflict and ambiguity in complex organizations. *Admin. Sci. Quart.,* 15(2): 1970.
Schlenker, B. R. Self-presentation: managing the impression of consistency when reality interferes with self-enhancement. *J. Personality Social Psychology,* 32(6): 1975.
Thibaut, J. W. and Kelley, H. H. *The Social Psychology of Groups.* New York: Wiley, 1959.
Thornton, R. and Nardi, P. The dynamics of role acquisition. *Am. J. Sociology,* 80(4): 1975.

# Chapter 6
# Patients and
# Patient Care

The overall goal of both the individual and the organization in nursing is quality patient care. The earlier chapters of this book have been concerned with the organization, the individual nurse, and the interrelationships of the two. This chapter, on patients and patient care, examines the product of the efforts of both the organization and the individual.

One of the characteristics of moving from the school world to the work world is more extended contact with patients and their families. Such contact resulted in increased awareness and concern for the overall quality of patient care. The first section, Quality of Patient Care, examines experiences and perceptions voiced by new graduates in the seminars with respect to how well the goals of quality care were achieved by both the individual and the organization.

One area of patient care of particular concern for the newcomers was the quality of dying and death, the subject of the second section of this chapter. Confronted with dying patients, new nurses had to come to grips with their own feelings about death and dying and with the impact of their feelings on the quality of death for the patients under their care.

## QUALITY OF PATIENT CARE

> The patients just aren't getting good care. I can't give the kind of care that I want to and that patients need. It's not that I'm incapable of doing it; I'm very capable, but because of circumstances of a political type, or being understaffed, patients are not receiving the care they should. You've got to compensate in some way and it usually winds up as frustration for you and poor care for the patient. (9:3C:7)

The chapter deals with the effects on the patient of the issues of concern to the new graduate that have been presented in this book so far. The subject area, quality of patient care, deals with the dynamics of the hospital's output and with the factors which influence the rendering of that patient care.

Most of the literature on hospitals that is concerned with the product of hospital services—patient care—is limited to how well the patient liked or was satisfied with the care he received[1, 2]. Here we will look at another side. How satisfied were the new graduate nurses with the quality of care that patients received? If the patient did not receive good-quality care, what prevented it? What could the nurses have done and what did they do about it? These three questions represent the major themes identified in the new graduate seminar discussions on patient care.

Concerns about the quality of patient care ranked sixth in the new graduate seminar discussions and were of interest nationally, occurring in all medical centers participating. Occurrence of the topic followed the usual pattern of other major concerns, with 46 percent of the discussions occurring in the early seminars, 38 percent in the middle, and 16 percent in the later ones. The rankings for frequency of occurrence of this subject ranged from fourth to eleventh, with rank clustering between fourth and sixth at six of the medical centers. The three medical centers that ranked the subject ninth to eleventh were A, H, and I. No common factors among these medical centers differentiated them from the others to account for the difference in importance they accorded the subject.

Emphasis in the subject area of quality of patient care was on the patient or his family, rather than on the effect of any factor on the nurse. The themes in this subject area fell into three main categories with subthemes as follows:

1.  Patients do get quality patient care because
    a.  (of general reasons—nothing specific).
    b.  I can get involved with them.
    c.  there is continuity of care.
    d.  I can see them make progress.
    e.  I or others had the skills they needed.
2.  Patients don't get quality care because
    a.  (of general reasons—nothing specific).
    b.  they don't complain enough.
    c.  I or the staff lack the needed skills.
    d.  there is not enough time.
    e.  there is not enough staff or there is maldistribution of staff.
    f.  there is lack of continuity of care.
    g.  they're forgotten.
    h.  people learn or practice on them.
    i.  of certain characteristics of the patient.
3.  I do something to improve the quality of patient care.

The first theme accounted for only 8 percent of the total number of discussions, while the second theme encompassed 89 percent. There were only four discussions in which new graduates talked about things they did to improve the quality of care for a specific patient. This should not be interpreted as meaning that the new graduates generally saw patients as not receiving good-quality care, but rather that poor-quality care was of primary concern to them.

## Perspective on Patient Care

The way in which hospitals go about producing their product—patient care—is unique in comparison to the production process of any other kind of organization. Patient care as a product emerges as a composite that is beyond the exclusive control of any of those who contribute to it. The patient care outcome results from a negotiated system of inter-actions which yield accommodative consequences[3]. It cannot be said that nursing alone, or medicine alone, or dietary care alone produces patient care. All departments within a hospital must negotiate together to accommodate and to produce patient care. This is quite different from what is found in other production organizations. Take, for example, General Motors Corporation, where a car emerges as a product of the production department. Other departments, such as research, design, procurement, marketing, and sales, are all part of the organization, but it is one central department which produces the product.

Hospitals are unique organizations in another way as well. In most organizations, the workers at the lower levels are further removed from each other than are those people on the policy-making or management level. By contrast, in hospitals the workers on the lower levels, staff nurses, dietary aides, interns, housekeeping maids, floor pharmacists are in much closer contact with one another than are their bosses with one another. A given housekeeping maid will see and interact with the head nurse of a unit far more often than the head of housekeeping will interact with the director of nursing service. In fact, the front lines of a hospital literally converge on the patient care units, as the workers converge there physically. Work must be integrated around a living but physically sta-tionary client.

These unique structural characteristics affect the product, patient care, in several ways. First, this functional convergence demands negotiation and accommodation. Not all workers can serve the patient, at the same time, that is, put their part into the production of the product. Not only is there competition for the resource of time, but there is competition for space and for the patient's very physical being. The X-ray department cannot have the patient at the same time that the physical therapist has him. The convergence of function in the patient care process requires almost continuous interdigitation of functions and people. There must be sufficient overlap in functions so that nothing is left undone, but it is not effective or efficient in terms of survival of the organization if there is too much overlap.

Not only does the uniqueness of the hospital structure affect the quality of the product; so also the separate, unique, and distinct ideologies that are apparent in the patient care process affect the outcome—patient care. An ideology is the rationale which justifies tasks and functions; it explains why certain things are done in certain ways, why people function in specific ways. Ideologies determine not only tasks to be done, but also the process and reason they are done in certain ways.

Mauksch[4] describes three major process systems of patient care, each with its own at least partially defined ideology: cure, care, and core. The *cure* process places primary emphasis on recovery. Direct intervention to promote healing is its mainstay. The structure and processes of care within a hospital are manifested most clearly through the medical practice. The mandate of cure is singular and unidirectional. The patient will be healed, his life saved, function restored, and health reestablished. Cure as an ideology is capable of complete success, but of course, is also capable of complete failure. The death of a patient is an example of the latter.

Whenever a mandate or an ideology is potentially capable of complete success or failure, the ideology is likely to have more power and to be more influential then functions or systems not subject to these two extreme positions. This is clearly dramatized in hospitals by the ascendancy of any kind of life-or-death consideration, that is, the likelihood of that consideration's being taken as a paramount over all else.

The *care* system and ideology argues for the needs of the whole human being, his family, and his situational needs. This ideology calls for the active participation of the individual to be cared for, in contrast to the cure ideology, where functions are performed for and on the recipient. Complete care can be given only to inanimate objects, so that complete care is as inconceivable as the complete absence of care. Rather than the either-or bimodal quality of the cure process, the results of the care process have a much more central distribution—rather like a normal distribution on a bell-shaped curve.

The third process and corresponding ideology are those processes devoted to institutional survival and self-maintenance, to the maximization of resources, and to the maintenance of managerial order, stability, and control. Mauksch calls these the *core* processes. These processes and characteristics are needed to keep the organization solvent and functioning in an efficient manner.

Some of the ideology or rationale underlying these process systems has been identified. For example, the mandate to heal underlies cure; the mandate to support the patient underlies care; and the mandate to maintain institutional survival underlies the core process. If these ideologies were further delineated and explored, we would learn a great deal more about the product of hospitals and how to improve that product. These ideologies tend to be associated with the different occupations and different groups within the hospital which converge on and at the patient bedside with their functions. "Patient care, in a significant way, is a dramatic interaction, negotiation, and encounter between the ideologies of medicine, nursing, and other health occupations"[5]. Although these occupations are interdependent and complementary, they are not linear and cumulative (that is, one does not build directly upon the other in a sequential fashion); nor are they given to identical priorities in the accomplishment of their respective functions. Furthermore, as any nurse well knows, medicine, nursing, housekeeping, and so on do not participate in patient care with equal power, social mandate, or institutional support.

Ideologies affect patient care in different ways. For example, the efficiency and cost accounting ideology that would be markedly consistent with the care system might be expected to be of more concern to the hospital administrator than to the physician or nurse. But it is still there and is represented at the patient bedside under considerations of whether to keep the patient in the hospital an extra day, whether to use for suctioning sterile gloves which must be charged to the patient, and so on. It affects the climate of effort, relationships, and service. Another example is the work ideology of the repair shop which can be seen to be the method of the operating room. Here the patient appears as an inanimate work object, a faulty product to be repaired, improved, and made functional again, usually without his participation and active involvement. Further examples of the influence of these various ideologies on patient care can be found in Taylor's discussion of the nursing, medical, and hospital care of "Red Carpet" patients[6]. But the major point to understand is that both structure of hospitals and the ideologies held by different work groups have an effect on and converge in some way on the product of the hospital-patient care. The following excerpt from one of the new graduate seminars illustrates this convergence:

> First of all we're set back an hour doing all our a.m. care because they tear the floor apart between ten and eleven for cleaning. And so we could really use another person just to make beds and to help people ambulate because you can't ambulate anyone during that time. You can't do a dressing change or a rectal irrigation in the middle of the hall so you just get behind. And besides, they have rounds today, and our psych counseling session is in the morning. And in the afternoon, there are nursing rounds. And so our head nurse gets bent out of shape because everybody can't make it to all these things and you certainly can't get your work done. And I had the worst weekend of my life. I'm still bent out of shape about that. (4:4:12)

In the following excerpt, we see an example of how a patient's ideology of the care process differed from that of his physician and nurse and affected the quality of his care.

So many patients are overwhelmed when a doctor comes into the room. It's like this one patient I had who was complaining about all these different things, and I said, "Why don't you tell the doctor about them, so he can take care of them?" And the patient said, no, that the doctor was so smart and the expert and all that, that he was supposed to know everything that was wrong with her, and that he was to tell her. Well, I think you have to reeducate patients to demand more of the doctors. So I told her, "I'll be in here when the doctor makes his rounds, and you ask him those questions and I'll remind you." Well, she couldn't do it. They won't complain to the doctor; they are afraid. They are afraid that their care will be jeopardized or that they will not be thought of as highly. (2:1A:25)

In this incident, it would seem that the patient accepted the *cure* process ideology, much like the physician. The nurse perceived a problem because she was more attuned to the *care* process. The patient may not have perceived that she was receiving poor care, but from the nurse's perspective, the quality of care was lower than it should be.

In the next excerpt, we can see clearly that the quality of care of a patient about to be discharged from the hospital was affected by a conflict between the cure and care ideologies.

It was really bad. I had this lady who had been in over a month, with cancer, and she was terminal, but not immediately. We were getting ready to discharge her and the doctor told her he wanted her to go to a convalescent home. This was after he had told her the day before that she was to be discharged home. And she was so upset and I was upset. I told the doctor that she wanted to be discharged home, that she wanted to die at home among her family. It's not like she's bedridden or anything. She's dependent but she gets around. I don't think she can take care of the house and cook and all that, but she has sons and daughters at home that can do that. She can take care of her personal hygiene and so on, and I explained all this to the physician. And he says that it wasn't her decision to make; that if he let her go home, she would die faster than if he discharged her to a convalescent hospital. (6:2A:13)

The quality of care from the physician's point of view may have been improved by the discharge to the convalescent hospital; but for the patient, the outcome was not as satisfactory as a shorter life at home.

One might assume that within occupational groups there would generally be common ideologies. This is true to some extent, but not completely. It is fairly common knowledge that within medicine, general practitioners are probably more oriented toward the care process than are their colleagues in surgery, who for the most part, are cure process oriented. The same kind of ideological split can be found in ICU nurses versus, say, rehabilitation nurses. Even within a single unit staff group, you can find members of the same occupational group with different ideologies. Take for example, the following excerpt:

That's something we have a problem with on our floor that really affects patient care. Some of us really go for continuous patient assignments so we can get to know our patient better, but then there're others on the staff who say, "Well, I don't want that patient two days in a row. I learn everything I need to know from him in one day." It really bothers me because their care is jeopardized because of the staff's selfishness. (2:1A:30)

Here we see that some of the nurses were more care-oriented, while others appeared to be "learning-cure" oriented.

With this overview as background, let us now take a look at the new graduates' comments concerning quality of patient care. How satisfied were they with the quality of care the patients were receiving?

On our unit we are usually able to give really good patient care. We have some really good nurses who can talk to patients about dying and such. And we give pretty good emotional care too. (7:3B:26)

I find I get a lot more attached to the patients now as a worker than when I was a student. I see them every day and have a lot more patient contact and get to know the patients. The thing that really makes for the quality of care is the continuity. Because you know the patients that you have, and by the second day that you take care of them, you end up knowing them because you're in the room so much you can get to know them real well. And they respond to you, and I think that really makes for good care. (1:6C:8)

And really, you know, some patients I really get superinvolved with and I really care a lot about them. Like, I've cried at deliveries because they finally got what they wanted, so they really know, too, that I care. (2:2B:27)

When I first started working I'd just had my psych nursing, so I really got off on psych nursing and felt that that was the only real *good* nursing. But I've found that you can give good nursing care in other areas too and you can combine types, if you know what I mean. Like if I'm going in to prep a gal for a hysterectomy, I say, "OK, tell me all about the horror stories that all your friends have told you," or "Who do you know that's had a hysterectomy who's been different after surgery?" And that gets them to come out with all their fears about being a eunuch and not being able to have sex and all that. Stuff like that that no one else had been able to get them to talk about, I was able to help with. That's really rewarding—more so than team leading or pill pushing. I think carrying my tray with all the junk on it— that's just my prop that I have when I go in and talk with my patients—it's a prop both for the patients and the rest of the staff. If they see you with a tray, they think you're really working. [laughter] I can get lots of things done with this thing in my hand or an IV bottle hanging off my other finger and that's the thing that I really get off on, is talking with my patients. (9:1A:17)

It's very gratifying. We have several patients who have come out of things and who are getting out of bed. I find it very gratifying to take care of someone so long and see them get out of bed. Okay, they are not like they used to be and they never will be, but at least they are alive and are better than before we started working with them. That's giving good care. (2:1A:33)

As we can see from these excerpts, the nurses felt that the quality of patient care was good for a variety of reasons: the nurses had the skills needed, they used them, became involved, provided continuity of care. We can see that these nurses were quite satisfied with the quality of care being provided.

The same cannot be said of the nurses in the following series of excerpts. All of these are negative responses to the question of whether the patients received a high quality of care. First, let us take a look at some general comments, wherein no reason for the poor quality was given.

I haven't felt like I've given good care in a long time. Sometimes when I'm specialing, maybe, but then I usually have other patients too; it's not fair to the patient you're specialing. (7:3B:20)

I think we give poor care to patients; I really do. And I feel like the patients are really getting shafted. (7:6B:27–28)

It's bad and it's frustrating. Granted they're chronics, but they shouldn't have as many exacerbations as they do. If they were properly cared for, it wouldn't happen. Instead of waiting till it's to such a point that they have to be hospitalized, if we taught them while they were in the hospital the last time, it wouldn't happen. And they wouldn't deteriorate to such a state that they have little chance of getting back to a healthy state. (3:4C:16)

Sometimes our patients get really lousy care. There are times, I admit, when they get lousy care. You deliver them in bed; you catch the baby just as it's coming out. (9:2A:15)

Patients don't get the care they need. They don't complain enough. If they did, maybe they'd get it. There's so much more to nursing than what we are offering the patients. (5:3A:41)

As is clearly evident, nurses from virtually all the hospitals participating were open and frank about conditions of "lousy" nursing care. The previous excerpts can be taken as general expressions of feeling, and they might, in fact, be little more than that: expressions of frustration. More helpful was when the new graduates gave some specific indication as to what was causing the poor quality of patient care. The following series of excerpts do that. In the first one, we see that the nurse has identified the lack of consultative skills as the problem.

We had a post-op patient who went off her rocker—went into a psychotic depression. She thinks she's dead. We try to convince her that she isn't. It's very frustrating. I'd like to give her good care but I don't know what to do. We had a psych consultation, but the psych nurse gave us no suggestions as to what to do with her. (7:3C:9)

A major factor to which many new graduates attributed poor quality of patient care was lack of time. This reverberated in several different ways.

> I just don't have time to do the nursing. I enjoy taking care of the patients, talking with them, and trying to see them and work with them as a whole person but I just haven't had as much time as I need to do that. I'm only taking care of pieces of them.    (3:4C:16)

> The thing I feel bad about is when I get really hurried and rushed. I tend not to be as nice and as kind to the parents and even to the kids as I want to be. I mean, when you've got IV's that are infiltrating—about 10 of them, you know—and all your meds are late, you don't have time to take the extra minute with the parent that makes for good care. At least I don't. I wish I did, but I feel like I don't and that I have to rush to get the routine procedures and stuff done. And I feel bad about that and the kind of care I'm giving. Patients lose out.    (8:4:16)

> You know that the care they were getting is just lousy because you need to talk to your patients and we just don't have the time to stand there and talk with them. Like, one couple I really, really wanted to talk to, but I stood in there and talked to them for two minutes and I felt like, "Oh, what are the others doing while I'm in here?" and the whole time I was thinking, "I've got to get out of here; I've got to get out there." You never know what's going on with your other patients. And you just feel like, "Wow, what a mess!" I need more time to give really good care.    (2:3B:13)

> I've had eight or nine patients to care for, and it's been very difficult and frustrating because you just can't spend the time with the patients that would mean they were getting the right and complete kind of care. And then they'll say, "Gee, isn't there anyone else to help you?" And you don't want to sound as if you're overworked! So you say, "Oh, no, this is fine!"    (3:3A:10)

As might well be expected, shortage of staff or maldistribution of staff came in for its share of blame for poor quality of patient care. It was the third most frequently cited source of poor-quality care. The examples were all very much alike, so only two will be presented here.

> The floor was just swamped; we were so busy. So they floated a nurse down from E3, but they were busy too, so they said I could only have him for an hour. And I felt really bad, because I'm sure they felt the loss on their floor, and I could have used him for the rest of the evening . . . Even the supervisor felt sorry for me; she tried to get somebody to come pass medications for me . . . we do all our own meds and IV and blood pressures and checks. I just can't believe that they have seven people on days and then they hand it over to me, just me, on evenings. And they were running around; they said they had a bad day. It's no wonder that our floor is not known for the good quality of care. It's bad, really bad. The patients really lose out.    (6:6B:15–16)

We had so many patients and so few staff that I couldn't get going on even one patient. I had accomplished hardly anything and one of the other nurses came back and said, "Come on, let's get going." Boy, I just couldn't get myself in gear. I just kept thinking how bad the staffing was and the poor care the patients were going to get. And there's no excuse for it. They could have their babies better out in the fields. It's really discouraging to see poor care, no support, no communication; it makes delivery hard instead of a beautiful, positive experience for them, because we don't have enough staff.   (6:3A:14–15)

The second most frequently cited reason for poor quality of nursing care was lack of continuity in care assignments. Interestingly, this was also one of the reasons cited for good quality of care.

Because some of the team leaders like to switch sides pretty often, the team members have to switch sides. Then the patients ask you, "Well, are you new?" or say, "I've only seen you once or twice," and you've been there all along. There's no continuity, and it's hard on the patient, seeing a new face every day.   (2:4A:30)

Shifting from south to east to west and not staying with patients over a longer period of time is awful for the patient and frustrating for the nurse. You spend so little time with a patient as it is over eight hours that you don't really get to know them and appreciate them and care for them as people.   (3:1C:16)

A good example of lack of continuity and what it does to patient care was one patient who was getting a dressing changed. Every day, someone else did it. So one day we were in report, and the doctor comes and says to the head nurse, "Has the wound improved?" And four of us say, "I don't know, I never saw him before. I only did it that one day." We didn't know whether he had improved or not. We didn't know what it looked like before. If someone had done it every single day, there would have been continuity.   (5:2B:23)

And this patient established a really good relationship with you when all of a sudden you're not there anymore. You're not his nurse; you're not even in the area where you are ever going to see him. The fact is that it's important to the patient that he sees someone he knows.   (4:1:3)

Lack of continuity of care is likely a result of differences in ideologies between the new graduates and the nurses making assignments.

The quality of patient care was also noted to suffer because sometimes patients who had been hospitalized for long periods of time got lost in the shuffle.

Poor thing. She's been having spasms ever since she had the surgical fusions done. The doctor has been debrideing the wound every day. And I've gotten just like everyone else in saying, "Oh brother! She's been here for so long; don't even worry about her." But she's really actually got something troubling her; I can tell. Something's holding her back; she's got a bad problem but she's been here for so long that people kind of forget her and don't make the effort to really find out.   (1:2B:6)

The emphasis on learning that is frequently found in large, complex medical center hospitals was also noted to be a factor lowering the quality of patient care.

I don't mean to sound like I don't think this is not a really good hospital, because I think it is, but it's a teaching hospital. And a lot of people are learning, and they're learning on the patients. Some of the patients suffer from the people that are *just barely* learning.   (2B:10–11)

The teaching services are pretty shaky. When the doctor asks you how to do what they're doing!!! "Is this the right way to suction this kid?" Brother!   (2:4A:37)

I have to be really careful when I sit down with a student nurse in the morning to make sure that I know exactly what she's going to be doing with the patients. The first week students were on, we had problems. Some of them didn't take their vital signs; they didn't do a lot of things before they went off, and the patients missed out.   (4:4:2)

That's the hardest thing about being in a large teaching hospital. A lot of the patients aren't really getting good *care*. Anybody comes in, pulls open the curtains, rips down the dressings—never really addressing you, and then walking out. It's really humiliating.   (3:2A:24)

We have new interns on the floor and one of them, it was his first time at starting an IV. Anyway he was successful and got so excited that he just left the thing totally open and the whole thing went in in about an hour and a half. That kind of thing can be really scary.   (1:3C:3)

In school, we got "holistic man" preached to us for three straight years. You know: see the patient as a whole, don't separate the mind from the body . . . When physicians or teams of people come in, they look at the feet, they look at the stomach, and they walk out again. And they talk in front of the patient. I could punch some of them, I really could. So many times, I felt like leaving nasty notes, or talking to the physicians privately. I just wonder what kind of things they go through as students that they're so insensitive.   (3:2A:25)

The quality of patient care seemed to suffer even more from the insensitive and undignified nature of the care rendered when the student was absorbed in the learning and not attentive to the patients' needs than from poor technique. The last two excerpts also illustrate ideological differences between care and cure processes and point up the necessity of integrating these two processes for most effective patient care.

In addition to clear-cut discussions about whether patients get good-quality care, there were a large number of discussions which emphasized some discrimination in the extent to which quality patient care was received by the patient. In the following excerpt, a nurse is saying that sometimes patients received the care they needed, and at other times they did not.

> If you have a heavy load, you just can't do it. Patients get rotten care. But then sometimes the load is more reasonable or patients don't need as much physical care, and then you can do it. One of the problems, though, is that you get into a set thinking you can't give good, whole, complete care, so then even when you can, you don't. (8:2B:12)

The next two excerpts illustrate that patients receive good care in some areas, but not in others.

> When you're short on time and staff, you can't do patient teaching. You're lucky if you can run in there and run out, and tell them what they're going to have done the next day. You're lucky if you can do that. I mean, just name it, you don't have time to sit and explain anything or to go back and reinforce; you're lucky if you get there the first time. They get good physical care, but that's pretty much all. (5:2B:3-4)

> We had at least four little old confused biddies. One kept coming up to me and crying; she was lonely and confused and she needed me to come and talk to her . . . The floor was total chaos. I got the orders done, the meds out and the IV's checked—but taking care of the psychological need of patients? (9:1C:34)

In the next five excerpts we see that the new graduates are distressed because they perceive that some patients get proper care while others do not. This is a particularly troublesome area for new graduates, since most of them through their school socialization process were subtly taught that all patients have needs, and all must receive whole-task care. Many newcomers find that this school teaching comes into direct opposition with daily practice and with their newfound perceptions of patients' needs. When they do not spend as much time with or do as much for ambulatory patients as they do for bedfast patients, they perceive that the ambulatory patient is not receiving adequate care.

> By the time I get through, I find that I spent most of the evening with maybe four critical patients, while the rest of the people, I really know nothing about except their vital signs and if they're going to die. Here I am in charge of the whole shift and I don't know most of the patients. And then families call to see how the patient's doing!! I hem and haw. (4:1:2)

> Patients, especially if they're ambulatory, don't demand your time. And I feel in a way that they're missing out on something they should be getting. (3:3A:30)

> The patient had to lie in a wet bed all night because the loop bag was leaking. The patient said everyone was in with the lady who was having the heart attacks all night. So now, the docs are unhappy about the poor care the man received. (7:3B:10)

> Some days when it's busy, I find I have to neglect some of my patients. I feel guilty, but I have to do it to give to others. Have to pull the curtain to

be with them and let them cry. There was an obvious need and I couldn't ignore it. I follow my own instincts and do what I think is right at the time—and then go apologize to the ones I neglected. (3:2A:16)

The fifth excerpt also concerns fairness and justice. Patients should not only receive quality care, but the care should be in proportion to cost. Patients are paying a lot but are not getting the care they are paying for. The care ideology opposes the core ideology.

> On the daily census sheets that come up, it says right on there, next to each bed number, how much each patient gets charged. It varies from private room to semiprivate room to ward. When you think about what the patient's paying all the money to come in here for care, and you're so short-staffed, they're not getting half the care they should be getting. (4:4:15)

## Characteristics of the Patients

Although this factor affecting the quality of patient care is being presented last, it was the one most frequently mentioned by the new graduates. Certain kinds of patients had characteristics which inhibited the nurse from providing good-quality patient care. The characteristics can be divided into three categories: general patient types, ideology of the patient, and personality characteristics or differences.

Certain types of patients had characteristics which aroused feeling states or behaviors in the nurses which the nurses felt inhibited them from providing good-quality care to the patient. These included dying patients, quadriplegics, drug addicts, the chronically ill, retarded patients, patients having abortions, lesbians, and registered nurses who were patients. Sometimes it was the high social value of the patient (for example, a child with a terminal illness) that made it difficult for the nurse to work with the patient.

> All my kids are dying! They all have brain tumors or cancer. I can't stand it. Such a loss. The sickest ones are the brightest, most charming ones.

> I could never be a pediatric nurse. I can't go for that. It's bad enough with adults.

> I don't know. I'm on 7 central with the quads. I don't know if it's worse, like emotionally, for the patient. You might adjust to it, maybe, but I can't even talk to them about it. They're all my age. I've sorted out my feelings some about it, because you have to go in there day after day and try to help them work through their feelings and work through their anger and work through their depression and it's just constant bashing of your head all the time. Yeah, I think that's harder to deal with than dying patients, with quads. (3:3A:18)

> I can't stand to work with RN's who are patients. We have one right now; she hasn't worked for two years and she told the administration that the PM shift didn't like her at all. That they never did what she wanted and it all came up over Kerlix that she wanted but she couldn't get because we

had looked on the floor and couldn't find any. It just slipped somebody's mind to call Central . . . RN's are superdemanding; they know too much of what to ask for. They know a lot and that type of patient is really hard to care for.   (9:3C:21)

It's the chronic and hopeless patients that make it a pit. We had an oldtimer who was supposed to die on Tuesday and they called the family and all. Everybody got themselves all set and now he's better; he's putting out urine again. So they'll send him home—but he'll be back. It's not just the chronics, but the hopeless chronics.   (3:5B:6)

It was common for the nurses to realize that their personal feelings about the patient or the group of patients that the individual patient represented was getting in the way of their being able to provide really good and complete nursing care.

A second characteristic of patients inhibiting the delivery of good-quality care involves a patient's having an ideology of the care process widely disparate from that of the nurse. An ideology frequently held by patients is the care process includes hotel services such as providing newspapers, ice water, personal laundry services, and so on. When patients believe the hospital care process should include these functions, both the patients and the nurse will perceive the quality of patient care as low. Generally, the nurse will not provide the function, but at the same time will feel that she is not giving good care because she is not meeting the patient's needs or demands.

Sometimes you get patients who are very belligerent. We have a young man on the floor now who uses very foul language if he doesn't get what he wants. I was taking care of him and I finally had it up to *here,* so I said: "I don't have to be talked to like that and you're not going to talk to me like that. If you want me, put your light on and I'm sorry if I don't get to see you right away because I don't always know when your light is on because I'm in another room." That may not be good care, but that's what I do.   (2:1A:33)

I really agree that you have to do that because people just have you running all over, like sending you for ice for the water or for tissues. This one guy can get up out of bed; he's perfectly capable, but he demands all these little things. And you're so busy, you don't know which end is up. The other day I was going to walk all the way down to the kitchen wing, so I said to everybody, "Hey, I'm going to the kitchen; anybody want anything?" I got all the way back and this guy asks for orange juice.   (3:3A:32)

I'm in there doing something with the patient and the girlfriend of this other one comes up and says that he wants a 7-Up, and I'm going, "Just a second and I'll be with you." They don't look to see that you're busy; they are self-centered. They aren't thinking about what you are doing for the other patient. I'm really getting tired of patients who tell you to do this and do that, and they never say please. I've noticed, the whole floor, everybody avoids this kind of patient; nobody wants to take care of them, so they get less care than if they weren't so demanding.   (2:2A:8)

This kind of difference in ideology between patients and nurses is also what is at the bottom of patients being labeled as "good" patients and "bad" patients. Although there were no discussions in which the graduates used this terminology or from which it could be inferred that they held such stereotypes, stereotyping of patients is not infrequent in nursing practice. It almost always represents differences in ideologies. Numerous examples of the qualities and characteristics of "good" and "bad" patients are provided by Taylor[7].

Quality of patient care is also perceived to suffer from "the human element": both patients and nurses are human and sometimes they simply "get on each others' nerves." The nurse may be aware that a certain patient is "bugging" her and may try to do the best she can, but she still recognizes that the quality of patient care is decreasing because of it.

> We're still fighting Florence Nightingale. We're human beings, and we're not going to get along with everybody. And you hit times when you're going to run into a patient that just rubs you the wrong way, or you him. I think the trick for me is to know it, and to know that's the way it's going to be, and just go ahead and do whatever I have to do, and get it done. I try to get it done at the same level that I would do it for any other patient. Maybe I might not add the TLC that I would to someone that I do get along with, but hopefully my standard of care will not drop too much. Just get it done and get out of the room, which is not fair to the patient either, I guess. (7:2C:4)

> We have a little boy and he's a perfect example of poor care because people are avoiding him. He's about eight, but he's retarded, and he's very, very affectionate. He wants so much to help, and he wants things to do. And just when you're the busiest of the whole day, he comes up to you and he's pulling on your uniform: "Can I help? Can I help?" "Not right now, Timmy, come back a little later." Then he goes to the next person on the staff and right down the ladder. Poor kid, he's a pain in the neck; everyone runs the other way when they see him coming. (5:2B:1)

> Tonight I felt like strangling one lady. I have a hard time assessing whether she's in pain or not. Every 20 minutes she asks for pain medication, and I know I should work with her on reducing tension and all, but she irritates me so that I get tired and then just sort of ignore her. It's really hard to be nice to that kind of patient. (7:2C:1-3)

## What Can Be Done to Improve the Outcome?

Besides the obvious suggestions such as increasing and improving staffing, and allowing more time per patient, the new graduates came up with two specific ideas for handling the bad effects of insufficient staffing.

> It seems like the less staff you have, the more frustration you have, and the patient is the one that gets slighted. When you have more patients, you have more responsibility, more things to do for the patients, more care, and psychological needs are slighted. It's the patient that suffers for it. I find I

simply have to make decisions as to what I'm not going to do in this type of situation. You have to set your priorities and get the most important things done. You have to organize your day really well if you're going to give good care. Plan to get the most important things done, sit down and plan what you're going to do first and second and also what you're not going to do at all, and what you're going to do if you have time.    (6:2B:13)

When we're short-staffed, I tell the doctors, "Look, I cannot take vital signs on the patient every 15 minutes. If you want that done, you'll have to get a special or transfer him to the unit." Number two, I call the supervisor and tell her what's going on and what I can and can't do. If she won't send me anybody and says, "You'll have to fend for yourself," I fill out an incident report so the lawyer and administrators will know. If you fill out enough of these incident reports which go through the nursing office, eventually you may get more staff.    (9:3A:19)

As one might imagine, not all of the newcomers agreed with the solutions proposed by their peers. Of the last two excerpts, there was considerably more agreement with the first than with the second, which was seen to have some possibilities, but also some serious drawbacks and consequences. No other kinds of solutions were proposed besides these two.

### Suggestions for Handling Concerns about Quality Patient Care

In addressing the issue of how to improve the quality of patient care there is a terrible tendency simply to say: get more staff; schedule staff more appropriately. That utopian answer certainly is not satisfactory; surely someone has thought of it before.

To the extent that virtually all of the reasons cited for poor quality of patient care have been covered in some other section of this book, there is very little that can be added in the way of suggestions for improving patient care. The one suggestion that can be made, however, is that we simply must put forth more effort in nursing to ascertain what are the predominant ideologies of the people who are our clients. Very little research has been done in this area; that which has tends to be outdated. Unless we know the patient's ideology regarding the health care process, what he expects when he comes to us for service, we are neither in a position to help him effectively, nor to work with that ideology in helping him to make needed adjustments in his life style to improve his own health. We cannot assume that because we, as nurses, have predominantly a care ideology that this is what is prevalent among patients. We know the difficulties encountered when the healing ideology of the physician comes into conflict with the care ideology of the nurse; even more serious consequences can and do prevail when the nurse does not know what motivates and guides her patient. With increasing emphasis and sophistication in assessment skills, there is truly no reason why this kind of ideological assessment cannot be done. Once the patient's ideology has been assessed, effective measures to change the attitudes of clients to their care can be utilized, as explicated in *Path to Biculturalism*[8].

## QUALITY OF DYING

From an ideological perspective, death is failure of the mandate to cure and of the ideology of healing. It is, however, one of the areas of patient care in which quality is directly related to the caring process. In the dying process, rather than the techniques and instruments and tools inherent in the curing process, the nurse as a person is the chief instrument or tool of care. What she feels, says, and does has a direct and instrumental effect on the quality of dying. "We have to take a good hard look at our own attitudes toward death and dying before we can sit quietly and without anxiety next to a terminally ill patient . . . For the patient death itself is not the problem, but dying is feared because of the accompanying sense of hopelessness, helplessness, and isolation"[9]. These two messages from one of the leading authors on working with dying patients, Kubler-Ross, capture the essence of the problem of death and dying as discussed in the new graduate seminars. Coming to terms with one's own attitudes about death and dying and the effects that such a state has on one's ability to be of help to dying patients was a major preoccupation of the neophyte nurses. Vying in importance with this was a concern with various aspects of the process of dying—timing, degree of awareness, uncertainty, and so on—and opinions and feelings as to the quality of death because of these factors.

The subject area of death has the appearance of a minor theme because of its low frequency count—only 59 discussions out of the total 2,163, for a rank of 12. However, the occurrence of the 59 discussions distributed throughout the medical centers. In many ways death was like the subject area of change except that the topic did not occur as frequently, although discussions of it were longer in duration. Unlike the usual pattern of occurrence, discussions of death occurred with almost equal frequency throughout the six seminars: 36 percent in the early seminars, 30 percent in the middle, and 34 percent in the late. The topic of quality of death ranked from eleventh to fifteenth in all medical centers except one, medical center G, where it was third. There is a logical explanation for this higher rank. Medical center G was the only place where a large number of nurses were working in special care units (ICU, CCU, and so forth); death occurs in these units with a higher degree of frequency than on the general medical-surgical units.

The focus of discussions of the quality of death was on the nurses' feelings about death and dying itself, and how these feelings affected the quality of care. Themes centering around the nurse's feeling incompetent about dealing with death, or not living up to her own or others' expectations in dealing with the events of death are not included here. The excerpts are simply statements of fact or feeling about the event of death itself.

### Discussions of the Quality of Dying

There was little, if any, disagreement among the new graduate nurses as to what constituted a high quality of care in dying, and what was low. See for example, the following two excerpts, the first of which indicates a high or positive quality; the second a negative or low quality:

> I like dealing with dying patients, although it's very draining. I have nightmares about dying myself, but I'm working on that and working it through, and it's been a satisfying experience to work with the dying. There's a patient who is dying of leukemia, and he came back to the hospital, after I had finished taking care of him, to see me and some of the others. And I went back to see him and it was one of the more satisfying experiences I've ever had. He was dying but he really, really talked to me a lot about it. And I found that I could sit and listen. It helped him; it really helped me. And it was just such a beautiful relationship. And I think, because of it, I've worked through more and will be able to help others who are dying. (3:2A:7)

> There's a patient on my side—I didn't see this patient when he was admitted because he's been here that long but when he was admitted they said he was perfectly healthy—well, you know, not perfectly, obviously, but for a 72-year-old man, he looked real good. But he's had repeated and repeated surgery and now, he's just nothing. I mean, he has no personality anymore at all. And they said that before he was operated on so many times, he would joke with you and everything, and now he's nothing. They did a urethral reconstruction on him and now he has no sphincter control and he's constantly wet . . . And he's just lost all dignity, you know. He did have cancer and he still has cancer. Sometimes I can't see the point of doing all this great surgery. These last couple of months have been sheer torture for this man. I mean, he's going to die of cancer anyway. It's very plain that they did more harm than good on a patient like this. You know, he could have been home and walking around normally instead of lying in a wet hospital bed like this. I feel so strongly about this and so outraged at what they've done to him that I have difficulty taking care of him. I can't bear to look into his eyes and see the indignity there. And the family too. His wife just sits with him constantly and she gets on the staff's nerves, you know, because she has to have everything just perfect. But you can see her point too, because she saw him come in healthy and this was supposed to help, but it's done nothing but drag him down, and now it's just a matter of time before he dies.   (1:2C:3-4)

One thing that is readily apparent in both of the preceding excerpts is that the nurse's feelings and attitudes about death had important consequences both for the nurse emotionally and for her ability to be effective in maintaining the quality of a relationship with the dying patient. In the following excerpt we see that even though one of the major conditions was the same—that is, frequent, "unjustified" surgeries—*because* the feeling of the staff was good, the consequences for the dying patient were much better.

> We have a little old lady who's been on our floor for at least a month, maybe a little more than that, and she's going to die on our floor. She has really extensive cancer, and they've opened and closed her several times, which is really unnecessary and ridiculous in my book. They did a laparotomy, thinking that they would get the tumor out, and now she has a drain. It's supposed to be just a safety valve, but it's draining horribly and it's a real mess. And they just don't have any of the tension, the angry feeling about her. It's too bad that they ever did operate on her, and so many times. I regret that they did that. But so far, the feeling about her has been really good. People seem to be able to accept that she's going to die on us. People like her and don't run away from her, and everybody seems really dedicated to making her as comfortable as possible. Of course, she's still getting pain meds and stuff like that, and they haven't officially declared her DNR [Do Not Resuscitate] yet. There's a whole different attitude toward the patient before and after they do that.   (7:2C:8)

From the preceding excerpt, it is very evident that one of the factors that is instrumental in triggering expressions of feeling and subsequent interactions with dying patients is the "No Code" or DNR directive. Such a directive is an overt and definite signal to everyone—family, nurse and physicians—that the inevitability of death has been established and that the time of death is virtually known.

New graduates expressed a variety of feelings about the dying process in their seminar discussions—many of them triggered by DNR directives.

> I was really disgusted. The code went on for an hour and it was really obvious that the guy wasn't going to make it. They finally let him go . . . We have a lot of cases where we get patients that just aren't going to make it and they keep doing all this stuff; using all these expensive drugs. That guy was getting bicarbonate every five minutes for an hour, times three, at five dollars a shot and that's just really small compared to all the other drugs and things that we used on him. I was really upset about the whole thing and I was just really disgusted because I just don't agree with doing that.
>
> Didn't the Kardex indicate "DNR"?
>
> No, see that's just the point. The question of him being a DNR patient had been raised, but the doctors kept saying—and I hate this word—kept saying, "He's salvageable"!   (1:2C:2)

The nurse in the following excerpt expressed more ambivalent feelings about whether a patient should be coded or not.

Today I saw it on the Kardex. Somebody had written "Resuscitate." I meant to erase it but I forgot to. Because I just don't think you should write *to resuscitate* a patient. Anybody's resuscible unless they have DNR written. Sometimes DNR bothers me and sometimes it doesn't. I have different feelings about death now that I've had some experience. Sometimes I get involved with a patient and it bothers me; sometimes, I don't and it doesn't really phase me.    (1:2B:7)

For this nurse, the extent of her emotional involvement seemed to be the factor determining how she felt about death and the DNR directive. For other nurses, the deciding factor was one of the following four.

1.  High social loss:
She was so young—only 18. She had her whole life ahead of her yet.    (5:2:7-8)

2.  Quality of life if person should live:
It really bothers me when I think about what it will be like for her and for the family if there is brain damage. She was anoxic for so long; I think there's just got to be.    (7:3C:5)

3.  Aloneness:
He was all alone and had no one. He didn't have anyone with him the whole night and he died all alone. That was very frustrating.    (6:2B:5)

4.  No way to help:
It was terrible. We couldn't do anything to make him comfortable. The pain put him in a vicious, vicious mood. He was put through such misery; it was wicked. It just drives you crazy to see people suffer like that, and there's just no way for you to help.    (3:2A:10)

For other nurses the DNR directive evoked one kind of feeling for the patient and another for the patient's family.

You have to keep in mind what's best for the patient. Sometimes it's just death, really, if the pain is that bad. We had a girl on our floor that hung on for three months; we thought she would go at any time but she hung on and hung on and hung on. She had cancer that had metastasized a long time ago and she had a chordotomy done on her left side. We were medicating her with morphine eight milligrams every hour and a half or so. And when you get in a situation like that, she had "DNR" orders and it didn't bother me at all. I got real close to her family and it bothered me because of them, but, as far as she was concerned, it didn't.    (1:2B:7)

Often the appearance of the DNR directive is the trigger which seems to enable the staff to express their feelings overtly about death or a particular dying patient.

We have this patient who is critically ill, but they just DNR'd him. I think it's OK; there are just *so* many things wrong with him. Nobody really wants him to die, and maybe I shouldn't say this, but one of the other girls was saying this morning, nobody really wants to see him live either. There's just *too* much wrong with him.    (1:2C:3)

It is obvious from all of the foregoing excerpts that the DNR directive appears to be an external manifestation and signal to everyone that death is inevitable and its time is certain—at least certain to the extent that the patient will definitely be dying on the unit. The DNR directive appears to sanction the overt expression of feelings regarding the impending death. The newcomers did, in fact, have some very strong feelings about DNR directives in particular and death in general. They also commented on other aspects of the treatment of death and dying in hospitals.

> It's rough. We see a lot of cancer cases and if it's that far gone, it's usually a very radical procedure that's done and that's kind of hard to take. Especially the radical mastectomies. I guess because I'm a woman and it really hits home. There are a lot of breast biopsies done on young girls but we had a young girl who was 23 who had a radical mastectomy and it really hit home. I think cancer is what scares me the most.   (6:2B:5-6)

> I get depressed and scared—all in one. We had one girl who had Hodgkins and they expected her to go any time. And she was only like 25 or 26, and that just really got to me. I went home and sat down and really started thinking about it, you know, death and all. She was just terrified; you could see it in her eyes. And it terrified me! I couldn't give her good care because I didn't have my own feelings under control.   (5:1B:7)

In their seminar discussions the new graduates showed not only an awareness of their own feelings about death, but also of the direct relationship between their feelings and their ability to care for patients who were dying. The following excerpt shows that some nurses still are prone to coping with death through avoidance, a strategy that has been widely documented in the literature[10].

> I find it impossible to lie to terminally ill patients, but I'm not comfortable in dealing with it either. I don't know; maybe I'm just protecting myself, but when I have to care for them, I talk with them hardly at all.   (7:3B:28)

Some of the nurses gave beginning signs of working through their feelings about death. In the following excerpt, the nurse seems to be in the process of doing this. She seems to have come to grips with the avoidance strategy, is now in the cognitive defense stage, but is aware of having eventually to deal with her feelings about death.

> I used to run away, but now I can stay and deal with the child. I find talking to the parent is more traumatic than talking to the children that are dying. The parents express what they are seeing. And I have to sit there and say, "Well, she's going through this phase now; and next she'll go through that phase." In my head, I know I should be talking with the parents about how they're feeling about losing their child, but I can't do that. Talking with them about the physical stuff and signs and all is the only way I can separate myself and not go crying. Crying wouldn't help anybody . . . What I do seems to work because the people don't really care what you say to them as long as you listen and you're there. And you can make appropriate

remarks, and at the same time, keep yourself together enough so that you
don't fall apart and start crying on *their* shoulder. That doesn't help
anyone.    (3:2A:4)

One cannot help but emphathize with a new graduate nurse such as the
one in the preceding excerpt who is expressing so many feelings with
which she is having to learn to deal in a very short period of time. One
feels inclined to say, "That's OK. Get involved."

Getting involved is what the new graduates in the following two
excerpts did. In the first one, the involvement and subsequent inability to
be with the parents and child at the time of death led to feelings of guilt.
In the second excerpt, the involvement led to criticism from some of the
staff.

She'd been on the bypass so long that 99 chances out of 100, she wouldn't
make it. Which made me more nervous. I had taken care of the child for
several days and I'd really gotten to know the parents, and I wanted to be
there. It was time for me to go off, but I didn't want to go home because I
knew how bad she was; I wanted to stay with the parents and try and comfort them. But I also wanted—I had to go home. So finally, I decided I
would go home and come back. I had to make sure my own children were
OK and had something to eat, and then I'd come back. When I got home, I
called and they had put her on the bypass for the third time, which is bad.
So I said, "OK, I'm on my way back in." And I just got ready to walk out
the door when Lizbeth called me and said, "She didn't make it; she's
gone." I really felt bad not being there. Getting so involved and not being
there at the end. I have to deal with my own feelings about that. I had to
think about it a lot; I think it's something we'll all come up against.
(2:3A:2)

Three of us went to the funeral of one of the patients who died on our unit,
and we got a lot of negative feedback because of that from the staff on the
unit. The other staff told us we shouldn't get so involved; that we were
taking it too hard. They said we needed to build up our defenses and be
hard core.    (7:3B:37)

Particularly in the situation cited in the last excerpt, the seminar served
as a forum where the new graduates could sort out whether it was really
necessary, in fact, to build up defenses, or whether involvement with
patients was a beneficial expression of caring.

From the foregoing, we see that the nurse's own attitudes and feelings
about death and dying are a major and highly instrumental factor in
determining the quality of care the dying patient and his family will
receive. The new graduates were quite cognizant of their feelings, and
there was a fairly high level of awareness among them that they had "to
deal with [their] own feelings," "sit down and do a lot of thinking,"
"come to terms with [themselves] before I [they] could help others."

The importance of attitudes and feelings toward death, and their
instrumental impact on the process of caring for the dying patient, have

been receiving increasing attention in the medical and nursing literature, in seminars, workshops, and so on. Despite this attention the psychological aspects of dying have still been given as much attention as the physical. Strauss et al.[11] note the relation between this situation and accountability. They make the point that while doctors and nurses are held accountable for the technical aspects of their work with the dying, these same people are not required to report to each other, or to their superiors, what they talked about with dying patients.

> I really felt good about this one lady that I did sit down and talk to. She was really worried. She has cancer and she is putting up a big fight, but she needs somebody just to talk to about dying and all. When she doesn't have a lot of medical treatment, or when she isn't going through tests, or when I don't have to do a dressing change or watch an IV, the kind of "go-and-do" things, then I have time to sit and talk with her, and I felt really good that today I had the time to do that. Because it's as important as the "go-and-dos"—but it's not something that somebody can see or that they're going to check up on you about. It's "Did you do the dressing change that was scheduled at 11:00?" but never "Did you sit and talk for 15 minutes?" (4:1:11)

Perhaps when nursing and medical staff are held as accountable for the "sit-and-talks" as for the "go-and-dos," the quality of patient care and of dying will be enriched. We have seen from the foregoing that one of the factors that makes it more comfortable for one to "sit and listen" to the dying is coming to grips with one's feeling and attitudes about death. Another important factor is an understanding of the "dying trajectory" of the patient.

**Dying Trajectory**

Dying trajectory is a term used by Strauss and Glaser[12] to describe the duration and shape of the pattern of dying for a particular patient. Duration refers to the length of time from awareness (usually the staff's awareness) to the actual demise. It can range from instant death to months. A second property of a dying trajectory is shape. A given pattern can plunge straight down, it can move slowly downward, or it might vacillate or spiral. A short-term reprieve pattern, for example, is a death trajectory in which an individual who was expected to die within a period of time suddenly begins to recover slightly or to linger in one phase longer than expected.

In the following excerpt, the nurse describes a dying trajectory and her reactions to different trajectories:

> Oh, that kind is horrible. When you spend eight hours with a patient and really get to know and love that patient and his family. Especially in Mark's case. That was the longest I've been in continuous contact with someone who was dying in the unit. And he was doing better for a while. But I don't

know, his condition is really irreversible and they should have quit a long time ago, I mean, a *long* time ago, after his first admission. But they didn't, so he's just lingering on, although every now and then he's better for a while. But we still have to take care of him; we still have to see him suffer; we still have to see him just shiver when you touch him because it hurts so bad and we can't give him anything for the pain because his pressure's not high enough . . . If somebody comes in and dies in a week, I can handle that. But somebody that we've seen get better, get worse, get better, even get up in a chair and laugh and wink at us and then get worse, that's horrible. (7:2C:6)

Clues to expected dying trajectories emanate from the patient's diagnosis and past medical history (cancer, of course, being one of the prime offenders), and from physical signs and symptoms and bodily condition (age, white blood count, weight, and so on). In combination, clues from these sources lead care providers to expect a certain kind of dying trajectory. If the death goes according to expectations, then everyone— including the patient sometimes—can prepare himself for the various events in the trajectory. If the dying trajectory does not follow schedule, then both staff and family members are caught off guard and unprepared. Expectations are crucial to the way in which the dying trajectory is handled by all involved.

What are some of the fundamental elements of the expectations of death? There are two basic questions that a seriously ill hospitalized patient poses for the staff: "Is this patient going to die here?" and "If so, when?" Although of course, death is inevitable for everyone, the first question raises the question of certainty or uncertainty of death; the second question refers to time of death. This last factor has two aspects: "When will the certain death occur?" or "When will the uncertainty about death be resolved?" The relatively recent practice of issuing DNR directives for certain dying patients makes clear and overt the perception of *certainty* of death, and it generally indicates when—at least it conveys the message that the time of death will be sooner than with a non-DNR because heroic, life-saving measures will not be employed. Therefore, if the person providing care is in touch with her feelings about death and there is agreement with the mandate of DNR, with this kind of dying trajectory, it should be possible to increase the quality of care of the dying.

In the following excerpt, we see the effect of expectations on the preparation and management of death:

She was really young, but she had cancer all over her. She did die; it happened really quickly. Because she was fine two days prior to that and then all of a sudden everything just went down hill . . . she was on our unit because she'd come in to get fitted for braces; the cancer had hit her bones. PT was working with her and then they were going to send her to medicine and then home . . . They had expected it—that she would die—but not right now. They didn't expect it to be all of a sudden, and no one was ready—the staff or the patient. She hadn't even said goodbye to her kids, because they didn't expect that she would die *now*.   (2:5A:1-4)

We see, therefore, that the certainty and timing of death affect expectations which enable adequate preparation for death. When looking at death expectations, one of the first questions to come to mind is: "Who's doing the expecting?" Is it the nursing and medical staff, the patient himself, the family? What is the extent of awareness of the various people involved in the care to be provided to an individual during a death trajectory?

In a groundbreaking piece of research in this area, Glaser and Strauss[13] have formulated a substantive theory of "awareness," based upon the foregoing questions. What follows here is abstracted from the results of their research and various writings.

The problem of awareness is crucial to what happens both to the dying patient and to the people who give him care during the dying process. Although, of course, many people are potentially involved in the death process for any one single patient, and it is possible for each of these people to have different levels of awareness and expectations of death, for our purposes we will focus only on the four different awareness contexts that emanate from the dyadic interaction of the patient and the hospital staff. (Glaser and Strauss discuss all 36 potential types.)

*Closed awareness* is the situation where the patient does not recognize his impending death even though everyone else does. If the decision is made to keep the patient from realizing, or even suspecting his impending death, then the problem is one of maintaining the context. This is done through maneuvers such as the construction of a fictional future biography ("When you go home, you'll be able to sit out in the garden"), the withholding of information, not allowing patients to see their records, physical isolation in a private room so the impending death will not be disturbing to others, depriving the patient of allies who would help him increase his awareness, and adroit management of the assessment that the patient makes of his own physical appearance, signs, and symptoms.

The closed awareness context tends toward instability because there are so many places where the preceding maneuvers and conditions can and do break down. The patient's physical signs might worsen to the point where even the patient, with limited understanding of medicine, can no longer deny what he sees or how he feels. The worsening condition or the perplexing and alarming symptoms generally move the patient into the next context: *suspicion*.

In the suspicion context the patient suspects what the hospital staff knows, and he therefore attempts to confirm or to invalidate his suspicion. Often this is done by attempting to detect crucial signs or by getting outright confirmation through inquiry and questioning. Nurses often find themselves suddenly confronted with such queries, as did the nurse who is quoted in the following excerpt:

> I had a patient who greeted me first thing in the morning asking me if she had cancer, and was she going to die? I hadn't had her as a patient before. I found it very difficult because I didn't know what she'd been told or what her family or anyone else wanted her to know. I hated beating around the bush, because she really wanted to know. The way she felt about it was that she'd rather know and deal with it, than not know. Now, maybe when she knew it, it would be something else, but nevertheless . . . After going out to the desk and asking what she did know, I was told, "Well, don't say anything; don't tell her." I wouldn't mind talking or discussing with someone if you knew ahead of time just what they knew, and what the family wanted, but I hate to jump into it with both feet and then find out that no one wanted her to know.   (3:2A:5–6)

From the preceding excerpt, we see that because of kindness—misguided, perhaps, but nonetheless kind intentions—the patient was unsuccessful in getting direct confirmation of her suspicions. It is quite possible that the nonverbal behavior and affect of the nurse caught off guard did provide the information needed to confirm the suspicions.

The following is an instance of more indirect seeking of confirmation by a suspicious patient:

> The patient had a wretched medical history. She was 65 and had a lot of psychological problems as well as physical. When she said to me, "What am I living for? I want to die," I couldn't think of anything to say. What should I say? I know she was trying to find out how bad off she really was, but I didn't know what to say. I doubt if I even should say something to cheer her up. I mean, if I was that old and miserable and lonely, I would want to die too. I couldn't handle those questions, so I found myself avoiding her as much as possible. She didn't get the care she needed from me. (7:4B:5–8)

Again, it would appear as though the patient was unsuccessful in converting the suspicion awareness to the desired open awareness context. Furthermore, we see that the patient's suspicions also affected the quality of care she received.

Unlike the preceding apparently unsuccessful attempts by patients to gain information about their fate, the following excerpt shows a suspicion context being changed into an *open* context.

> I mean it was terrible to be hit like that. " Am I dying?" he says to me. So I answered, "Yes." The family didn't want him to know, but he *knew* it. So he goes, "I knew it. Thank you." You know, he could see it; he could pick it up. It was crazy not to tell him. He could see he was bleeding. I mean, he

couldn't understand why he had all these intestinal obstructions from the tumor, but he could see he was bleeding continually. It was ridiculous. And the family had a priest come in every day. So he knew. The family could not handle it; that's what it was. They just didn't think they could handle it if they told him . . . But after I told him, at least he and I could talk about it.   (3:2A:7)

Most often, suspicion moves directly into a condition of open awareness, but sometimes a context of *mutual pretense* goes on for a while, at least with some of the functionaries in the interaction. In mutual pretense, the personnel and the patient both are aware that the patient is dying, but each pretends that the other does not know. The mutual pretense context can be stable if both parties want it to be, but pretending takes quite a bit of energy—a commodity often lacking in the dying patient. It often leads to very awkward communication patterns, as can be seen from the following excerpt:

Well, we had this lady that was dying from cancer and the doctor gave her two weeks. They were going to keep her in the hospital and let her die in bed. The way the doctors did it bothers me because they would just go in and stick their head in the door and leave. They would not go in and sit and talk with the family or give the patient any consolation. They didn't really come out and tell the patient, "You're dying." They just kind of talked all around it and over her head. She knew that she was dying, but they would not come out and say, "You're dying; we can't do anything for you." They would say, "Well, wait until tomorrow and we'll see, and then after it seems that you're getting better we'll see what we're going to do from there." They went all around it with her. And she knew that she was dying, but they evaded the whole thing and they never really did get that close to the family. It put a strain on the nurses, because we weren't allowed to tell her anything because they didn't want her to know. And she knew and we knew, and she knew that we knew, but what else could we do? That kind of communication pattern can put you in the middle. It can get really awkward.   (1:2C:6)

The last awareness context, and the one generally most conducive to a good-quality dying trajectory, is that of open awareness. In this context both the staff and the patient are aware that he is dying and they act on this awareness relatively openly. Of course, even with this awareness, there are still ambiguities associated with time and mode of death. Although the patient knows he is dying, he may think or, as in the following excerpt, be deliberately led to believe that the time is still months away.

The patient came right out and asked the other nurse, "How long have I to live?" And she said one or two years. That was an outright lie: he has maybe six or eight months. And he has a right to know; he asked.   (9:3B:31)

He also may not know the extent to which he might deteriorate in the process, so these aspects may well remain closed. Nonetheless, the probability for increasing the quality of care in the dying process is augmented if there is at least the minimal degree of open awareness. In general, the new graduates felt quite strongly that patients had a right to know.

> The hardest thing for me to understand is what right the doctor has to withhold that kind of information.
>
> Yes, I agree with that too. Because the woman, after the whole thing got settled, gained a lot more peace with herself than before. I really feel like the patient should be told no matter what. And then if the patient chooses to deny it, that's up to her, not me. I really feel that we have the responsibility to present the patient with accurate information.    (3:2A:6)

Very often, open awareness context involved the family and relatives but not the patient, because the patient was a child, comatose, or insentient in some way. In the following excerpt, we see the benefit derived from an open awareness interaction with a man who not only knew that his wife was going to die, but also was made aware that death was almost immediately imminent.

> They knew she was going to die that night. I had called the doctor and told him that I really didn't think she was going to make it. And he agreed and said that he'd call the husband and tell him. So I guess around 8:00 o'clock he came and told me he was going to go home to arrange some things, and we had talked about it before, and he was getting pretty well adjusted to it. So he went home and then when he came back about 9:30, we just sat down and talked. And he was in tears. But that was the easiest way for him to express himself at that point. Her sister was there; he had called her. And they were all in tears, but it was very calm and beautiful. Everything was sort of ready and taken care of . . . During the night, it happened, and the husband came out and actually told the night nurse, "Well, she has just stopped breathing."    (2:5A:1-4)

From this excerpt, we see that the open awareness of the impending death permitted sufficient time and coping strategies for needed preparation. Such preparation is denied to both patient and family when aspects of the events in the death trajectory are deliberately withheld.

In the following example the new graduate is relating to her seminar colleagues her experiences with a young couple who were just told by the resident that the doctors thought their baby had died in utero. The resident leaves the room and the nurse is left alone with the couple. The new graduate goes on to relate how, over time, from the first knowledge of the death until the time of discharge, she worked with the family in helping them come to terms with their own guilt about the baby's death, their fear of future childbearing and having abnormal children, why the doctors did not do a C-section, what the stillborn infant looked like, and the mother's separation from the baby. The new graduate's dialogue with her colleagues continues around the issue of whether the parents should be shown the dead fetus. She says:

> I think how you handled that—to show the parent the dead baby or not— depends on their wishes, but also on whether the baby is normal to start with. When there's an obvious defect, there's a different reaction. And it's different for the nurse too. What I mean is that after this thing with Carol and I, I went into NICU and talked with the other nurses about babies who were dying or had died. And they were telling me different ways families cope and nurses cope with their feelings. I did a lot of thinking about that, and if the baby that's died is normal or not, and if the parents know ahead or not. So I felt I dealt with that, those feelings, too.
>
> Yeah, that is something that you really have to work out.
>
> Yes, if you don't work it out, you can't be of any help to the family. (2:5B:29-37)

This example illustrates how the combination of an open awareness context and of the nurse getting in touch with her own feelings helps make a potentially devastating experience for both nurse and patient into a growth experience for both.

In summary then, the quality of dying is affected by two main factors: the attitudes and feelings of the staff toward death and the degree of awareness concerning expectations in the dying trajectory. Given this understanding, what can be done to improve the quality of dying for the patients under our care?

### Suggestions for Improving Quality of Dying

Much has been written with a view toward helping those who are concerned with and who interact with the dying to cope with their own feelings about death and to understand and to help others cope with death. That advice and those suggestions will not be repeated here. What is strongly suggested, however, is that after a couple of significant experiences with dying patients, new graduates should go back and reread some of the material they read while in school. Although schools of nursing are increasingly incorporating into their curricula material on dealing with the psychological aspects of death, this material tends to be theoretical and abstract. Real, clinical experience with dying patients is exceedingly difficult to provide to students. Furthermore, it is unlikely that as a student the new graduate would have become very involved with a dying patient or gotten to know him well before the end of his life. For these reasons, unless the new nurse had a significant personal or family experience with death, it is unlikely that she will have worked through her own feelings and attitudes toward death. The first death experiences in the new job will probably provide the needed stimulus to do that. The material read as a student should be reread; it will probably make much more sense and be much more meaningful and helpful now than it was then.

Although there have been gradual improvements in the care of the dying during recent years, much more still needs to be done to ensure for the dying the very basic right to good-quality care and a dignified death. Establishing a means of holding nursing staff accountable for the psychological aspects of care of the dying, as well as for the physical aspects, would do much toward improving the quality of such care. The quality of care for the dying could also be enhanced by taking the time and making the effort to ascertain particular skills and abilities of various staff members, and then to make a deliberate and conscious effort to use those skills to the best advantage of the patient. One of the authors of this book, because she had encountered and had learned to deal with some very significant death experiences in her personal life, was particularly adept at working with the patients and families of the dying. Recognizing this, her own head nurse called upon her to utilize these special skills in providing the good-quality care to the dying that other staff could not provide. This is not to say that it would not be desirable for all staff to learn to work effectively with the dying, but just as some of us are particularly good at starting IV infusions, others are particularly skillful in working with the dying.

Another way that would help immensely in improving the quality of care for the dying would be for health professionals to get a realistic perspective on their own and their colleagues' attitudes toward death. Let us talk about the nurse trying to understand the physician's perspective. The interactions between doctors and nurses are often characterized by disagreements on various aspects of the psychological care of the dying patient—say, for example, whether the patient should be told he is dying or not. Understanding the possible perspective of the physician will enable the nurse to know, at least, the arguments that she might use to convince the physician to alter his approach to the dying if that is what is desired. For example, in the 1965 paperback edition of a little book entitled *The Meaning of Death* that is widely used in schools of medicine, Aronson, a psychiatrist, cites three goals for the physician who is working with dying patient[14]. The first goal deals with the issue of whether or not to tell the patient of his impending death. Aronson advises that the physician be guided by the following four rules. 1) Do not tell the patient anything which might induce psychopathology. 2) Hope must never die too far ahead of the patient. 3) The gravity of the situation must not be minimized, but this can be conveyed through a serious demeanor. 4) Tell the patient about his impending death in such a way as to avoid just idly sitting around, awaiting death. The second goal is to "Look steadfastly at the patient as a failing machine, at the same time as we psychotherapeutically, or with common sense, try to persuade ourselves and him that he is still a human, with a role and an identity"[15]. The third goal cited by Aronson is to counter the patient's drift toward madness and disparity, to mobilize whatever resources you can to neutralize the patient's grim awareness of the fatal disease process that is overtaking his body.

Many nurses will find that these potential goals of the physician for working with dying patients are directly in opposition to those promulgated by the caring ideology. Take for example, the second one. The caring ideology would turn this goal around so that it read, "Look steadfastly at the patient as a person with rights and dignity, at the same time as we realize that his body is a failing machine." In spite of possible distaste for the perspective of the curing ideology, learning what this perspective is and whether, in fact, a particular physician with whom you are working subscribes to it will do much to provide you, the nurse, with some idea of where to start, if you wish to try and interject more of the caring ideology into the dying process.

Concomitant with the foregoing suggestion is another idea which nurses may wish to consider—using the framework of the awareness context as a way of dealing with other health professionals. This framework readily provides a pattern that can be used to communicate intentions, goals, behaviors, and attitudes that one professional group or a single individual may hold in an instance of impending death. For example, if the nurse encounters what she perceives to be a patient's suspicion that he is dying, she can communicate with others by describing the behavior that led her to that conclusion. She can also communicate to other professionals the consequences of such an awareness context, and try to foster a collaborative goal of moving toward open awareness.

## REFERENCES

1. Julian, J. Compliance patterns and communication blocks in complex organizations. *Am. Sociological Rev.,* 31: 382, 1966.
2. Mauksch, H. and Tagliaozzo, D. "The Patient's View of the Patient Role" in Gartley, J. E. (Ed.) *Patients, Physicians and Illness* (2nd ed.). New York: Free Press of Glencoe, 1972.
3. Strauss, A. et al. "The Hospital and Its Negotiated Order" in Freidson, E. (Ed.), *The Hospital in Modern Society.* New York: Free Press, 1963, pp. 147–169.
4. Mauksch, H. O. Ideology, interaction and patient care in hospitals. *Social Sci. Med.,* 7: 817–830, 1973.
5. Mauksch, H. O. 1973, p. 820.
6. Taylor, C. *In Horizontal Orbit.* New York: Holt, Rinehart and Winston, 1970, pp. 63–75.
7. Taylor, C., 1970.
8. Kramer, M. and Schmalenberg, C. *Path to Biculturalism.* Wakefield, Mass.: Contemporary Publishing, 1977.

9. Kübler-Ross, E. *On Death and Dying.* New York: Macmillan, 1969, p. 269.
10. Glaser, B. and Strauss, A. *Awareness of Dying.* Chicago: Aldine, 1965, p. 5.
11. Strauss, A., Glaser, B., and Quint, J. The nonaccountability of terminal care. *Hospital,* 38: 73–87, 1964.
12. Strauss, A. and Glaser, B. *Anguish: A Case History of a Dying Trajectory.* Mill Valley, Calif.: Sociology Press, 1970, chap. 1.
13. Glaser, B. and Strauss A. Awareness contexts and social interaction. *Am. Sociological Rev.,* 29: 669–679, 1964.
14. Aronson, G. J. "Treatment of the Dying Person" in Feifel, H. (Ed.), *The Meaning of Death.* New York: McGraw-Hill, 1965, pp. 251–258.
15. Aronson, G. J. 1965, p. 255.

## BIBLIOGRAPHY

Cassem, N. H. Death with dignity: Confronting the decision to let death come. *Critical Care Med.,* 2(3): 1974.
Davitz, L. and Davitz, J. R. How do nurses feel when patients suffer? *Am. J. Nursing,* 75(9): 1975.
Moran, M. C. Grief and dying. *Hospital Prog.,* 55(1): 1974.

# Chapter 7
# Effectiveness
# of the Seminars

Content analysis attempts to characterize the meanings in a given body of discourse in a systematic and quantitative fashion[1].

Up to this point, we have concentrated on examining and interpreting the discussions recorded in the new graduate seminars. Now we will turn to an evaluation of the results and outcomes of the seminars as a process for the easing of the adjustment of the new graduates to their initial work experience.

What were the outcomes of the seminars? The effectiveness of the seminars will be weighed by 1) evaluating attendance as an indicator of success and 2) comparing the expected and the actual outcomes of the seminars. The material describing the actual outcomes will be drawn not only from the seminar discussions, but also from evaluations of the seminars by the new graduates and comments made by the satellite directors during interviews at the termination of the research project. The final area to be addressed in this chapter will be the factors which affected the success of the seminars.

## ATTENDANCE

Attendance can be an indicator of success in that the more one is benefiting from participation in an event, the more likely one is to continue to come. The modal response in terms of the number of seminars attended by each participant was five. In two of the medical centers, there was a wider range of the number of seminars attended. For these two medical centers, there were more participants who attended only two or three seminars than in all of the other medical centers combined. One was a large medical center and one a small medical center; in neither did the type of education of the new graduates differ from the overall picture, nor were these medical centers the ones reporting the lowest amount of support from head nurse. The time of the day that the seminars were conducted in these medical centers was not different from the others. The only thing unusual about these two medical centers is that they were the last two medical centers added to the study; perhaps the difference in attendance at seminars is related to the length of lead time for the study. These two medical centers, not having quite as much time to prepare, may not have had the procedure and mechanics of the program worked out as well as those having more time. No other reasons were apparent.

## EXPECTED VERSUS THE ACTUAL OUTCOMES

In Chapter 1 four expected outcomes of the seminars were explicated. The first was that new graduates would realize that reality shock was a normal growth process and was to be expected and that there was nothing "wrong" with them. In essence, the new graduates would not feel alone in this experience. The following excerpts from the new graduate seminars show that this first expected outcome was achieved:

> The only thing that makes me feel good is the coming to this escape. I like to come here. I like to gripe. It's very therapeutic for me.   (6:4B:12)

> I think they've been good. My head nurse asked me yesterday and I told her I had a meeting to go to and it was my day off but I was coming. And she said, "Boy! Coming in on your day off. They must be pretty good." They really have been good. Sometimes things just get so muddled in your mind that if you can talk about it, things get somewhat organized. And it's always good to get feedback from other people who are more objective about the situation.   (4:6:22)

> I think the seminars have helped to ventilate your feelings and know that you're not the lone ranger in the crowd, that other people are having the same problems. It helped me immensely to know that I wasn't the only one going through the frustrations and the changes.   (1:6B:9)

> I think it's been kind of good in that I better realize that other people are going through the same thing, and that they're worse off than I am in some of their problems. You get ideas on how to do things and improve things and change things, whereas you might not have thought of these things by yourself.   (6:6A:19)

Additional data on the first outcome comes from an evaluation form completed by the new graduates at the time of the final workshop two and one-half months after the seminars had been completed. One of the reasons for delaying administration of the evaluation form until that time was to assess the long-range effects of the seminars. It's one thing for a participant to say that she finds the seminars helpful at the time they are going on; it's another if she still believes the seminars to have been helpful two and one-half months after their conclusion. Eighty-four of the 113 new graduates in the program completed and returned the form (a 75 percent return). The questionnaire asked the nurses to list the major, if any, benefit they received from the seminars. All respondents reported at least one benefit; some reported more than one. See Table 7-1. The 106 responses represent the most frequent responses. The remaining 24 responses all had a frequency of one or two. The most frequent major benefit reported, "I learned that others were feeling like I was," further supports the expected outcome that new graduates would not feel alone in their reality shock experience if they attended the seminars. With the exception of two comments, all of the responses to the question of major benefits were positive. Two individuals indicated that the benefit of the seminars was being able to leave duty. Although this may not be a totally negative comment, this was not a goal of the seminars.

TABLE 7-1.
WHAT WAS THE MAJOR BENEFIT YOU RECEIVED FROM THE SEMINARS?

| Number | % | Response |
|---|---|---|
| 59 | 45.3 | I learned that others were feeling like I was. |
| 21 | 16.2 | I saw ways of dealing with problems, feelings, or conflicts. |
| 16 | 12.3 | I was able to express both positive and negative experiences. |
| 5 | 3.8 | I recognized feelings I had regarding the transition. |
| 5 | 3.8 | Comparing myself to others helped me to feel better and gave me support. |
| 106 | 81.4 | |

Two additional questions to determine the value of the seminars, "Were the seminars helpful?" and "Would you recommend them to another new graduate?" allowed the new graduates to indicate clearly if the seminars were helpful enough to be worth continuing. See Tables 7-2, 3. As can be seen from the new tabulations of the responses to these questions, the new graduates found the seminars helpful and would recommend them to other new graduates. These data provide additional indication that the seminars were helpful to the newcomers.

TABLE 7-2. WERE THE SEMINARS HELPFUL?

| Number | % | Response |
|---|---|---|
| 78 | 92.85 | Yes |
| 1 | 1.19 | No |
| 3 | 3.58 | Yes and no |
| 1 | 1.19 | Undecided |
| 1 | 1.19 | No answer |
| 84 | 100.00 | |

TABLE 7–3. WOULD YOU RECOMMEND
THE SEMINARS TO ANOTHER NEW GRADUATE?

| Number | % | Response |
|---|---|---|
| 78 | 92.85 | Yes |
| 2 | 2.39 | No |
| 4 | 4.76 | Undecided |
| 84 | 100.00 | |

Space was also provided on the evaluation form for general comments on the seminars. The comments written in by the respondents indicated both positive and negative aspects of the seminars.

I had felt lost for some time and could not get any comments from my head nurse. I had no idea how I was doing. It helped to know that others were having the same problems.   (D)

They were helpful to a point, but they became repetitive.   (F)

Very helpful. We could have discussed more resolutions of problems or suggestions for solutions to problems brought up.   (D)

It was a good time for me as I was hitting my peak of disillusionment with the job. It was good to be able to air my feelings and begin to understand what was going on.   (H)

Many of the feelings expressed in the group discussions were experienced by us all. It was more comfortable knowing that we weren't the only ones to experience reality shock.   (H)

I had too much else to learn and do to concentrate on the seminars.   (E)

Needed the bitch sessions. It took six weeks to compile a list of gripes and then we had time to go back to the units and recheck perceptions and try alternatives.   (G)

The seminars were marvelous. The knowledge and personal experiences shared helped me through a lot of difficult moments and inspired me to try a lot of solutions I would have been insecure about if I had been trying on my own.   (B)

I like listening to the others talk. They weren't good at first, but after we got to know each other it really helped. Everyone was supportive.   (C)

The program allowed me to see that I was not the only new graduate that was having difficulty transforming roles.   (B)

Despite negative comments indicating that the seminars at times were repetitive and there could have been more effort to dig for solutions to problems, the overwhelming direction of the comments by the participants was positive.

The last source of information regarding the outcome that new graduates would not feel alone in the reality shock process was the satellite directors who led the seminars. When interviewed, the directors indicated that they saw the major benefit of the seminars was that the new graduates could safely ventilate their feelings and not feel alone in their experiences.

The seminar comments, new graduate evaluations, and the interviews of the satellite directors provided evidence that the first expected outcome was successfully met. The seminars do provide the new graduates with the opportunity to share their experiences with other new graduates, hence gaining a sense of support because others are in the same leaky boat.

The second expected outcome was that the new graduates who participated in the seminars would be better able to hold onto their values and ideals while having those same ideals tempered by reality. There are basically three sources of information which feed into the determination of the effectiveness of the seminars with respect to this outcome. Besides the seminar comments, additional data emerge from one of the questions asked in an interview conducted with the new graduates nine months after they began work. The purpose of the interview was to determine the degree and effectiveness of change agent activity. The respondents were also asked if their ideas and attitudes about nursing had changed since they first started in their jobs. If new graduates reported little or no change in ideas and attitudes about nursing, it can be expected that they did in fact maintain the ideals with which they had entered practice. Likewise, change activity can be viewed as an indication that the new graduates were working towards their ideals of nursing practice. Data obtained from the interview questions must be considered to be results of the total Role Transformation Program and not just the seminars. How much is due to seminars alone is unknown. The data must be viewed with this in mind. The third source of data is the professional role conception scores of the new graduates nine months after they began work. The same reservation exists with this data as exists with the interview data. Results obtained must be attributed to the total program and not just the seminars.

The first and only information unique to the seminars regarding maintenance of values and ideals comes from the seminar discussions themselves.

> But it's really hard when a patient wants to talk and maybe she wants to talk for two or three hours. You really can't stop and talk. And you can't pull out in the middle of a conversation when she's starting to open up, because that could be bad too.

> Sometimes, if you can set limits, I don't think it's wrong. If you sense someone needs to talk, you can say fine, I only have so much time that I can sit and spend with you. I don't think that it's wrong to let a patient know exactly how much time you have.

I used to stop and talk with this lady when I would get a few minutes, but somehow, I should have spent more time.

I would have tried to arrange the rest of my work for the rest of the shift by talking to the other people. Then I could tell the patient "I can't right now, but I'll be back at a certain time." Or if I could organize my own work accordingly, I could talk with her and let her know how much time I could spend.   (9:3C:14)

I find time to teach the patients. There are some things like bed teaching that I can do very quickly. And if a patient is scared, I just go through and tell him what we are going to do as a prep, and that he'll be up about two hours after the procedure and his IV will come out.

Let me ask you this. How do you handle the patient whom you try to give this quicky teaching, which is really not what you are supposed to be doing, and the patient just keeps going on and on? You don't want to be rude and turn around and walk out if the patient really needs more.

Well, it depends. Sometimes I'll tell him to come out to the desk and talk to me while I'm charting. I say, "I don't have time right now, but in ten minutes come down to the desk and talk to me."

Really? They come to the desk to talk to you?

Yes. I'm always there for about an hour and I'm just charting the medication.   (6:6B:21)

You try to go really fast; a lot of people do.

Well, I don't think that that is such tremendous quality. Because you are rushing so fast to get done that you don't necessarily do the best for that patient. Maybe taking your time with them would end up better.

It would be, but sometimes you just can't because there's pressure.

No, but what I'm saying is that I know you think it is your fault because you aren't fast enough. All hospitals are like this. It's not the nursing staff. Every nurse everywhere is too slow because all the hospitals have the same problem. I don't really think it is the fault of the nurses. I take my time and I don't care. If someone wants to pressure, let them pressure. I'm doing all that I'm supposed to be doing.

Well, in my opinion, you have two choices. You can get everything done but not well, or get a little done right and leave the rest for the other shift. You can't really do both.

I've found that I do the things necessary and pertinent to nursing so that my patient care is given. The excess stuff like filling water pitchers, I won't do if it is going to cut into my time with the patients. I'll get an aide to do it.

Sometimes there is nobody else there to do it. Then you have to.

I'm sorry, I feel the care I have to give my patients is very important and that what I want to have done comes first and the nonessential things I'm not going to worry about because there is just so much you can accomplish.   (5:2B:16)

Sometimes I start telling patients and they start asking questions. I can't tell them exactly about the procedure so I tell them that the doctor will be in today or tomorrow.

You use the doctor as an excuse?

Yes, you have to; the doctor ordered it. And it's the quickest, easiest way to get away from an explanation.

That really upsets me. I . . . we were taught never to use the doctor—that the nurse should explain things to the patient—what the procedure is, what it's for, and why, what will happen afterwards. You don't have to tell them exactly what they're looking for physically but you do need to give a general explanation.   (6:6B:23)

The preceding conversations excerpted from the seminars illustrate how the new graduates constantly reminded each other of the values they were taught in school. It is unknown if the steadfast way that some of the new graduates spoused and practiced their values actually had an effect on the others, but certainly if there were no reminders of what "we were taught," there would be less chance of retaining those values. At the same time, the new graduates indicate that they were not completely ignoring the real world. Although one should talk to the patients, it can't be for three hours. Treatments cannot be ignored in providing the kind of care desired, but avoiding such chores as filling water pitchers certainly will not be terribly disruptive to the real world of nursing. The seminars thus provide data that the values and ideals of the newcomers were more likely to be retained as a result of their seminar discussions.

Another source of data for determining the achievement of the second expected outcome is the interview data. New graduates were asked if there had been any changes in their ideas and attitudes about nursing as a result of their first job. A preliminary analysis based upon frequency distributions and categorization of the responses indicates that 78 percent of the new graduates who participated in the seminars experienced a change in ideas and attitudes about nursing by the time of the ninth month of employment. Of the 106 nurses interviewed who participated in seminars, 122 comments in regard to the changes in their attitudes were given. The comments were categorized as representing 1) congruent changes (in the same direction as original ideas), 2) neutral, or 3) incongruent changes (in opposition to original ideas). The congruent changes accounted for 19 percent of the changes and the incongruent for 18 percent. The remaining neutral comments are not of concern here. Examples of congruent changes described by the nurses are: "I've become more strongly committed to what I originally believed"; "I've become more conscientious about the details of the care for the patients"; and "I've become more aggressive in meeting my patients' needs." Examples of incongruent changes are: "I've had to become very task-oriented"; "I'm compromising the ideals I learned in school"; and "I'm becoming more cynical and less caring than I was before." The results found here are not totally unexpected as some change was anticipated. The fact that 18 percent were incongruent changes would seem to indicate that the new graduates are able to maintain the majority of their ideas and attitudes about nursing.

Another aspect of the interview data which provides insight into the new graduates' values and ideals is the change agent data. Change activity is used as an indicator of retention of values and ideals because it is assumed that if new graduates were making changes in the system, then the values and ideals which they held must have been the driving force. If the new graduates had lost their ideals and had fused with the system, then little or no change agent activity would go on, as there would be no need for change. The data indicated more change agent activity and more effective change agent activity for the new graduates who participated in the seminars as well as the rest of the program. Thus, it served as evidence of retained ideals and values.

The last source of data to support the second expected outcome are the scores on the professional role conception scales. If the new graduates still held the professional ideals measured by the Corwin Role Conception Scale, the scores should remain in the high professional range. At nine months of employment, the mean professional role conception score for the participants was 30.08. When compared to the scores of many other groups of nurses, this is a high professional score and would indicate retention of loyalty to the ideals and values which the new graduates held upon entering the work world[2].

The third expected outcome of the seminars was that the new graduates would feel better as a result of being able to compare themselves with others at the same level of ability. Direct data to evaluate this expectation was sparse. There was only one very overt reference in seminars which indicated the comparing of self to peers was necessary.

> I think it is a good support system. Sometimes it's very hard to talk to another nurse that's been here maybe a year or two because although she can remember, she's grown from her experience and has other concerns and abilities.   (3:5C:17)

The numerous "war stories" told by the new graduates during the seminars provided considerable opportunity for indirectly assessing attainment of this expectation. It is highly probable that while listening to another's experiences a listener sizes herself up in comparison to the teller and to the other listeners who comment on the story. The listeners' verbal expressions of how they would have handled various situations is the behavioral evidence of this comparison.

In other instances, particularly in the areas of competency and self-concept, seminar excerpts clearly indicate that the new graduates are comparable in terms of the way they perform and their feelings about themselves, but there was no overt indication that the new graduates were comparing their own abilities to the abilities of the others. New graduates would discuss their sense of insecurity in the performance of their role or say that they felt dumb when they asked questions of others. Rarely did the new graduates actually indicate, "I don't feel quite so bad when I hear that the rest of you didn't know what to do either." Perhaps the words weren't necessary; the evidence does indicate some support for the achieving of this outcome.

The fourth and final expected outcome was that experiences would be shared through discussions which would prepare the newcomers to meet possible upcoming events.

We have this little boy on our floor, and the day before yesterday he was in halo traction, which is where you have these wires around him and a cast all the way down. Well, Monday night I walked into his room and he was *blue*! He shocked and arrested very nearly. I felt very incompetent and very unprepared. Because I froze totally. I had no idea how to get to this kid because he had this cast on, all the way down. What could we do? It was a very, very frightening, horrible, terrible experience. I can't go into how horrible it was. The kid was blue and I thought we were going to lose him and oh, it was horrible. Afterwards I felt as though I hadn't been trained at all. I had never been shown anything. Nothing like this had ever happened to me. I had to really look at myself and say, "Hey, you can't do everything. You can't know it" . . . [interrupted]

Well, how did they get to him?

Well they didn't have to. I ran to get the saw. And then I ran back and the arrest page was on. It was horrible. They suctioned him and they got the mucus plug and it had interfered with perfusion. He was missing $C_2$ and they had done a fusion. They were worried about respiratory distress. He had come back from ICU just the day before. So, here he was blue. So they suctioned him and it was like a 30-second apneic period and his heart kept going, but they were afraid he was going to arrest. But it was awful. It seems as if we have all the theory but when it came right down to it, I froze. And I never thought I ever would freeze and I sure did. I didn't feel as if I had met what I thought I should do—be supernurse. I ran fast for the saw. If I had done something different I could have done better. Thank heavens there were enough other people around who knew what they were doing.

Boy, I don't know. They can't teach you everything. Who'd expect something like that?

What to do in an arrest with a full body cast? I wouldn't know.

Scream and panic!

We need a "how to" book. (5:4B:4)

"War stories" served to allow the person relating an incident to receive from the other new graduates suggestions of other approaches which might be used should the incident occur again while helping to prepare the others to deal with similar situations. Many of these stories of bad experiences centered around death scenes, codes, and emergency situations. Others dealt with more everyday problems such as violating a sterile technique. Many of the stories of more common everyday events which prepared the listener for things to come can be seen in the section on backstage reality. Based on this evidence it would appear that the fourth expectation was met.

An unanticipated outcome, accountability to the group, surfaced in relation to the problem solving that went on in the seminars. As was noted earlier, the new nurses' narratives of experiences at times served as a basis for seeking alternative suggestions. At other times, when the nurses provided a fellow seminar participant with an idea about how to handle a situation, the participants expected to be informed of the results of their suggestion at a future seminar.

> Well, last week after I talked about the problems with the ten-hour shift I went back and talked to one of the girls that works on the floor. She's not there often but I think she is a clinical specialist or something. Well, she was real concerned and said that she would look into the problem. Like I said, I think the head nurse knew about the problems but didn't think things were serious enough to do anything about it. But now I think something is going to get done about it.   (4:6:1)

A sense of group accountability sprang up as the new graduates inquired just how successful their fellow nurses had been if an attempt was made at all. Although not expected, this was an important outcome as the new graduates are more likely to act on suggestions made if they know that at a subsequent meeting they will be asked to let the group know how things worked out.

Overall the evaluation of the seminars shows that three of the expected outcomes were substantially supported by seminar comments and by new graduates' as well as satellite directors' evaluations. One expected outcome—peer comparison—did not show the same extent of direct support.

## FACTORS AFFECTING THE SEMINARS

Four primary factors affected the success of the seminars: the timing of the seminars, situational circumstances, head nurses' support of the seminars, and the leaders' abilities. Each factor will be described separately.

The seminars in all of the medical centers were slated to start five or six weeks after the new graduates began working. The choice of time of day was left to the individual satellite directors. In order to be most effective, the seminars should have begun when the new graduates entered the shock phase of reality shock. The new graduates were asked to evaluate the appropriateness of the timing. Only 49 of the 84 new graduates who returned the evaluation form answered this question. The percentage of respondents indicating that the timing was correct ranged from a low of 30 percent to a high of 85 percent at the different medical centers. A follow-up question asking if the timing should be earlier or later indicated that 75 percent of the 49 answering the question believed the seminars should start earlier. Because of the small number of responses to the question, it is difficult to assess accurately their meaning. It can be said that the medical centers generally would do better to begin the seminars a week to two weeks earlier. This would mean that the seminars should start in the fourth or fifth week of employment rather than the fifth or sixth week.

The new graduates' assessments and the satellite directors' assessments of the appropriateness of timing of the seminars were quite different. All but two of the satellite directors indicated that the timing seemed appropriate. One director indicated that the seminars began one week too soon, whereas the other felt that perhaps the seminars should begin a week earlier. Based on the information available, it is difficult to say what the best timing actually would be.

The timing is likely best determined by establishing the appropriate starting schedule for each individual institution. Keeping in mind the symptoms of the shock phase of the reality shock process, it is necessary that a hospital observe when the new graduates seem to hit the shock phase, and begin there. It may be that trying a five-week start and then asking the new graduates about the timing will provide the best direction of establishing the most appropriate timing.

Seminars were scheduled at all times during the day, ranging from early morning until late evening. With the exception of the two medical centers mentioned earlier, all had high attendance records. No one time of day seemed more appropriate as long as the principle of conducting seminars at a time when new graduates are either on shift or not required to make a special trip in to the hospital (right before or after the shift) is kept in mind in setting the time.

A second factor affecting the success of the seminars was the situational circumstances at the given medical centers. Two of the satellite directors indicated that the lead time between their training session and the start of the seminars did not provide adequate time to enlist the aid of the persons involved in the scheduling of the new graduates to make sure that the newcomer would be on duty during seminar time; thus, the level of attendance was affected.

One of the other major factors complicating the seminar success was the level of staffing on the units. At times, the full complement of staff positions for a unit was not filled, and thus the new graduates had difficulty getting away for the seminar. In other instances, the hospital's patient census went way up, increasing the need for staff and interfering with the new graduates' attendance. Additionally, many new graduates had not yet begun their rotation patterns when the seminars were first set up. As their schedules changed, it became more difficult for them conveniently to attend the seminar.

One medical center experienced a rather severe financial strain during the course of the seminars and withdrew overtime pay and compensation time for attendance at seminars. It may be that this affected the new graduates' attendance at the weekly meetings.

Support for the seminars by head nurses was a third factor affecting the success of the seminars. Because of the research nature of the program of which the seminars were a part, it was difficult to obtain the full support of the head nurses. We wanted the head nurses to feel that both the experimental program and the control program would be beneficial in helping new graduate nurses make a successful role transformation. Varying degrees of support were attained. The perception of support from head nurses ranged from 100 percent of the new graduates in some medical centers feeling support to a low 62 percent of the new graduates in other hospitals indicating they felt support from head nurses. The new graduates commented in seminar on behaviors which indicated support.

> My head nurse has turned out to be one of the all-right people. She makes out my assignment so that realistically, I can get it done before I come. It's not a problem. She says, "You're committed to this. You've got to go. Don't feel guilty."

> It's the same on my floor. My head nurse is really good.   (3:4A:37)

New graduates also indicated on the evaluation form some ways in which their head nurses showed support to them for going to seminars:

> Scheduled my time so I could go.

> Encouraged me to attend.

> Gave me assignments so I could go.

> Reminded me to go.

> Provided compensation if I went during off-duty time.

> Asked me how I was doing.

> Provided positive reinforcement for going.

Upon interview, the satellite directors provided confirming information as to how the new graduates were supported by the head nurses.

The new graduates were also asked to give examples of behavior indicative of lack of support from their head nurses. They listed the following behaviors as nonsupportive:

Showed no interest.

Made negative comments.

Scheduled me so that I could not attend.

The satellite directors added one additional nonsupportive behavior for head nurses and other staff nurses as well. The satellite directors indicated that some head nurses made it uncomfortable for the new graduates to come usually by pressuring the new graduates to feel as though they were deserting the unit.

The last but not the least important factor in the success of the seminars was the leaders' ability. Some people have certain characteristics and abilities which facilitate leadership; others do not. It was not possible to evaluate systematically or objectively the leaders' behavior in the seminars. The data to be presented here were provided by the new graduates and the seminar leaders themselves.

There were comments from only two new graduates on the evaluation forms indicating any kind of evaluation of the leaders. One new graduate stated that more solutions to problems could and should have been sought, and another indicated that at times the seminars were dominated by a few of the more vocal members. The absence of other negative comments would seem to indicate that for the most part, seminar leaders were perceived as providing adequate assistance in problem solving and the opportunity for all to participate. All other comments, a number of which were provided earlier, indicate that the leaders were successful in helping the new graduates to ventilate their feelings.

The satellite directors reported experiencing a number of difficulties in leading the seminars which may have affected the success of the seminars. The major difficulty encountered by the satellite directors was remaining in the facilitator role. For a number of the seminar leaders, this difficulty stemmed from past experience as a teacher rather than as a leader of a loosely structured group. A tendency to slip back into the teaching role was often expressed. Seminar excerpts at times indicated that when new graduates referred to content from the instructional materials, there was a tendency to focus in on the content of the materials rather than on how the materials related to the new graduates' experiences.

At times, the new graduates raised issues for which the satellite directors felt they themselves could effectively provide interventions outside the seminars. The contract prevented them from assuming this intervention role. The leaders found that restraining themselves from intervening was particularly difficult when the new graduates revealed practices on the unit which the satellite directors thought jeopardized the patient's safety. Although it was difficult for many of them to do, the seminar leaders concentrated their efforts on helping the new graduates to intervene and did not take any direct steps to solve the problems discussed by the new graduates.

Emotional reactions to some of the issues raised in the seminars provided an additional source of difficulty for the seminar leaders. Several of the satellite directors indicated that material such as level of staffing and incompetence of the supervisors whom they knew may likely have created some nonverbal responses which could have inhibited the free discussion by the new graduates. The satellite directors indicated that in most instances they thought they were able to refrain from making verbal comments; the new graduates may or may not have picked up on subtle nonverbal cues. The seminar typescripts reveal no indication that the new graduates felt inhibited in discussing material.

One last area which the seminar leaders found difficult but which probably did not affect the success of the seminars was the lack of an in-house support system for themselves. Although the leaders were in contact with the project director, it was not the same as having someone at the institution who could listen and satisfy the satellite directors' own needs to ventilate their feelings after the seminar discussions. As indicated earlier, the formation of an in-house support system is strongly recommended.

The overall evaluation of the seminars in terms of attendance and comparison of expected and actual outcomes indicates that the new graduate seminars provided a helpful experience. The new graduates were able to express their concerns in a wide range of areas and to realize that they were not alone in their initial reactions to the role transition from student to staff nurse. The support and suggestions from the other participants in seminars allowed them to recognize and deal with their feelings.

Although there were negative factors which affected the potential success of the seminars, these factors did not seem to outweigh the benefits. With more experience, it is expected that the leaders will be more comfortable with the seminars and their role in them. As a result of the initial program, the medical centers which participated can now individually determine the best time frame and elicit the needed support from head nurses to gain even more effective results from the institution of temporary new graduate referent groups.

## CONCLUSION

As the tree is fertilized by its own broken branches and fallen leaves, and grows out of its own decay, so men and nations are bettered and improved by trial, and refined out of broken hopes and blighted expectations[3].

The new graduates came together to share their experiences and to support one another during a time of situational crisis. The living through of this event created an experienced group of people whose sharing will undoubtedly help those to follow with their adjustment to their first job. However, the new graduates' experiences have further implications.

The new graduates' comments have provided us a stimulus for systematic examination of the concerns they expressed. In the explication of the subject areas of the new graduates' concerns, we have made every effort to provide suggestions which would be helpful to all of those in nursing—the educators and service individuals alike. At times, suggestions were more heavily slanted to one group or another, depending upon the nature of the concerns. One of the suggestions in the section on change was the formation of an insider-outsider change agent team to work on suggestions and ideas. An equally viable team would also be formed by the joining of nursing education and nursing service. Each could act as an insider and each as an outsider in helping to make improvements in both the educational process and practice of nursing.

As many readers may have discovered in reading the experiences of the new graduates in practice, a common reaction might have been, "I know just what they are talking about" or "I've been there before." Such a reaction to these experiences forms the basis for an important implication. For each of us, the question must be raised, "What have I done about some of these same problems and concerns?" Although global suggestions and attempts can be made to deal with the concerns of the new graduates, the most important action begins and is moved forward at the individual level. The new graduates have been encouraged to let the experiences of those who passed before act as a driving force in preparing for and meeting their first job. Let us accept their experiences as a challenge to all of us in nursing to systematically address and to work out constructive resolutions to the problems and concerns of nursing.

## REFERENCES

1. Berelson, B. "Conflict Analysis" in Lindzey, E. (Ed.), *Handbook of Social Psychology*, vol. 1. Reading, Mass.: Addison Wesley, 1954, p. 489.
2. Kramer, M. *Reality Shock: Why Nurses Leave Nursing*. St. Louis, Mo.: C. V. Mosby, 1974.
3. Robertson, F. W. "Broken Hopes" in *Leaves of Gold*, rev. ed., Lythe, C. F. (ed.). Williamsport, Pa.: Coslett, 1948, p. 15.

# Index

# Index

BELMONT COLLEGE LIBRARY

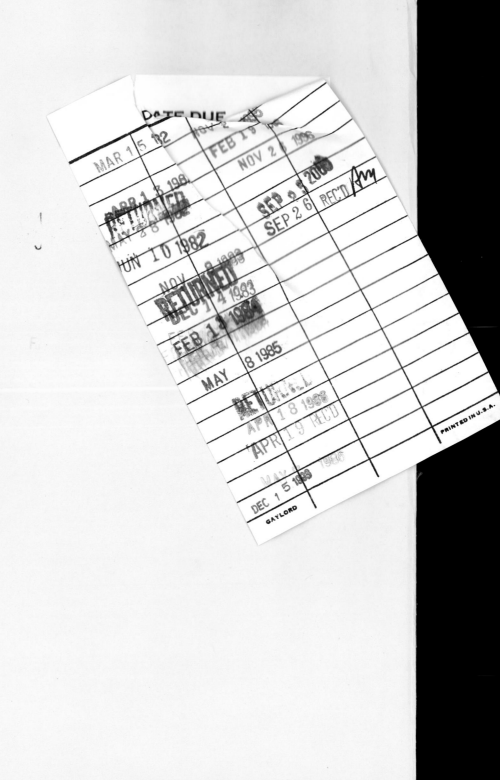
DATE DUE

| | | | | |
|---|---|---|---|---|
| MAR 15 82 | NOV 2 | FEB 1 | NOV 2 3 1986 | |
| APR 1 8 1982 | | SEP 5 2000 | REC'D *Amy* | |
| RETURNED MAY 2 8 1982 | | SEP 26 REC'D | | |
| JUN 10 1982 | | | | |
| NOV 8 1983 RETURNED DEC 1 4 1983 | | | | |
| FEB 1 8 1984 | | | | |
| MAY 8 1985 | | | | |
| RETURNED APR 1 8 1986 APR 1 9 REC'D | | | | |
| MAY 1 5 1986 DEC 1 5 1986 | | | | |

GAYLORD            PRINTED IN U.S.A.